Medical Library

Queen's Univer:
Tel: 02?
E-mail

For due dates

QUB borrowers see 'N
http://library.qub
or go to the Library

HPSS borrowers see '
www.honni.qu

This book must be
than its due date
earlier if ir

Fines are imposed on overd

Gerodontology

Gerodontology

Edited by

Ian Barnes BDS, PhD, FDSRCS
Professor of Conservative Dentistry, Prince Philip Dental Hospital, Hong Kong

and

Angus Walls BDS, PhD, FDSRCS
Senior Lecturer in Restorative Dentistry and Honorary Consultant, The Dental School, Newcastle upon Tyne, UK

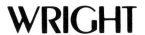

Wright
An imprint of Butterworth-Heinemann Ltd
Linacre House, Jordan Hill, Oxford OX2 8DP

ℜ A member of the Reed Elsevier plc group
OXFORD   LONDON   BOSTON
MUNICH   NEW DELHI   SINGAPORE   SYDNEY
TOKYO   TORONTO   WELLINGTON

First published 1994

© George Warman Publications (UK) Ltd 1994

British Library Cataloguing in Publication Data
Gerodontology
 I. Barnes, I. E. II. Walls, Angus
 618.97

ISBN 0 7236 2159 4

Library of Congress Cataloguing in Publication Data
Gerodontology/edited by Ian Barnes and Angus Walls.
 p. cm.
 Includes bibliographical references and index.
 ISBN 0 7236 2159 4
 1. Aged—Dental care. I. Barnes, I. E. (Ian E.), 1939–
 II. Walls, Angus.
 [DNLM: 1. Geriatric Dentistry. WU 490 G377 1994]
 RK55.A3G49 1994
 618.97'76—dc20
 DNLM/DLC   93–41499
 for Library of Congress   CIP

The articles on which this book is based were first published in *Dental Update* a publication of George Warman Publications (UK) Limited, Warman House, 20 Leas Road, Guildford, Surrey GU1 4QT, England

Typeset by Keytec Typesetting Ltd, Bridport, Dorset
Printed in Scotland by Cambus Litho Ltd, Glasgow

Contents

Contributors

S. Baillie BSc, MBBS, MRCP
Consultant in Geriatric Medicine, North Tyneside District General Hospital, Tyne and Wear

I.E. Barnes BDS, PhD, FDSRCS
Professor of Conservative Dentistry, Prince Philip Dental Hospital, Hong Kong

R.M. Basker DDS, LDSRCS, MGDS
Professor of Prosthetic Dentistry and Honorary Consultant in Restorative Dentistry, Leeds Dental Institute, University of Leeds

J. Christensen DDS
Associate Professor, Department of Gerodontology and Oral Gerontology, Royal Dental College, Copenhagen, Denmark

J.R. Drummond BMSc, BDS, PhD
Lecturer in Dental Prosthetics and Gerontology, Dundee Dental School, University of Dundee

J. Fiske BDS, MSc, FDSRCS
Senior Lecturer in Dental Public Health and Community Dental Education, King's College School of Medicine and Dentistry, London

R.J. Ibbetson BDS, MSc, FDSRCS
Consultant in Restorative Dentistry and Honorary Senior Lecturer, Eastman Dental Hospital, London

R.B. Johns PhD, LDSRCS
Emeritus Professor of Restorative Dentistry, University of Sheffield School of Clinical Dentistry

E.A.M. Kidd BDS, PhD, FDSRCS
Reader in Conservative Dentistry and Honorary Consultant, United Medical and Dental Schools, Guy's Hospital, London

I.D. Murray BDS, MDS
Lecturer, Department of Restorative Dentistry, University of Newcastle Dental School

J.P. Newton BSc, BDS, PhD
Senior Lecturer in Dental Prosthetics and Gerontology, Dundee Dental School, University of Dundee

J. Ralph DDS, FDSRCS, HDD
Consultant in Restorative Dentistry and Honorary Senior Lecturer, Leeds Dental Institute

J. Scott BDS, PhD, FDSRCS, FDSRCS(Ed), FRCPath
Professor of Oral Diseases, Department of Clinical Dental Sciences, School of Dentistry, The University of Liverpool

C. Scully PhD, MD, MDS, FDS, FFD, FRCPath
Professor and Honorary Consultant, Eastman Dental Institute for Oral and Dental Healthcare Sciences, London

D.J. Setchell BDS, MSc (Mich), FDSRCS
Senior Lecturer in Conservative Dentistry and Honorary Consultant, Eastman Dental Hospital, London

R.A. Seymour BDS, PhD, FDSRCS(Ed)
Professor of Restorative Dentistry and Honorary Consultant, Department of Restorative Dentistry, Newcastle upon Tyne Dental School

A. Sheiham BDS, PhD, DHC
Professor of Dental Public Health, Joint Department of Dental Public Health, University College London and the London Hospital Medical College. Department of Epidemiology and Public Health, University College and Middlesex School of Medicine, London

B.G.N. Smith BDS, MSc, PhD, FDSRCS
Professor of Conservative Dentistry and Honorary Consultant, United Medical and Dental Schools, Guy's Hospital, London

D.G. Smith BDS, DRD, FDSRCS (Ed)
Consultant in Restorative Dentistry and Honorary Lecturer, The Dental Hospital, Newcastle upon Tyne

C.J.R. Stock BDS, MSc
Senior Research Fellow, Eastman Dental Hospital, London

A.G.W. Walls BDS, PhD, FDSRCS
Senior Lecturer in Restorative Dentistry and Honorary Consultant, The Dental School, Newcastle upon Tyne

P. Ward-Booth BDS, MBBS, FRCS, FDSRCS
Professor of Maxillo-facial Surgery, University Department of Oral and Maxillo-facial Surgery, Bristol Dental School and Hospital

R.W. Wassell BDS, MDS, PhD, FDSRCS
Lecturer in Restorative Dentistry, University of Newcastle upon Tyne Dental School

K. Woodhouse MD, FRCP
Professor of Geriatric Medicine, University of Wales, College of Medicine, Wales

Preface

No dentist will be unaware of the increased interest being taken by the dental profession in the care of the elderly. There are several reasons for this. First, in many countries people are living longer, keeping their natural teeth, and wishing to keep them longer. We might think that this steady increase in demand would have been quietly accommodated by the profession without ado. Yet gradually, a speciality – Gerodontology – has evolved; why?

The cynic might say that this interest in the elderly has come at an opportune time; for academic departments in the dental schools who have found a revived area for research and publication; and for practitioners, who may view the transfer of the dwindling work load required by the young to the burgeoning of the old, to be providential. Indeed, is 'Gerodontology' really a speciality? The treatment of the older patient is simply an extension of well-established practice, using techniques that the caring dentist will, largely through common sense, have developed over the years. Whatever view you hold, the fact remains that old people do have particular problems, and special needs.

This book brings together specialists, to explain and discuss those parts of their discipline that relate to the elderly. We have tried to relate these different expertises one to the other, so as to paint a coherent picture of the problems and practicalities of offering dental care to the elderly. The book cannot be a complete text of all the clinical conditions that will be met and the operative techniques that will be used. For example, the treatment of tooth wear, endodontics, oral pathology and surgery, or the provision of full dentures, warrant books of their own. Nevertheless, we hope that practitioners will feel it helpful to read of the principles that underlie what in many cases will be their practice; and that perhaps some of the techniques described may augment their practice. As for undergraduates, those in vocational training and those who are in their early years in practice, some of the lessons that the authors have learned, many through trial and error, may perhaps more painlessly and more quickly be absorbed.

Ian Barnes; Angus Walls
Newcastle upon Tyne
February 1994

Acknowledgements

This book is the sum of the experience of several experts in their fields. We have simply built a framework, then persuaded, chivvied and finally edited so as, hopefully, to develop a homogeneous and non-repetitive house-style. Thanks must be given to all the authors, for their contributions; and for their tolerance and patience, which was also shown in good measure by our Departmental Secretary, Miss Claire Grainger. Professors Roger Watson and James Soames have given helpful advice.

The basis of many of the chapters was a series of articles published in *Dental Update*, who kindly agreed that they could be republished in book form. Professor Ted Renson and Andrew Baxter were always helpful in the original preparation. At Butterworth-Heinemann, Dr Geoffrey Smaldon and the production team have been very supportive.

All photographs of patients have been reproduced with informed consent.

1

Gerodontology: A condition and a problem?

Angus Walls and Ian Barnes

This chapter discusses the numbers of old people in the population. Many of these people retain their teeth. The dental management of the old person can be considered to include management, treatment and treatment planning. The combination of an increase in numbers and an increase in the complexity of treatment will have an effect upon the practice of dentistry in the future.

In the Preface to this book we have discussed briefly whether the concept of Gerodontology as a separate branch of dentistry is valid. It cannot, however, be denied that the pattern of the dental treatment of the older patient has changed over the years, and continues to change. In Britain the traditional 'dental image' of an old person has, until recently, been that of a toothless person who lost his or her teeth a number of years previously and who wears complete dentures with varying degrees of success. This perception is now changing because of an increased dental awareness and an improvement in the dental status of older people (Fig. 1.1a, b).

There has been a concurrent increase, within the dental profession, in awareness of the dental problems of the elderly. In some parts of the country this may have been focused by the reduction in caries in children. The patterns of change are essentially the same in 'developed' countries throughout the world, although the methods of the delivery of care may differ.[1,2]

Why is gerodontology of increasing relevance?

Two factors are principally responsible for the increasing relevance of 'Gerodontology'; namely, alterations in the structure of the population, and changes in the patterns of dental health. The increase in the public's awareness of the need for dental health which we have considered earlier also plays a part.

Alterations in the structure of the population

The population of the United Kingdom is slowly increasing (Fig. 1.2). This is not true of all other 'developed' countries; although in most, if not all, the structure of the population is changing.

At the turn of the century, the population of the UK could be represented diagrammatically as being approximately triangular in structure. There was a broad base of young people, and rapidly diminishing numbers of older individuals. The projected profile for the year 2001, based upon population trends in 1983, is more rectangular in structure. There are approximately the same number of young people as in the past, but a greatly increased proportion of ageing and elderly individuals (Fig. 1.3).

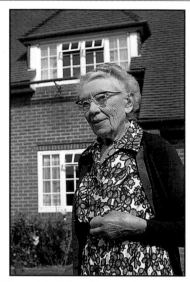

Figure 1.1a This 88-year-old retained nearly all of her teeth until the time of her death at the age of 96. She remained independent, though in a sheltered home, until the age of 94

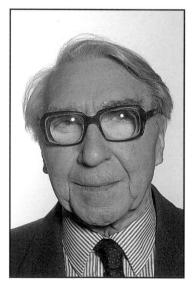

Figure 1.1b This senior academic was 87 years old when this photo was taken. He retains most of his teeth and five years later still runs a farm successfully

the distribution of the ages. The proportion of 'old' people over the age of 75 will increase, whilst that of 65–75-year-olds will decrease (Fig. 1.4). This will have an impact upon the pattern and delivery of social, medical and dental care within this age-group.

These alterations in structure of the population during the twentieth century can be accounted for by improvements in the economic status of individuals, social environment and in health care. Thus, there has been a significant reduction in mortality in the perinatal period, childhood, and adolescence.

This reduction in mortality is reflected in the progressive increase in the life expectancy of different age-groups over the century (Fig. 1.5). In 1988 the life expectancy of a male child at birth was 75 years, compared to 48 years in 1901. The figures for a female child are 80.5 years and 51.6 years respectively (Fig. 1.6). Interestingly, there has not been a similar increase in life expectancy for 65-year-olds during the century, the increase being only 2.4 years for men and 5.3 years for women over the same time.[3] The explanation for this apparent paradox is simple. If you lived to be 65 in the early years of the century, much of the risk, for example of tuberculosis or diphtheria, was overcome and behind you.

The practical consequence of these statistics is that many more people are living to enjoy their 'old age'. Anecdotally, admittedly, but of particular interest to one of the authors is that in considering his four closest schoolfriends, excluding one parent who was a pathologically heavy smoker, the averaged ages, at death and currently of the four surviving parents is 85 years. All were or are edentulous.

Despite this upbeat message, the overall life span is unlikely to increase significantly. The reasons for this and the biological significance of the ageing process will be considered in the next chapter.

The altered population profile has been accompanied by a change in the structure of the family unit, and this has had an effect upon the provision of health care to the aged. Families in Victorian and Edwardian England tended to be large by today's standards. The younger family members were available to look after the fewer surviving elders. This and social convention favoured the 'extended family'. Nowadays, the pattern of family life is

There will be some growth in the total number of people over the age of 65 between the present day and 2031. However, within this group there will be significant changes in

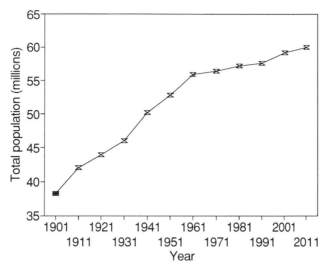

Figure 1.2 Growth in the population of the UK 1901–2011 based on 1983 data[3]

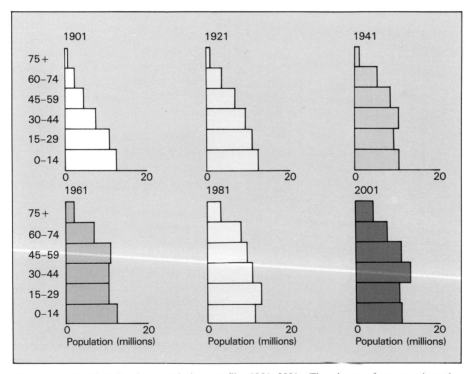

Figure 1.3 Alteration in the population profile 1901–2001. The change from a triangular structure in 1901, with a broad base of young people, to a more rectangular form in 2001 can be seen clearly

different. There are fewer children in the family unit, the average in 1988 being 1.98. The working wife, the decrease in size and relative expense of housing, and an unwillingness to accept the 'inconvenience' of crowded accommodation will have played a part in reducing the importance of the extended family. This is, however, an unrealistically harsh analysis.

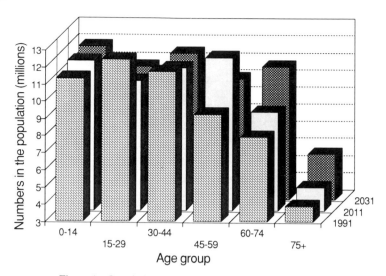

Figure 1.4 Population trends 1991–2031.[3] The number of people over the age of 60 will gradually rise with increases in both the 'young old' (60–75) and in the 'old old' (75 plus)

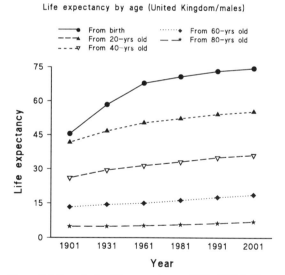

Figure 1.5 Trends in life expectancy 1901–2001.[3] There has been a steady increase in life expectancy at birth, but very little increase at 60 and 80 years of age

It is now largely realized that these dated stereotypes are not correct. Most old people lead active lives. They are happy to be independent, and wish to remain that way for as long as is possible. With modern medicine, the 'welfare state', modern household appliances and the like, the wish for independence is usually realizable well into advanced old age. Of those that need care, a high proportion are looked after in their own homes by a mixture of family, neighbours and 'professional carers'. Less than 10% of people over 65 live in institutions.

The increase in awareness of the need for dental health

[with Jim Ralph and Robin Basker]

There is a well-documented trend of a worldwide reduction in dental caries experience amongst children. Although not proved, a major aetiological factor is probably the widespread use of fluoridated dentifrices. There is also evidence that oral health is improving in the older age-groups.[4] In the United Kingdom, these improvements include a steady decline in the rate of edentulousness. The reduction in total tooth loss is shown in Figure 1.7, where it can be seen that major improvements have occurred amongst middle-aged people – tomorrow's elderly. The 1988 survey of adult dental health in the UK has predicted the future pattern by calculating optimistic and pessimistic estimates to cover the next fifty years (Table 1.1). The pessimistic view is based on the assumption that the rate of total tooth loss between 1978 and 1988 will remain

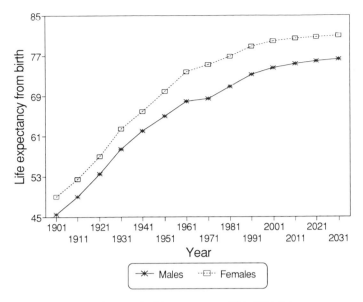

Figure 1.6 Changes in life expectancy 1901–2031.[3] A comparison between men and women

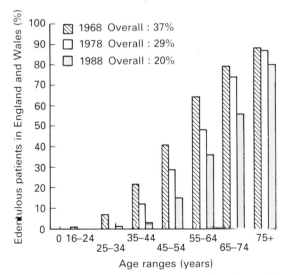

Figure 1.7 The proportion of the population of the UK with no natural teeth by age.[4] There has been a steady decline in the rate of edentulousness over the 15 years from 1968 to 1983

unchanged. The optimistic estimate assumes that there will be no further total tooth loss and that the future pattern will be a reflection of current levels of edentulousness as they feed through the age-groups. Depending upon the viewpoint taken, it is estimated that by the year 2038 either 94% or 100% of all adults

Table 1.1 Estimation of the percentage of the UK population that will retain some natural teeth in a given year

	Pessimistic estimate	Optimistic estimate
1998	86%	88%
2008	90%	94%
2018	93%	98%
2028	94%	99%
2038	94%	100%

will be retaining some natural teeth. In all probability the answer lies somewhere between these two figures.

Similar predictions have been made for those aged 65–74; they are shown in Table 1.2

Table 1.2 Estimation of the percentage of the age-group 65–74 in the UK that will retain some natural teeth in a given year

	Pessimistic estimate	Optimistic estimate
1998	59%	63%
2008	74%	83%
2018	84%	96%
2028	86%	99%
2038	86%	–

as the proportion of this age-group who will retain some natural teeth. Again, irrespective of whether one accepts the pessimistic or optimistic calculation, it is quite clear that more and more restorative treatment will be directed towards people who still possess some of their natural teeth.

The trend, described above, is not uniform, and there are variations according to the age and sex of the individual, and also according to the region of the country in which they live. At the same time that this improvement has occurred there has been greater demand for treatment. An increased proportion of the dentate population now attends for regular dental care.[4]

The problems

The problems, perceived or real, that we face in treating old people, can be considered under the three broad headings of management, treatment and treatment planning.

Management relates to the physical and mental deteriorations, and the increase in pathology, often associated with complex medication, that inevitably occur as we age. We might think, for example, of the extreme case of the patient who has suffered a stroke.

Treatment relates more directly to the need to maintain or repair the dental tissues, which have been damaged, sometimes to an exaggerated degree, sometimes minimally, as the patient has aged. Toothwear, root surface caries, and dry mouth, are all problems that are increasingly likely to be met.

Treatment planning, is perhaps the most difficult matter with which to come to grips, and relates both to management and treat-

ment. The dental needs of the ageing subject, if considered in isolation, may at first sight seem to be little different from those of the younger individual. For example, toothwear and root surface caries are amenable to routine dental care, even in an elderly patient. However, the complex nature of the work that is often required, when allied to the potential for poor tolerance of protracted dental treatment, either as a result of disease, frailty or senescence, can make treatment planning difficult. Thus, old people, especially the dentate elderly, form a distinct group in terms of the provision of care. In the long term, the nature of the treatment required by old people will probably not alter greatly. However, the call that this increasing cohort of dentate old people will make upon the dental services in the future is likely to be significant. This raises questions in relation to manpower planning and structure, which will be considered in Chapter 21.

This book considers the 'problems' of treating the elderly. However, those who have undertaken such treatment will know that although technical and management skills are required, dealing with old people is usually a pleasure.

References

1 Ed.: R.J. Simonsen, *Dentistry in the 21st century: A global perspective*, Quintessence Books, Chicago 1991
2 Ed.: W. Kunzel, *Geriatric dentistry in Eastern European countries*, Quintessence Books, Chicago 1991
3 *Social trends (18)*, Central Statistical Office, HMSO, London 1988
4 Todd J.E., Lader D., *Adult dental health*, HMSO, London 1991

Medical aspects of ageing: Facial and oral pain

Shelagh Baillie and Kenneth Woodhouse: with Crispian Scully on pain

Before considering the dental treatment of the elderly it will be useful to understand something of the nature of the ageing process, and the deteriorations that inevitably occur as we age. Some of these deteriorations are so usual as to be considered normal, others are associated with disease that may occur as the result of the deteriorations or by chance.

Mechanisms of 'normal' ageing

Theories of ageing abound, but none adequately explains the various manifestations of ageing throughout the body. It is likely that several mechanisms are involved. It may be that different tissues age in different ways.[1,2]

'Programmed' ageing

The concept of a decaying biological clock has been aired many times. Some lifetime events, such as growth, puberty and the menopause, are genetically determined, and it has been suggested that ageing is too. Certainly, 'normal' cell lines age when cultured in vitro. For example, the multiplication of fibroblasts decreases in cell culture and stops after 20–50 replications, depending on whether they are derived from embryos or adults. Only 'malignant' cell lines are immortal.

In the intact organism, the rate of ageing may be genetically determined, and is reflected in the lifespan. This difference is most marked between species. For example, one day for a mayfly, about 80 years for a human. However, differences are also seen between individuals of the same species. The expected lifespan in humans can be estimated fairly well from the age of parents and grandparents at death. 'Biological', rather than 'chronological', age in humans is an important and well-understood concept (Fig. 2.1). All physicians are familiar with the 'geriatric' 60-year-old and the 'middle-aged' 80-year-old. One of our own patients took up hang-gliding in his eighties!

Error accumulation and mutation

Mutation is a result of faulty transcription of DNA during cell division. It can result from irradiation, exposure to chemicals or other factors. Normally, mutations are corrected by complex DNA repair mechanisms, and it has been suggested that these are impaired with ageing. Mutation, or other errors in DNA, RNA, or protein synthesis, may result in the production of faulty enzymes or proteins. Some workers believe that such 'error accumulation' is the basis of the ageing process, although further work is required to establish the validity of this theory.

Reactive oxygen and free radicals

During normal metabolism, and the metabolism of foreign compounds, reactive oxygen species (peroxides and superoxides) and free

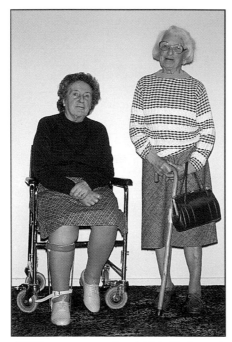

Figure 2.1 The woman on the right is 94, lives alone, is mobile, has no illnesses and is on no medication. She is biologically young. The woman on the left is 70, is disabled after a severe stroke, has seven diagnosed medical problems and will require long-term medical care. She is biologically old

radicals (highly reactive molecular fragments) may form. These may damage nucleic acids, proteins, membranes and other critical cellular structures. Repair mechanisms usually correct such damage, but 'error accumulation' may occur over a lifetime. Attempts to prolong the life of experimental animals by decreasing the production of reactive oxygen and free radicals, using antioxidants such as vitamin E, have been disappointing.

Immunology

It is well known that the thymus gland involutes with age. The number of circulating T-lymphocytes decreases, and tests of cell-mediated immunity are less likely to give a positive result. The decline in T-cells and T-cell function is associated with an increased incidence of cancers and infection. Interestingly, abnormal 'autoantibodies' directed against normal bodily tissues are more likely to be found in such circumstances. Whether these immune changes are fundamental to the ageing process or are simply a manifestation of it, remains unclear.

Bodily changes associated with ageing

It is important to distinguish between events that are a feature of 'normal ageing' and those that are a result of diseases which are more common in the elderly. For example, many old people suffer cerebrovascular disease, but it should be recognized that this is a pathological rather than an inevitable physiological event. Similarly, many old people have heart failure, but this is a result of heart disease, not 'normal ageing'. Thus, both cerebrovascular disease and heart failure are age-related phenomena.

Changes of 'normal' ageing

Skin and appendages

Changes in the skin are the most visible manifestation of ageing. The skin wrinkles and sags due to reduction in subcutaneous fat, increased collagen and fragmented, inelastic elastin. Blood capillaries are more fragile and may rupture, leading to senile purpura. The hair greys as a result of decreased pigment production by the follicle, and nail growth rate is reduced by almost one-half.

Heart and blood vessels

As in the skin, the amount of collagen in the vessel wall increases, and elastin becomes less elastic. The arteries become stiffer, and systolic blood pressure and pulse pressure tend to rise. Arteriosclerosis is commonly seen. The heart itself may hypertrophy, and some fibrosis develops. The heart valves tend to become stiffer. If coronary artery disease is absent, however, cardiac output can be well maintained.

Lungs

Changes in pulmonary physiology occur, even in non-smokers with no history of respiratory disease. Vital capacity tends to fall, with an increase in residual volume. Thoracic compliance is decreased, and these changes lead to a fall in maximal respiratory capacity. Coughing is not so efficient, and ciliary function in the bronchial epithelium may be decreased, leading to a greater incidence of lower respiratory tract infections.

Gut and liver

Decreased acid output in the stomach is so common as to be almost 'normal'. The effect of this on the absorption of foodstuffs is probably of no major importance. Absorption is generally adequate, although that of iron and calcium, and active sugar uptake, may decline. Malnutrition, if it occurs, is usually a result of illness, socioeconomic problems or confusion, rather than malabsorption. Oesophageal motility may be disorganized and lead to swallowing problems, and hiatus hernias are frequently seen. Stomach and small-bowel movements undergo only minor alterations, but large-bowel motility may decline and constipation and diverticulosis are frequent. The liver tends to shrink and its blood flow falls, although significantly impaired liver function is not seen.

Kidneys

Renal function declines with age, with a fall in nephron numbers of between 30% and 40% from age 25 to age 85. Renal blood flow, glomerular filtration rate and tubular function decline proportionately. Serum creatinine, however, does not rise, because of lower production from the reduced muscle mass. Renal drug excretion decreases.

Blood

Blood volume and red cell survival do not alter with age, and anaemia, if present, is the result of iron or vitamin deficiency, or disease. Immune changes have already been mentioned but, apart from T-cell changes, white blood cell numbers and differential count are unaltered. Platelet function is still under investigation. There is, however, no good evidence of hyper- or hypocoagulability.

Muscles and bones

Muscle mass and power decline with ageing. Arthritis, especially osteoarthritis, is common. Osteoporosis is extremely frequent, especially in women, and leads to increased fracture rates. This is most common in the hip and wrist, but the possible presence of a fragile mandible must always be borne in mind when extracting teeth in an older individual. Oestrogen replacement may prevent or ameliorate osteoporosis, but the condition is difficult or impossible to reverse once established.

Endocrine glands and metabolism

Serum thyroxine does not inevitably decrease with age. Nevertheless, thyroid disease is frequent. Thyroid-stimulating hormone (TSH) levels and TSH response to stress are maintained. In women, the menopause results in decreased oestrogen levels, which accelerate the development of osteoporosis, and in high levels of pituitary gonadotrophins. Changes in male gonadal function are less marked. Glucose tolerance is impaired, the response to a glucose load is reduced, and diabetes mellitus of the non-insulin-dependent type commonly occurs.

Nervous system and senses

Nerve cells are not replaced when lost. While the weight of the brain does not change significantly, studies of brain pathology demonstrate a loss of neurons in some cortical areas and a loss of cellular interconnections. Cerebral blood flow probably declines significantly. Cognitive impairment is a frequent but not invariable accompaniment of ageing, with poor memory and slower thought processes. It can be difficult to separate very mild dementia and 'normality'. However, many if not most old people remain intellectually normal until death.

Senses tend to fail with ageing. In the eye, the lens becomes thicker and less pliable, and people who previously had good sight require spectacles for near vision in the early forties. Hearing, especially for high tones, fails, particularly in men over 60. Smell, taste and touch all decline. Pain fibres appear to remain intact, and suggestions that there are changes in the pain threshold are controversial.

Disease and ageing

While age itself is not a disease, there is no doubt that many common illnesses become increasingly frequent with advancing years. Many of these are relevant to dental practice, and are considered here.

Disorders of the nervous system

The most important age-related disorders of the nervous system are cerebrovascular disease, extrapyramidal disease, dementia, depressive illness and facial pain.[3,4]

Cerebrovascular disease

Disease of the cerebral arteries is the third most common cause of death in developed countries and is responsible for significant mortality and morbidity in the elderly population. Although the manifestations of this condition are legion, the most common abnormality seen in clinical practice is that of hemiparesis (Fig. 2.2). All motor and sensory functions may be affected to a greater or lesser degree. The effects of motor derangement include facial palsy, and arm and leg paresis.

The disability resulting from a hemiparesis will restrict mobility, making it difficult for the patient to attend a clinic or surgery, and will impair activities of daily living such as basic hygiene and self-care. Appropriate physiotherapy, occupational therapy and social services help may ameliorate these problems. A frequent accompaniment, particularly of a right hemiparesis, is language impairment. This may involve a receptive dysphasia in which the patient is unable to comprehend what is being said to him, an expressive dysphasia in which he is unable to find the words to express himself, or a mixture of the two. Communication may be difficult or impossible.

Facial palsy will impair the manipulation of dentures, and frequently leads to the accumulation of food and debris between teeth and cheek on the affected side. It may be difficult

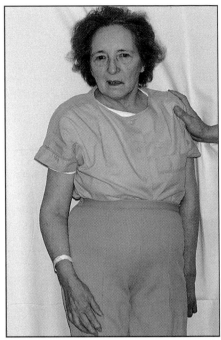

Figure 2.2 A patient with a dense left hemiparesis as a result of cerebrovascular disease. She cannot use her left arm and cannot stand without support

or impossible for the patient to maintain dental hygiene. Swallowing may be sufficiently impaired to affect dietary intake.

Dementia

Dementia is a progressive and irreversible impairment of cognitive function. It usually, but not invariably, occurs in those over the age of 65. The two commonest causes of senile dementia are Alzheimer's disease and multiinfarct dementia (a form of cerebrovascular disease). The illness is characterized by fading memory, poor concentration, followed by intellectual impairment and, later, self-neglect and incapacity for self-care. Dental hygiene usually deteriorates in these patients, and poor oral health is a frequent finding.

Psychological illness

Psychological illness in old people is frequently ignored or neglected, and may be misdiagnosed as dementia. Depression is common in the geriatric population. The clinical features are similar to those experienced by the young and include feelings of misery, sleep disturbance, poor appetite, anorexia, weight loss, self-neglect and social isolation. Pitt[3] has reviewed depression in the elderly in a very readable chapter.

Depressive illness in the elderly frequently responds well to antidepressant therapy, although this may result in oral complications. The often used tricyclic antidepressants have anticholinergic effects, which may lead to a dry mouth with associated dental problems. The new selective 5-HT uptake inhibitors are particularly useful in agitated depression in the elderly and have many fewer side effects.

Extrapyramidal disorders

Parkinson's disease becomes more common with advancing age.[5,6] It is a clinical syndrome caused by degeneration of pigmented neurons in the basal ganglia. The characteristic triad of clinical signs includes bradykinesia, rigidity and tremor. Disorder of posture is frequent, and hypersalivation may occur. Drug treatment is highly effective, although one of the most frequently recommended agents for mild parkinsonism (orphenadrine) can cause a dry mouth as a result of its anticholinergic effects. Preparations containing L-dopa do not have this side effect and are probably more effective.

Many extrapyramidal disorders are drug-induced. It has been suggested that the condition is a drug-induced or drug-associated disease in as many as 50% of elderly patients with parkinsonism. The most commonly implicated agents are the antipsychotics such as phenothiazines, thioxanthines and butyrophenones. These drugs can produce a tardive dyskinesia with long-term use and this may occur in 20–40% of patients who receive the drug for more than 6 months. The characteristic picture is of dyskinetic orofacial movements, including lip-smacking and tongue protrusion. Such orofacial movements can hinder dental hygiene and the management of dentures. The treatment is to withdraw the drug, but at least 40% of patients never improve. Orofacial dyskinesias may occur spontaneously in a small proportion of otherwise 'normal', drug-free elderly patients.

Age-related disorders of the nervous system can cause facial pain, and this is discussed at the end of this chapter.

Cardiovascular disease

Cardiovascular disease becomes more common with advancing years. The main disorders to consider are: valvular heart disease and endocarditis; hypertension; hypotension; ischaemic heart disease and heart failure.[7,8,9] Cardiovascular disease is also a cause of pain.

Valvular disease and endocarditis

Although the incidence of new cases of rheumatic fever has become less over the past few decades, cases of residual rheumatic heart disease are frequently seen in the elderly population. A variety of non-rheumatic, degenerative valve diseases occur with age, and increasing numbers of patients with prosthetic valves are reaching the geriatric age range. Endocarditis may result, and prophylactic cover is important.

National guidelines for antibiotic prophylaxis have been published in the current *British National Formulary*. Patients with abnormal, or prosthetic, valves who have not suffered from bacterial endocarditis and who are to undergo dental treatment with or without local anaesthesia, should receive oral amoxycillin, 3 g, 1 hour before procedure — provided that they have not received penicillin more than once during the previous month. Patients who are allergic to penicillin, or have received penicillin more than once in the previous month should receive oral clindamycin, 600 mg, 1 hour before procedure. Patients who have had endocarditis should receive amoxycillin and gentamycin as detailed below.

For dental procedures which are to be done under general anaesthesia, where there is no special medical risk, patients who have not received penicillin more than once in the previous month should receive i.m. or i.v. amoxycillin, 1 g, at induction, then oral amoxycillin, 500 mg, 6 hours later. Special risk patients (those with prosthetic valves, or those who have had endocarditis) should receive i.m. or i.v. amoxycillin, 1 g, and i.m. or i.v. gentamycin, 120 mg, at induction, then oral amoxycillin, 500 mg, 6 hours later. Patients who are penicillin-allergic or who have received a penicillin more than once in the previous month should receive i.v. vancomycin, 1 g, over at least 100 minutes, then i.v. gentamycin, 120 mg, at induction or 15 minutes before procedure.

No particular antibiotic prophylaxis is needed for dental procedures following coronary artery bypass grafting, but in general, anaesthetics should be avoided for four weeks post-operatively if at all possible.

No dentistry should be performed within 6 months of prosthetic valve surgery, to allow the valve to endothelialize. If essential, such work should be performed in a hospital environment.

Hypertension

Blood pressure rises with age. A study by Danner *et al*. in 1978 showed that, in a healthy group of individuals aged over 90 years, half the men and three-quarters of the women had systolic blood pressures over 160 mmHg. Suggestions have been made that blood pressures in excess of 160/90 in elderly men and women should be considered abnormal. The European Working Party on 'Hypertension in the elderly' produced results which indicate that some benefit in the prevention of stroke may accrue from treating hypertension in the 65–75 age-group. However, there is little evidence that treating hypertension in the over-75s with drugs affords significant benefit.

Hypotension

Orthostatic or postural hypotension may be defined as a fall in systolic blood pressure of greater than 20 mmHg between the lying and standing positions. It is a significant cause of morbidity in the elderly. An important factor is impairment of the autonomic nervous system with age, which results in a failure of the normal baroreceptor response to postural change. Diabetic neuropathy, polyneuropathy, cerebrovascular disease and Parkinson's disease have all been implicated. Once in the upright position, the decreased baroreceptor response causes blood to pool in the periphery, resulting in postural hypotension, dizziness, or even collapse. A variety of drugs, including antihypertensives, antidepressants, neuroleptics and diuretics, may exacerbate the condition.

Treatment of mild hypotension is simple, and includes discontinuation of the offending drug or drugs; the use of elastic stockings; and changing position gradually rather than suddenly. This has obvious implications in respect of the speed at which the dental chair is tilted. In more severe cases, treatment with drugs such as fludrocortisone may be necessary. Benzodiazepines have been shown to impair postural blood-pressure control in young patients, and it is possible that this effect is even more marked in the elderly. Thus, particular care should be taken with an elderly patient during the recovery phase from sedation with benzodiazepines.

Ischaemic heart disease and heart failure

Ischaemic heart disease becomes more prevalent with age and is accompanied by an increased incidence of cardiac failure. This has important implications for elderly people undergoing dental treatment, particularly if intravenous sedatives or a general anaesthetic are to be used. Myocardial infarctions are frequently 'silent', and patients can be afflicted by severe coronary artery disease without any history of angina pectoris or any form of chest pain.

Treatment of heart failure or of angina pectoris in eldcrly people follows the same lines as in the young. Calcium antagonists are more often used, because of their relative lack of adverse effects. Diuretics are well tolerated by most elderly people, but some complain of dizziness and a dry mouth.

Cardiovascular conditions can cause facial pain in the elderly, and this is considered at the end of this chapter.

Musculoskeletal disease

Musculoskeletal disorders are important in the elderly because of their frequency and the high degree of associated morbidity.[10] The two most common disorders are osteoarthritis and rheumatoid arthritis. Polymyalgia rheumatica, calcium pyrophosphate arthropathy and other connective tissue disorders also occur. Impaired mobility may profoundly affect life-style and hinder attendance at clinic and surgeries. Painful or reduced joint function in the hands will affect not only dental hygiene, but also diet. Difficulty in shopping, food preparation and eating can lead to a soft, often sweet, low-roughage diet, with subsequent vitamin deficiencies and resultant oral problems.

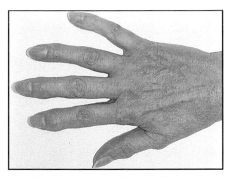

Figure 2.3 Deformity of the interphalangeal joints in a patient with osteoarthritis. (The swellings are called Heberden's nodes)

Osteoarthritis

Osteoarthritis is present in the joints of 75% of the over-65s. It most commonly causes pain followed by enlarged joints, and particularly affects the knee, hip, or first metacarpo-carpal joint. Joint movement is often reduced with obvious deformity (Fig. 2.3). The diagnosis is confirmed by radiographs. Management is supportive, with physiotherapy and occupational therapy playing important roles. Treatment can be supplemented by drugs such as simple analgesics and non-steroidal anti-inflammatory agents, although adverse effects are common, particularly with the latter. A history of joint replacement with a prosthesis is a not uncommon finding in an old person seeking dental treatment and dentists are often concerned about the need or otherwise to prescribe prophylactic antibiotic cover. Whereas it is courteous to seek the advice of the patient's orthopaedic surgeon, a recent paper from a working party on the need for such cover suggests that the risk is small and outweighed by the potential disadvantages.[11]

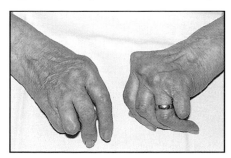

Figure 2.4 Severe deformity of the hands in a patient with rheumatoid arthritis. The skeletal changes are bilateral and can cause the sufferer some difficulty with oral hygiene

Rheumatoid arthritis

Rheumatoid arthritis affects 2.5% of the population and its onset may occur in any decade. It is a chronic systemic disorder which symmetrically affects the peripheral metacarpophalangeal and proximal interphalangeal joints. The articular cartilage erodes and the supporting structures degenerate, causing characteristic joint deformities (Fig. 2.4). Flexion contractures of the elbows and knees may occur. Temporomandibular joint arthritis can also occur. The disease may vary in severity, from mild to severe, to destructive, and completely disabling. Symptoms include pain and stiffness. Rarely, in the late stages, self-care becomes impossible.

Polymyalgia rheumatica

Polymyalgia rheumatica is related to giant cell arteritis and is characterized by pain, stiffness and tenderness, particularly of the shoulder muscles, although other muscle groups may be involved. Severe pain and stiffness around the shoulder girdle will impair daily activities, including oral hygiene. Laboratory findings include a characteristically elevated ESR. The disease can be disabling and is easily treated by the prescription of systemic steroids.

Disorders of nutrition

Ageing is associated with decreased requirement for food as a consequence of decreased physical activity and energy expenditure.[12,13] Appetite and food intake may well decrease. In 1979, a DHSS survey reported that 2.5% of the elderly population over 65 who were living at home were malnourished, largely as a result of social factors such as isolation, poverty and lack of awareness. Many of the medical conditions described above, particularly confusion and dementia, will contribute to impaired daily activities and poor dietary intake.

Symptoms and signs of malnutrition are often vague, and include low body weight, bone and muscle pains, and fatigue. Some vitamin deficiencies result in oral manifestations (Table 2.1), which may be noticed by a dental practitioner and should lead to further investigation.

Table 2.1 Vitamin deficiencies causing oral abnormalities

Vitamin	Oral signs of deficiency
Vitamin B$_2$ (riboflavin)	Angular stomatitis
	Cheilosis
	Cracked and fissured lips
	Glossitis
	Papillary atrophy
	Magenta tongue
Vitamin B$_{12}$	Glossitis
	Angular cheilosis
Folate	Occasionally tongue ulcers
Vitamin C	Gingivitis
	Bleeding, swollen, spongy gums

Ref: Oxford Textbook of Medicine, 2nd edn, Chs 8, 19. A.J. Weatherall, J.G.G. Ledingham, D.A. Warrel, eds. Oxford: OUP; 1987

Neoplasia

The elderly are at increased risk of neoplasia. The oral and facial implications of this will be covered in Chapters 4 and 18.

Orofacial pain

[with Crispian Scully]

Pain of any kind can be difficult to diagnose and treat in the elderly. They often have a high threshold for complaint, and many accept pain or illness as a part of old age. The three medical conditions that cause facial pain, and which are more common in the elderly, are giant cell arteritis, trigeminal neuralgia, and herpes zoster.

Trigeminal neuralgia

Lesions affecting the trigeminal nerve can cause facial pain which may be associated with a facial sensory deficit and impaired corneal reflex on the affected side. Idiopathic trigeminal neuralgia (benign paroxysmal trigeminal neuralgia; tic douloureux) is the most common neurological cause of facial pain.

Most patients are in the 50–70-year age-group and the pain usually involves the mandibular division of the trigeminal nerve. The characteristics include:

- Unilateral electric shock-like, brief, stabbing (lancinating) orofacial pains.

- Pain-free intervals between attacks. However, recurrence is common and very often the pain spreads to involve a wider area over time and the intervals between episodes tend to shorten.
- Pain of abrupt onset and abrupt termination.
- Triggering of pain from the oral or perioral region on the ipsilateral side in some patients. The trigger site bears no necessary relation to the painful area and may not be in the area of distribution of the affected trigeminal nerve division, but is always ipsilateral to the pain. Pain may be brought on by chewing, talking, swallowing, smiling or exposure to cold.
- No sensory loss in the trigeminal region or other neurological abnormalities.

The cause of trigeminal neuralgia is unclear, but it may be due to a vascular malformation pressing on the roots of the trigeminal nerve.

Management

It must be established that no abnormal neurological signs are present before drug treatment is started. Carbamazepine (Tegretol) remains the main treatment for trigeminal neuralgia. It is not an analgesic; it must be given continuously prophylactically. The dose should be increased until symptoms are controlled unless side effects (especially ataxia) become excessive. Most elderly patients respond to 200–400 mg three times daily. The blood pressure and blood picture should be monitored and electrolytes checked from time to time.

Local cryosurgery to the trigeminal nerve branches involved (cryoanalgesia) can produce analgesia without permanent anaesthesia, but the benefit is often only temporary. Surgical destruction of the trigeminal ganglion (radiofrequency ganglionolysis) or decompression of the trigeminal nerve may be required in the rare intractable cases.

Herpetic and post-herpetic neuralgia

Herpes zoster (shingles) is often preceded, accompanied and followed by neuralgia. Post-herpetic neuralgia causes continuous burning pain that affects mainly elderly patients and may be so intolerable that suicide can become a risk. Treatment is difficult but antidepressants or chlorpromazine may possibly help if analgesics are not effective.

Psychogenic causes

Atypical oral and facial pain is an ill-defined entity which includes:

- Atypical facial pain (or 'neuralgia')
- Temporomandibular pain-dysfunction syndrome (facial arthromyalgia)
- Atypical odontalgia
- The syndrome of oral complaints
- Burning or sore mouth (oral dysaesthesia).

Features common to all types include:

- Patients are often female
- Many are middle-aged or older
- Constant chronic symptoms
- The symptoms do not waken the patient from sleep.
- The location of the pain is ill-defined, may cross the midline to involve the other side, or may move to another site
- There is a total lack of objective signs
- All investigations are negative
- There are often recent adverse life-events, such as bereavement or family illness
- There are often multiple oral and/or other psychogenic related complaints, such as headaches, chronic back pains, irritable bowel syndrome or dysmenorrhoea.

Atypical facial pain is relatively common, usually in middle-aged or older women who complain of a dull, continuous ache, usually in the upper jaw. Despite this, sleep and appetite are only rarely disturbed, and analgesics are rarely tried by the patient.

Many such patients are depressed or hypochondriacal, and persist in blaming organic diseases for their pain. Attempts at relieving pain by dental treatment are usually unsuccessful. Some respond to prothiaden. However, many refuse psychiatric help or medication.

Facial pain

Several disorders in which the most obvious organic feature is vascular dilatation or constriction cause facial pain. The pain is usually obviously in the face rather than in the mouth.

Migraine

Migraine is a recurrent headache affecting women especially. It appears to be related to arterial dilatation which may be precipitated by alcohol, some foods (e.g. ripe bananas or chocolate), and stress. Classic migraine has the following features:

- Preceding warning symptoms (an aura)
- Headache which is severe, usually unilateral (hemicranial) and lasts for hours or days
- Photophobia, nausea or vomiting.

Migraine is usually managed with drugs, particularly sumatriptan. If attacks are frequent, prophylaxis with clonidine is the treatment of choice, but sometimes pizotifen, ergotamine or methysergide are used. In acute attacks patients usually prefer to lie in a quiet, dark room. Ergotamine given early may abort an attack.

Migrainous neuralgia

Migrainous neuralgia is less common than migraine and males are mainly affected. Attacks are sometimes precipitated by alcohol. The pain is unilateral, episodic, burning and boring in character, and localized around the eye usually. Generally, attacks last less than 1 hour, commence and often terminate suddenly, and often awaken the patient in the early morning (2–3 a.m.). This pain is associated on the affected side with profuse watering and congestion of the conjunctiva, rhinorrhoea and nasal obstruction.

Migrainous neuralgia is managed with sumatriptan, ergotamine, pizotifen or methysergide prophylactically. Sometimes corticosteroids or lithium carbonate are needed.

Cranial (giant cell) arteritis

Giant cell arteritis is sometimes called temporal arteritis. It is an autoimmune condition that leads to an acute or subacute arteritis which particularly affects the extracranial vessels. The intracranial vessels are also affected to a lesser extent. It is important that an early diagnosis be made for this condition, as, if untreated, it may lead to blindness and stroke. Headache is the prominent feature, and may be generalized intense and aching or localized over enlarged tender and non-pulsatile temporal arteries. Claudication of the muscles of mastication, especially the masseter, may occur during chewing. Ischaemic optic neuropathy may occur, and is a common, preventable, cause of blindness in elderly people. Diagnosis can usually be made from the characteristic clinical picture, and a very high erythrocyte sedimentation rate (ESR) or plasma viscosity. A temporal artery biopsy may sometimes be necessary, and will show the arterial elastic tissues to be fragmented with giant cells numerous in the region of the deranged internal tissues. Treatment with high-dose prednisolone is very effective, and is sometimes used as a diagnostic test. Treatment may need to be continued for 1 or 2 years, until the underlying pathology subsides.

References

1 Davies I., Biology of ageing – theories of ageing, in, *Textbook of geriatric medicine and gerontology*, ed. J.C. Brocklehurst, Churchill Livingstone, London 1978

2 Exton Smith A.N., Overstall P.W., Mechanisms of ageing, in, *Geriatrics*, MTP, London 1970

3 Pitt B., *Psychogeriatrics*, Ch. 7, Churchill Livingstone, Edinburgh 1984

4 Rossor M., Dementia, *Br. J. Hosp. Med. 1987*; 38: 46–50

5 Bakheit A.M.O., Drug treatment of Parkinson's disease, *Hospital Update 1990*; 6: 497–504

6 Stephen P.J, Williamson J., Drug-induced parkinsonism in the elderly, *Lancet 1984*; 2: 1082–3

7 European working party on high blood pressure in the elderly: Trial Report, *Lancet 1985*; 1: 1349–54

8 Danner S.A., De Beaumont M.J., Dunning A.J., Cardiovascular health in the tenth decade, *Br. Med. J. 1978*; 2: 663

9 Eds, Martin, Camm, *Heart disease in the elderly*, John Wiley, Chichester 1984

10 Ed, V. Wright, *Bone and joint disease in the elderly*, Churchill Livingstone, Edinburgh 1983

11 Simmons N.A., Ball A.P., Cawson R.A., Eykyn S.J., Hughes S.P.F., McGowan D.A., Shanson D.C., Case against antibiotic prophylaxis for dental treatment of patients with joint prostheses, Letters to editor, *Lancet 1992*; 33: 301

12 Eds, A.N. Exton-Smith, Caird, *Metabolic and nutritional disorders in the elderly*, Wright, Bristol 1980

13 *DHSS report no. 16*, Nutrition and health in old age, HMSO, London 1979

3

Orofacial ageing

John Drummond, James Newton and John Scott

A number of age changes affecting the orofacial structures are of clinical importance when treating elderly dental patients. Some of these changes will make certain clinical procedures more difficult and will reduce the prognosis. This is particularly true of prosthetic and restorative dental treatment. Other oral age changes need to be recognized by the dental surgeon as being a normal finding and not part of a disease process. Reassurance can be given to the older, worried patient if the dentist is familiar with these ageing changes.

A distinction must be made between a true age change and one that is related either to disease or merely to the passage of time. One definition of true age changes are that they conform to the following criteria:

- An age change is not necessarily deleterious
- The change is progressive
- The change is seen in all members of the species
- The change is not reversible.

Whilst some changes in orofacial structures can be regarded as true age changes, others are undoubtedly related to a disease process or are a combination of a pathological process and ageing. The following tissues will be considered:

- Bone
- Alveolar bone

- Temporomandibular joint
- Muscle and nerve
- Salivary glands   Whole saliva
  Submandibular gland
  Parotid ageing
  Minor glands
  Salivary function

- Oral mucosa
- Periodontal tissues
- The teeth.

Bone

Following the growth of the skeleton, there is a period of consolidation over about 15 years with further calcium accretion, decreased cortical porosity and increasing cortical thickening. Peak adult bone mass is attained at about 35 years. Subsequently, bone mass declines with age, with both cortical and trabecular bone being lost.[1]

In old age, particularly in women, an increased proportion of cortical bone is occupied by resorption centres, particularly in and near the endosteal surface. An additional factor in bone loss with age is an imbalance between resorption and replacement of bone in the Haversian systems. New Haversian systems are not completed so that the central canals remain permanently wider than normal. One of the results of continuing subperiosteal osteoclastic activity in old age is that there is a gradual increase in the diameter of some bones. The bones of the skull are similarly affected and this accounts, in part, for the changes in facial appearance which often take place in advancing years.

Ageing also affects the internal architecture of bone (Fig. 3.1). There occurs a decrease in cortical thickness which is greater in women than in men. Cross-sectional studies suggest a slow steady reduction in cortical bone mass throughout life, with a man of 75 years having a thickness of 90% compared to one of 25 years. In women, however, bone loss begins around 35–45 years of age and is much more rapid than in men, with a woman of 75 years having a cortical thickness of only 60% compared to one of 25 years.[2] This loss of calcified tissue, particularly in women, has been extensively studied but one must be wary of interpreting changes with age that are measured at one site, as reflecting what is happening in the whole skeleton or at another site. Certainly, total body calcium in women, as determined by neutron activation analysis, falls by 3% for 45–55 year olds, but by 9% per decade in post-menopausal women.[1,3]

It has been shown specifically that the density of mandibular bone decreases by around 20% between the ages of 45 and 90 and that throughout this age range, values for women were significantly lower.[4] In addition to being less dense, the bone is often more brittle, with increasing numbers of microfractures of the thinned trabeculae which heal slowly due to impaired remodelling. There is also an increase in bone porosity which is mainly the

result of an increase in vascular spaces.[1]

At a cellular level, resorption is usually not appreciably affected by age. Age-related changes in osteoclasts are more related to the status of the bone marrow than to the bone itself. Osteoblasts, however, are derived from bone-lining cells which, unfortunately, are severely depleted in number and activity by ageing. Thus, failure of osteoblast production and function to keep pace with resorption is thought to be a key factor in long-term changes in skeletal form. Although remnants of periosteal and endosteal precursor cells can be stimulated to produce osteoblasts, the overall bone-forming capacity of aged individuals is compromised.[3] The imbalance between osteoclastic and osteoblastic activity is exacerbated by the withdrawal of oestrogen during the menopause. As the oestrogen level falls, the balance between parathormone and calcitonin shifts in favour of parathormone, which significantly increases the renal excretion of minerals. There is also an age-related decrease in the circulatory level of hydroxylated vitamin D_3 which impairs intestinal absorption of calcium. Consequently, there is an increasing reliance on bone for the maintenance of adequate calcium levels. The elderly also have an impaired ability to increase calcium absorption in response to a low calcium diet.[5] In addition to changes in the supply and distribution of calcium salts, the blood supply to older bone may be impaired.

Changes may also be observed in the collagen matrix. Here, greater cross-linkage occurs, with the replacement of reducible cross-links by non-medullar and acid stable cross-links.[6]

Changes to particular bony structures in the oral cavity may be affected and even accelerated by other factors.

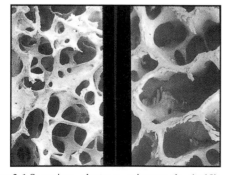

Figure 3.1 Scanning electron micrograph (×18) of a longitudinal section of sternum showing normal (left-hand side of illustration) and osteoporotic bone (right-hand side of illustration) in a 26-year-old man and a 73-year-old man, respectively

Alveolar bone

Alveolar bone participates in the general loss of bone mineral with age by resorption of the bone matrix. This process may be accelerated by tooth loss, periodontal disease and inadequate or inappropriate prostheses in genetically susceptible individuals or those with systemic disease (Fig. 3.2). Conversely, occlusal drift or over-eruption may stimulate alveolar bone deposition.

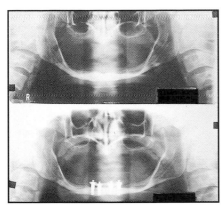

Figure 3.2 Grossly atrophic mandible (patient treated with osseointegrated implants)

Temporomandibular joint

The situation with regard to the temporomandibular joint is unclear. A number of abnormalities including arthritic changes and deterioration of the meniscus have been described, but the relationship to and relative importance of age, as distinct from local trauma and systemic disease, is uncertain.[7]

Muscle and nerve

Muscle function

There is evidence to show that there is a reduction in the total muscle mass amounting to about one-third over an 80-year period (Fig. 3.3). There is a relatively larger annual loss when subjects of 70 and 80 years are compared.[9,12,13] It has also been shown that

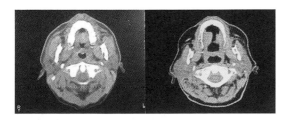

Figure 3.3 Computer tomographic scan of the jaw muscles, masseter and medial pterygoid, in a young subject (left-hand side of illustration) and an old subject (right-hand side of illustration). There is a substantial reduction in the cross-sectional area of these muscles in the older subject

there is no major reduction in muscle fibre size with age which reflects a decreased number of fibres.[8] Consideration must, therefore, be given to whether the age-related loss of fibres is due to the loss of complete motor units or whether each unit comprises a diminishing number of muscle fibres. Electrophysiological studies have shown a loss of motor units with age, particularly after the age of 60 years.[9,10,11] Progressive enlargement of the remaining motor units suggests that they are taking over and reinnervating muscle fibres that have lost their nerve supply.

Recent work on jaw-closing muscles has shown a prolongation of the contraction phase with age, which may either indicate a general age change of the muscle or the loss of faster twitch fibres.[12] However, any such preferential loss of one fibre type would have to be rather large to be identifiable with standard histological sampling techniques, and earlier electrophysiological studies have not shown discrete populations of fibre types. It has been observed that in certain arm and leg muscles of old subjects, fibre type grouping does occur but that the extent differs between muscles.

Other work on jaw muscles of the elderly has shown neither signs of atrophy nor a decrease in the population of type II fibres known to be fast contracting and to develop high tension.

With regard to the motor units of older subjects, longer contraction times have been recorded and in addition the threshold firing rates of these units are reduced. This reduction in firing rate may be regarded as being consistent with previous observations of a lengthening of the contraction time because a more slowly contracting muscle will develop a partially fused tetanic contraction at a lower frequency.[13]

It has also been found that there is a significant reduction in maximum tension and a loss of isometric and dynamic muscle strength in older subjects.[11,14,15] An important determinant of the maximum force which can be produced by a muscle is its cross-sectional area. Using computed tomography it has been found that there is a significant reduction of about 40% in the cross-sectional area with age in two jaw-closing muscles, the masseter and medial pterygoid. Also, changes in X-ray density of these muscles indicate an increase in the amount of fibro-fatty tissue with increasing age. These results are consistent with studies of the chest, abdomen, arm and leg muscles, and may indicate a general age change of the muscle tissue in the body as a whole. Specifically, they suggest that there is a reduction in the masticatory forces which can be utilized by ageing subjects. In all cases, female subjects exhibited significantly smaller muscles.[16] It has also been suggested that the elderly are able to employ less precision in the contraction of their masticatory muscles than young individuals.[17]

Superimposed on these changes, further reductions in jaw muscle bulk are found in edentulous subjects when compared to dentate subjects.[18] This supports evidence that the level of masticatory force and chewing efficiency in patients where the natural dentition has been replaced by an artificial one is greatly reduced.[19] However, complete denture wearers often regard their masticatory function as satisfactory.

Experimental studies have indicated that there is adaptation in muscle tissue, particularly in muscle fibre, following a change in functional conditions.[20] Also, it has been reported that there appears to be a reduction in Type II fibres in the jaw muscle of those who have an artificial dentition. It was suggested that this change might be attributable to altered functional demands, with atrophy of these fibres occurring as an early consequence of tooth loss.

It has been postulated that the underlying defect in the neuromuscular system during ageing is a progressive motor neuron dysfunction which is first manifested by an increasing inability of the motor neuron to maintain its colony of muscle fibres in a fully viable condition.[11] As the motor neuron degenerates, neighbouring ones may sprout and take over the supply of some of the muscle fibres. In this way the second neuron controls a larger motor unit. However, if the process of denervation progresses, the fibres in the larger motor unit will also lose their supply and become atrophic.

Nervous system

When reviewing muscle function with age, consideration must also be given to the nervous system because they are intimately related. It is well known that nerve cell loss is universal in old age and can therefore be considered a true age-related change. In the cerebral cortex, although there are considerable variations, nerve cell loss has been calculated at between 36% and 60% between the ages of 18 and 95 years. In the spinal cord, however, there is negligible loss up to the age of 60 years but thereafter there is a reduction of between 5% and 50%. Senile plaques and neurofibrillar tangles are also present in the ageing brain but it is still debatable as to whether they are a normal age change.[5,14,15]

Current research has also indicated that there are age-related changes in neurotransmitters, implying that there is a potential functional impairment in the elderly. It has been suggested that observed reductions in dopamine synthetic enzymes particularly, reflect impaired dopaminergic transmissions which in turn may be responsible for the motor dysfunctions characteristic of old age. However, the result of work on other transmitters is not so clear and requires further investigation.[15,21]

Peripheral nerve function usually declines with advancing age in that there are age-related changes which are universal, progressive and inevitable. There is a decrease in conduction velocity, increased latencies in multi-synaptic pathways, decreased conduction at neuromuscular junctions and loss of receptors.[5,9,15]

It has been postulated by some researchers that neural events are important with regard to ageing in other tissues, in that neurons exert a trophic influence on such diverse tissues as skin, connective tissue and bone. It is suggested that by withdrawal of its trophic influence the nervous system determines the onset and speed of the ageing process throughout much of the remainder of the body.[11]

Salivary glands

The investigation of salivary gland function can be problematical. Uncontaminated saliva can be difficult to collect from a single gland, such as the submandibular, and histological specimens of healthy gland are not easy to obtain. The use of computer generated tomographs is proving to be useful (Fig. 3.4).

It is widely accepted that a diminution in

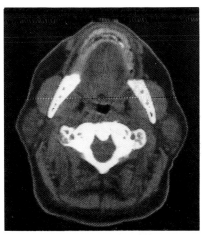

Figure 3.4 Computer generated tomograph through the parotid glands

salivary function is a normal concomitant of human ageing. Elderly people are assumed to secrete lower quantities of saliva both at rest and in response to the stimuli of talking and eating compared to mid-aged and young adults. At best, such notions oversimplify matters and with the development of clinical knowledge, as a generalization they become increasingly difficult to sustain.[24] It is true that complaints of xerostomia (dry mouth) are more common in the elderly than in younger age-groups. The current view attributes this more to the effects of intercurrent chronic illness and especially drug therapy in the elderly than to any intrinsic features of the ageing process itself. It has been estimated that 75% of drugs listed in the British National Formulary exert some degree of depression on salivary secretion. Most antidepressants and antihypertensive agents, for instance, have a marked hyposalivatory effect and these are drugs which are commonly prescribed for the elderly. Some of these agents are listed in Table 4.4, Chapter 4. Nevertheless, after due allowance is made for debilitating illness or iatrogenic causes of xerostomia in the elderly, there does remain an element of salivary reduction which is attributable to ageing changes in the glands themselves.

The principal functions of saliva are lubrication, buffering, and protection of the oral hard and soft tissues. Thus, any serious loss of salivary flow is likely to lead to difficulties with speech and swallowing, increased levels of dental caries and increased vulnerability of the mucosa to mechanical trauma and microbial infection. For example, such changes are regularly seen in irradiated patients where the salivary glands are severely damaged. However, such magnitude of oral disease is not commonplace in the healthy elderly which suggests that any reduction in salivary flow that does develop with ageing may not be of clinical significance.

Whole saliva

This term refers to the total pooled saliva in the mouth at any one time. Several studies of salivary function, using very strict criteria for selection which exclude drug therapy, chronic diseases or other likely causes of xerostomia, have shown that the resting level of total salivary secretion (that which is constantly present throughout the day between meals and unrelated to talking) is indeed reduced in the elderly. The important point to note, however, is that in these individuals there is little evidence of the severe drying consequences such as increased caries or the other disorders that are listed above. The conclusion that has tentatively been drawn is that such reduction in resting flow as does occur naturally in the aged is commensurate with the physiological demands of the oral cavity at this time of life. Sufficient saliva is still present at rest to adequately protect the oral hard and soft tissues. Thus a finding which is of statistical significance in a population, such as a reduced resting salivary flow in the elderly as a group, is not necessarily of biological significance in the individual patient.[24] One possible explanation is that the resting rate of clearance of saliva from the mouth may also be reduced in the elderly so that its level is equivalent to the reduced level of resting secretion. It is only when some additional reduction of flow is experienced, as in drug therapy or after irradiation, that the balance between flow rate and clearance is disturbed and pathological oral desiccation occurs.

It is also important to note that, in many of these studies of the healthy elderly, no diminution in stimulated total saliva could be demonstrated in comparison with young healthy adults. Thus, when physiological demand is made on the salivary glands in the healthy elderly, an adequate response can be elicited.

Whether such a response could be maintained over as long a period of time in the elderly as in the young has not been adequately tested. However, in view of the undoubted structural losses of salivary tissue which occur in old age, it is suspected this may not be the case.

Parotid ageing

The parotids are the largest salivary glands in man and contribute 20% of resting saliva and 50% of maximally stimulated saliva. Because the parotid duct orifice is accessible and easily isolated, salivary flow from this gland has been studied more extensively and more frequently than any other salivary gland. Several well-designed studies using geographically and socially different populations have repeatedly failed to demonstrate any differences either in stimulated or unstimulated flow rates with increasing age.[24] Many of the studies have employed large numbers of subjects and this is important because the normal rate of flow varies over a very wide range . For example, unstimulated parotid flow rates vary within a 100-fold range, whilst for stimulated flow rates the normal range is 20-fold. There is no evidence that these ranges differ between different age-groups.

Studies of parotid gland size have also shown no difference with age. This also is an important observation because total gland mass is one of the more important determinants of maximal salivary flow rate. Qualitative studies on parotid saliva indicate some changes with age but these are difficult to interpret and are not necessarily linear, that is to say they do not occur uniformly across the life span. There is some evidence, however, that in healthy males the concentrations of certain ions, for example Na^+, Ca^{++}, Cl^- and of total protein are reduced with age, as is the pH. Nevertheless, overall there appears to be little functional decrement in parotid saliva with age.

On the other hand, studies of parotid gland structure in relation to ageing have elicited some apparently conflicting evidence. Accurate quantitative histological analyses have indicated that as age increases the total amount of secretory tissue in the parotid gland is gradually replaced by fibro-fatty tissues (Fig. 3.5a,b).[22] This follows trends already well established for the human submandibular and labial glands which show a linear reduction in glandular parenchyma across the span of human adult life. The nature of these changes is described more fully below.

Submandibular gland

The submandibular is the second largest major salivary gland in man, and by anatomical position is readily accessible for surgical or post-mortem removal. Not surprisingly, therefore, it has been the subject of numerous structural studies in relation to ageing. However, its secretion is difficult to obtain in isolation, uncontaminated by other secretions pooling in the floor of the mouth. For this reason, much less study has been made of possible functional age changes in submandibular saliva. Moreover, from the few functional studies that have been reported to date, no uniform picture emerges. One group of investigators showed no change with age, while another group with apparently equally rigorous selection of patients showed over 60% reduction in stimulated and unstimulated flow in the elderly. Clearly, further studies are needed to clarify this situation. Certainly, there is evidence of a reduction in submandibular gland size occurring in the later decades of life. Also, quantitative histological studies, using techniques which can accurately estimate the relative volume proportions of different gland components, have shown that over the adult life span the secretory acinar tissue becomes depleted at a uniform rate which ultimately totals 40% of the initial mass. These losses are accompanied by degenerative histological changes in the secretory acini themselves, as well as in the ducts which appear to be more numerous and irregular. Changes also occur in the amount and type of connective tissue in the glands. Although fatty tissue only occasionally reaches the prominent amounts frequently seen in the parotid gland, it is generally more abundant in the submandibular glands in old age than in the young. The fibrous tissue is coarser and more abundant and appears to be replacing the secretory tissues of the gland. Furthermore, scattered foci of atrophy with limited amounts of chronic inflammatory infiltration become progressively more numerous with age.

Finally, it has been shown that small intraductal plugs of solid material which are

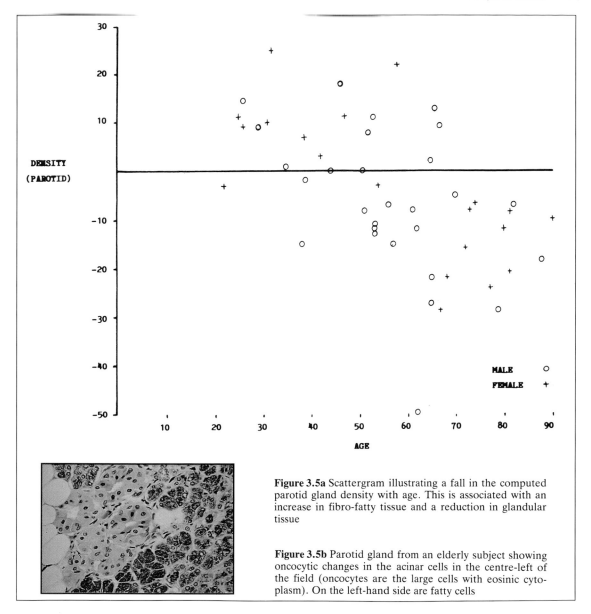

Figure 3.5a Scattergram illustrating a fall in the computed parotid gland density with age. This is associated with an increase in fibro-fatty tissue and a reduction in glandular tissue

Figure 3.5b Parotid gland from an elderly subject showing oncocytic changes in the acinar cells in the centre-left of the field (oncocytes are the large cells with eosinic cytoplasm). On the left-hand side are fatty cells

possibly the precursors of salivary calculi, also become more numerous with advancing age.

Minor salivary glands

The most frequently studied minor salivary glands in man are the labial glands.[26] However, studies have also been made of palatal and lingual glands in relation to ageing. In general, all of these glands show degenerative structural changes and losses of glandular epithelium in the later decades of adult life (Figs 3.6, 3.7).[24] The changes are usually more severe in the labial glands, possibly because their relatively exposed position renders them more vulnerable to repeated trauma. The ducts are often severely dilated, the acini are fewer and smaller than in younger glands and interacinar fibrosis is frequently present.

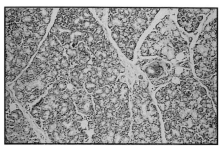

Figure 3.6 Young submandibular gland, showing lobular architecture and abundant secretory acini

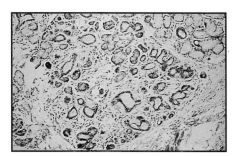

Figure 3.7 Minor salivary gland (labial) from an old subject. The lobules contain sparse numbers of acini composed of relatively few secretory cells separated by fibrous tissue

Functional studies of the minor glands are difficult to carry out because of difficulties of isolating groups of glands and then ensuring that all their secretions can be collected. Unlike major glands, minor glands discharge by numerous individual secretory ducts opening directly onto the mucosal surface. Pre-weighed filter paper discs can be used to absorb the secretion over a defined mucosal area over a given period of time in order to assess flow rate. Alternatively, these minute volumes of saliva can be collected in small capillary tubes. One of the problems with this approach is the accurate definition of the test area, for example on the labial mucosa, so as to ensure that comparisons between age-groups are made on a common basis. Using this technique it has been possible to demonstrate reductions in labial salivary flow but the few reported studies require confirmation.

A summary of salivary function

There is no doubt that salivary epithelial degeneration, atrophy, loss of acini and fibro-sis occur with increasing frequency and severity as age increases. These changes occur to a variable extent in all human salivary glands so far studied. However, the degree to which these structural changes are reflected in functional changes with age is much less clear. Certain individual glands, such as the parotid, show no diminution of function with age, whilst for others, the submandibular for example, there is conflicting evidence for reduced flow rates in old age.[23]

It is generally accepted that resting whole saliva is reduced in volume in old age whilst stimulated whole saliva is not. Given the undoubted structural changes present in the salivary glands in old age, the latter finding, especially, suggests that the salivary glands of old people are capable of working more efficiently than those of young people. It has been postulated that a salivary functional reserve capacity is present in young adults which is increasingly called upon with ageing to allow an optimal physiological response to be maintained for a given level of stimulation. Furthermore, the reduced level of resting whole saliva experienced in old age is probably commensurate with the resting physiological demands of the oral cavity at that time of life.

Most important of all, the xerostomia experienced so frequently by elderly patients is far more likely to be due to the side effects of medication than to any 'natural' ageing change in the salivary glands, despite the severe histological damage sustained by these glands in old age.[24,25,26]

Oral mucosa

Dental surgeons are familiar with the changes that may occur with age in the skin and oral mucosa. These changes may lead to a number of problems.

An unwrinkled skin does not imply that there have been no ageing changes in the epithelium; rather the aged skin is being supported by underlying fatty tissue (Fig. 3.8). Atrophic changes can also be found in the sebaceous and sweat glands and there is a reduction in mean skin epithelial thickness with age.

Some intra-oral changes may be noticed

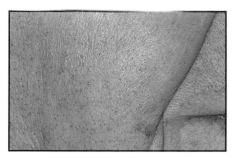

Figure 3.8 An 87-year-old man with relatively unwrinkled and unblemished skin

with the naked eye and these include prominent sebaceous glands and a smooth appearance of some mucosal surfaces. Sublingual varicosities are commonly found in many elderly individuals and are not now thought to be related to any systemic disease. Patients occasionally ask about prominent varicosities and should be reassured. In elderly individuals it is also noticeable that the sebaceous glands become more prominent, probably because of mucosal thinning. However, visible age changes are by no means usual, and as with the skin, it can be impossible with healthy old people to determine, by simple examination, any deterioration in the oral tissues (Fig. 3.9).

A number of studies have examined cell proliferation in the oral mucosa of elderly individuals and although some results are conflicting most suggest there is a decrease in proliferation with age. There is now good evidence in humans that there is a reduction in mean epithelial thickness with age.[28]

In the tongue, a reduction of epithelial thickness of around one-third from youth to old age can be measured. Although the progenitor layer appears to show no reduction

in width, there is a reduction in nuclear/cytoplasmic ratio. Another consistent finding is that there is an overall simplification in epithelial structure with age and the rete pegs become much less prominent (Fig. 3.10a,b).[28]

Although there is some information about the structure of the epithelium in old individuals, little is known about functional changes with age. There can be little doubt that some of the histological changes would suggest that the mucosa is more easily damaged in the elderly. This may account for problems such as burning tongue, and denture wearing, particularly when associated with dry mouth. Changes in the function of oral

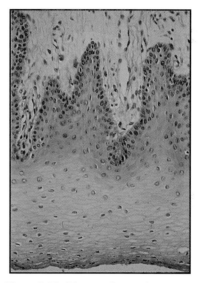

Figure 3.10a Mucosa from the ventral surface of a young tongue. Note the thickness of the epithelium and well-formed rete ridges in comparison to Figure 3.10b

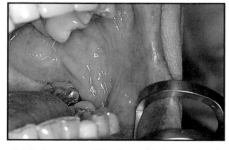

Figure 3.9 It is not possible from this 'macroscopic view' to make any valid judgement about the subject's age. In fact this healthy mucosa belongs to the same 87-year-old man shown in Figure 3.8

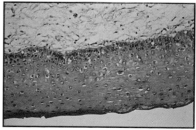

Figure 3.10b Mucosa from the ventral surface of the tongue of an old subject. The epithelial layer is reduced in thickness and a rete ridge system is lacking. Such mucosa may be susceptible to trauma

epithelium with age may be related to the development of certain oral diseases such as oral carcinoma. However, no firm evidence exists for this, and for the present this relationship must remain speculative.

The teeth

Whilst the teeth usually show some sign of changes with age these changes are not just a result of age but reflect, wear, disease, oral hygiene and habit. Toothwear is dealt with specifically in Chapter 7.

The enamel undergoes a number of significant age changes, including an increase in nitrogen and fluoride concentration with age. The increased fluoride content of surface enamel is particularly important as this may modify susceptibility to caries and affect the adhesive properties of enamel in older individuals following etching with phosphoric acid.

Changes that occur in the dentine pulp complex are familiar to all dentists because of the clinical effects they have. The continued formation of dentine with age causes a gradual reduction in the size of the pulp chamber (Fig. 3.11). The formation of secondary dentine is particularly prominent on the ceiling and floor of the pulp chamber; formation on the walls is considerably less. The other change that occurs in dentine is that of sclerosis by continued formation of peritubular dentine. This change may lead to a reduction in dentinal sensitivity in elderly patients. Sclerosis is often very marked in the roots which may be almost glass-like in appearance (Fig. 3.12).

As well as a reduction in the size of the pulp, the other change with which dentists will be familiar is an increased incidence of pulpal calcification. The calcification may be diffuse or in the form of pulp stones, and in the majority of cases is related to previous dentinal/pulpal injury. Extensive calcification involving the pulp chamber and root canals may cause problems with root treatment of these teeth. A change in the blood supply to the pulp is well documented and takes the form of a reduction in arterial supply by way of the root canal and a reduction in the numbers of capillaries in the pulp.

Changes in pulpal blood supply may alter the inflammatory reaction in the pulps of teeth of older people. Another marked change is the increase in the number of collagenous fibres, particularly in the coronal area (Fig. 3.13). On occasions the pulps of apparently healthy teeth may die as a result of bacterial invasion through furcal canals, or even the apical canal, as a result of periodontal involvement. This can pose diagnostic problems.

It is a common clinical finding that dental procedures that require the provision of local

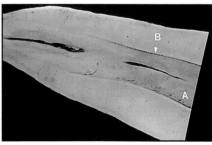

Figure 3.11 Ground section through a root showing marked secondary/reactionary dentine deposition (A), which can be distinguished from the primary dentine (B)

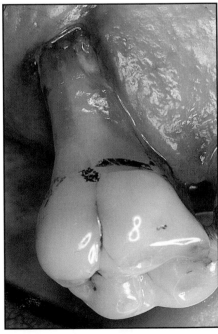

Figure 3.12 Palatal root of a periodontally involved tooth showing an increased translucency of root dentine associated with age

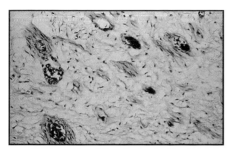

Figure 3.13 Pulp tissue showing decreased cellularity associated with age

anaesthesia in the young, require less or none in some older patients. This may relate to the greater thickness of dentine and to age changes within the pulp. It is unlikely to be as a result of reduced central perception and a raised pain threshold.

There is a progressive increase in the thickness of the cementum throughout life, and up to three times as much cementum may be found in individuals over 75 years when compared with young individuals. The progressive age-related laying down of cementum should not be confused with hypercementosis or cemental tumours which are pathological processes. An exaggerated deposition of cementum is seen in patients suffering from Paget's disease.

Some of the age changes are sufficiently consistent to enable single extracted teeth to be used to establish the age of the 'donor' to within five years.

It is often believed that old teeth are more brittle than young. There is no evidence that the crowns of intact teeth are any more susceptible than the young, other than as a consequence of fair wear and tear, particularly in those teeth weakened, iatrogenically, by intracoronal 'restorations'. The roots may, as a consequence of calcifications, be less elastic, and this combined with hypercementosis and localized changes in the alveolar bone may increase the difficulties of extraction, in which matter the fragility of the mandible should not be forgotten.

Periodontal tissues

Age changes in the periodontal tissues must not be confused with those seen in disease processes. The changes that occur in the periodontal tissues with age are considered in Chapter 7.

References

1 Woolf A.D., Dixon A. St J., *Osteoporosis – a clinical guide*, Martin Dunitz, London 1988; 215–21
2 Paterson C.R., MacLennan W.J., *Bone disease in the elderly*, John Wiley and Sons, London 1984; 17–30
3 Roberts W.C., Gonsalves M., Aging of bone tissue, in, *Geriatric dentistry*, eds, P. Holm-Pedersen, H. Loe, Munksgaard, Copenhagen 1986; 83–93
4 Wowern N.V., Stoltze K., Sex and age differences in bone morphology of mandibles, *Scand J. Dent. Res. 1978*; 86: 479–86
5 Kenney R.A., *Physiology of aging: a synopsis*, Year Book Medical Publishers, Inc. London 1989; 15–25 and 37–97
6 Shikata H., Utsumi N., Fujimoto D., Collagen in aging bone of the jaw, *Front. Oral Physiol. 1987*; 6: 85–95
7 Drummond J.R., Newton J.P., Yemm R., Dentistry for the elderly: A review and an assessment of the future, *J. Dent 1988*; 16: 47–54
8 Grimby C., Danneskiold-Samsoe B., Hvid K., Saltin B., Morphology and enzymatic capacity of arm and leg muscles in 78–82 year old men and women, *Acta Physiol. Scand. 1982*; 115: 125–34
9 Masoro E.J., Physiology of aging, in, *Geriatric dentistry*, eds, P. Holm-Pedersen, H. Löe, Munksgaard, Copenhagen 1986; 34–55
10 Brown W.F., A method for estimating the number of motor units in thenar muscles and the changes in the motor unit count with aging, *J. Neurol. Neurosurg. Psychiat. 1972*; 35: 845–52
11 McComas A.J., Ageing, in, *Neuromuscular functions and disorders*, Butterworths, London 1978; 101–8
12 Newton J.P., Yemm R., Contractile changes in human jaw muscle with age, *J. Oral. Rehab. 1990*; 13: 205
13 Newton J.P., Yemm R., McDonagh M.J.N., A study of age changes in the motor units of the first dorsal interosseous muscle in man, *Gerontology 1988*; 34: 115–19
14 Cunningham W.R., Brookbank J.W., *Gerontology – The psychology, biology and sociology of ageing*, Harper and Row, New York 1988; 81–105
15 Hubbard B.M., Squier M., The physical ageing of the neuromuscular system, in, *The clinical neurology of old age*, ed., R. Tallis, John Wiley and Sons, 1989; 3–26
16 Newton J.P., Abel R.W., Robertson E.M., Yemm R., Changes in human masseter and medial pterygoid muscle with age: a study using computed tomography, *Gerodontics 1987*; 3: 151–4
17 Yemm R., Newton J.P., Lewis G.R., Age changes in human muscle performance, in, *Current topics in oral*

biology, eds, S.J.W. Lisney, B. Matthews, University of Bristol Press, 1985; 17–25

18 Newton J.P., Yemm R., Abel R.W., Menhinik S., Changes in human jaw muscles with age and dentate state, *Gerodontology 1993*; 10: 16–22

19 Wayler A.H., Chauncey H.H., Impact of complete dentures and impaired natural dentition on masticatory performance and food choice in healthy ageing man, *J. Pros. Dent. 1983*; 49: 427–33

20 Eriksson P-O., Thornell L-E., Histochemical and morphological muscle fibre characteristics of the human masseter, the medial pterygoid and the temporal muscle, *Arch. Oral Biol. 1983*; 28: 781–95

21 de Groot J., Chusid J.G., *Aging, degeneration and regeneration in correlative neuroanatomy*, Prentice–Hall, London 1991; 215–21

22 Scott J., Flower E.A., Burus J., A qualitative study of histological changes in the human parotid gland occurring with adult age, *J. Oral Pathol. 1987*; 16: 505–10

23 Tylenda C.A., Ship J.A., Fox P.C., Baum B.J., Evaluation of submandibular salivary flow rate in different age groups, *J. Dent. Res. 1988*; 67: 1225–8

24 Scott J., Structural age changes in salivary glands, *Front. Oral Physiol. 1987*; 6: 40–2

25 Drummond J.R., Morphological changes in human salivary glands, *Front. Oral Physiol. 1987*; 6: 31–9

26 Baum B.J., Changes in salivary function in older subjects, *Front. Oral Physiol. 1987*; 6: 126–33

27 Scott J., Qualitative and quantitative observations on the histology of human labial salivary glands obtained at post mortem, *J. de Biologie Buccale 1980*; 8: 187–200

28 Scott J., Valentine J.A., St. Hill J.A., Balasooriya B.A.W., A quantitative histological analysis of the effects of age and sex on human lingual epithelium, *J. de Biologie Buccale 1983*; 11: 303–31

4

The pathology of orofacial disease

Crispian Scully

Pathological lesions of the orofacial tissues are more often seen in the old than in the young. Whilst the dentist may not be required to treat these diseases, he or she is often ideally placed to make an identification, if not a diagnosis, that will allow a speedy referral. Such intervention may be life-saving.

Oral pathology is far more commonly seen in the elderly than the younger population.[1,2] For example, one recent study of biopsy material showed more than a five-fold increase in prevalence, in the UK, in those over 65 years old, of potentially malignant and malignant disease, benign proliferative lesions and lichen planus.[3] Up to 10% of lesions biopsied in the elderly have a malignant potential.[4] Many other studies in Europe and North America have shown a prevalence of oral mucosal lesions in the elderly, particularly lesions associated with the wearing of dentures, of about 25%.[5-21] In the developing world the situation, not surprisingly, is worse, with nearly 60% of persons having mucosal lesions.[22]

Regular oral examination by a trained diagnostician is required for the elderly, whether dentate or not.

This chapter will discuss mainly the more common and serious problems in oral pathology seen in the elderly (Tables 4.1, 4.2). The more general causes of facial pain have been considered in Chapter 2 (Table 4.3).

Table 4.1 Relative prevalences of some oral mucosal conditions in institutionalized elderly persons

Lesion	% affected
Denture-induced stomatitis	20
Fibrous hyperplasia	12
Sublingual varices	12
Angular cheilitis	9
Keratoses	3
Carcinoma	1

After Jorge *et al.* 1991 (ref. 22).

Denture-related lesions

Denture-induced stomatitis

Denture-induced stomatitis is seen predominantly in the elderly (Fig. 4.1).[21,23] Commonly, though incorrectly, called 'denture sore mouth', it is often an asymptomatic infection, mainly with *Candida* species.[24] Micro-organisms are found on the mucosa and the denture-fitting surface and include not only *C. albicans* but also black-pigmented *Bacteroides* species, and occasionally *Staphylococcus aureus*.[25] The condition is induced particularly by wearing dentures continuously day and night. Host factors, such as haematinic deficiency or xerostomia, underlie a few cases. The evidence clearly indicates that denture-induced stomatitis is often chronic atrophic

Table 4.2 Main oral pathology in the elderly

Oral malignancy
Keratoses
Leukoplakia, erythroplasia
Traumatic ulceration
Denture-induced hyperplasia
Denture-induced stomatitis
Xerostomia
Lichen planus
Mucous membrane pemphigoid
Angina bullosa haemorrhagica
Pemphigus
Candidosis
Avitaminosis or anaemia-related mucosal disease

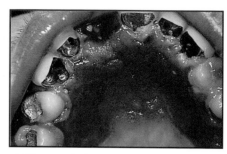

Figure 4.1 Denture-induced stomatitis; there is a sharp contrast between normal palatal mucosa and that of the denture-bearing area

candidosis, although other organisms and trauma may contribute. Hypotheses such as allergy to denture materials have been discounted. Nevertheless, it is unclear why only some denture wearers get chronic atrophic candidosis, because *C. albicans* is a common oral commensal. Factors that may be important include the local environment beneath a denture; the spectrum or type of organisms in denture plaque; and the host immune and other defences.

There is no evidence that host defences play an important role in predisposition to denture-induced stomatitis in most cases. A few patients are iron deficient, especially those with angular cheilitis (stomatitis), and correction of the deficiency may sometimes aid resolution of the lesions. Other deficiencies, for example, of folic acid or B-complex vitamins are occasionally found, especially in the few patients who also have angular cheilitis and/or atrophic glossitis. It is possible that local defences such as those mediated by saliva might be important, since xerostomia clearly predisposes to oral candidosis. The condition usually responds to scrupulous denture hygiene, including overnight storage in a fungicidal solution, for example Milton. Anti-fungal medications such as amphotericin, miconazole

or nystatin may be required, and should be applied (in a water-miscible base) to the fitting surface of the denture prior to insertion into the mouth.[24,26]

Angular stomatitis (Fig. 4.2) may be associated with denture-induced stomatitis. Both *Candida* species and *S. aureus* may be isolated from the lesions. It can occasionally occur alone, when it may signify the presence of underlying systemic disease. Treatment of any associated denture-induced stomatitis is an essential step in the management of angular stomatitis, although the application of topical antifungals such as miconazole to the commissures may also be required, together with prosthodontic advice.

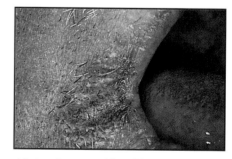

Figure 4.2 Angular stomatitis. Although usually caused by *Candida* species, it is also associated with staphylococcal and streptococcal species

Table 4.3 Orofacial pain in the elderly*

Neurological	Trigeminal and glossopharyngeal neuralgia
	Post-herpetic neuralgia
Psychogenic pains	Atypical facial pain
	Burning mouth syndrome
	Facial arthromyalgia
Vascular	Giant cell arteritis
Referred pain	e.g. Angina pectoris

*Local causes are by far more common.

Denture-induced hyperplasia

Overextended denture flanges may cause mucosal ulceration and eventual hyperplasia. Leaves of proliferative fibrous tissue may be seen, typically in the labial vestibule (Fig. 4.3). The initial treatment comprises the trimming of any gross denture overextension so as to remove the cause of irritation. This will often provide immediate symptomatic relief. However, the reduction of a denture flange can result in a decrease in the stability of the prosthesis, which in turn allows the denture greater freedom to move so causing further irritation. Temporary soft lining materials play a valuable role in stabilizing such denture bases by improving their adaptation to the alveolus. The mixed material is placed into the fitting surface of the denture in order to record an impression of the abused ridge. The patient is asked to close the jaws gently together to ensure that the occlusal relationship is maintained. Such relined dentures must be reviewed regularly. Surgery is sometimes needed.

Denture-induced ulcers (see below)

Potentially malignant and malignant lesions

In western countries oral cancer accounts for less than 3–5% of all malignant tumours.

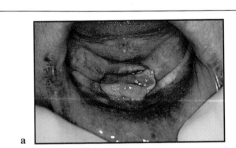

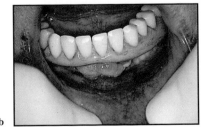

Figure 4.3a, b Denture-induced hyperplasia

Globally, it is a significant world health problem and is mainly seen in the elderly.[27] In parts of South East Asia, particularly India, some 40% of malignancy is oral cancer. In some countries, including the USA and United Kingdom, the incidence of oral cancer appears to be rising.[28]

Over 90% of oral malignant tumours are squamous carcinomas. Most appear to arise in apparently healthy mucosa, but a few cases are preceded by clinically obvious premalignant lesions, especially erythroplasia, leukoplakia, or speckled leukoplakia (Figs 4.4, 4.5, 4.6) and others. Erosive lichen planus, syphilitic glossitis, submucous fibrosis, iron deficiency or previous oral malignancy may also predispose to carcinoma.[29]

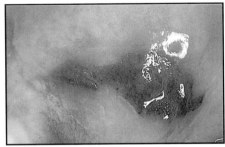

Figure 4.4 Erythroplasia

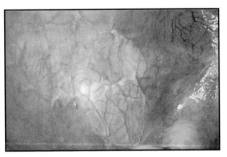

Figure 4.5 Leukoplakia

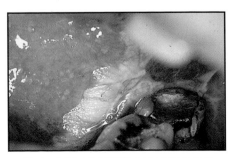

Figure 4.6 Leukoplakia and erythroplasia

In such an accessible site as the mouth, cancer should be detected at an early stage. Unfortunately, many are still detected only at an advanced stage and a diagnosis is frequently delayed by up to 6 months. Early detection and treatment is the short-term goal, though prevention must be the ultimate aim.[30] Some aspects of treatment are considered in Chapter 18.

History

The following paragraphs outline some of the features from the medical and dental history; and clinical features, that can lead to a diagnosis of oral cancer.

Age

Oral cancer, particularly in the West, predominantly affects those over 55 years of age. Facial skin malignancies, particularly basal and squamous cell carcinoma and melanoma, are also more common in the elderly.

Gender

Oral cancer is seen mainly in males. Over the past 50 years or so there has been a gradual decline in the overall incidence of oral cancer in the West, almost entirely due to a decline in the number of men affected. Recently there has been a trend towards an increased incidence of oral cancer in many countries.

General health

Chronic renal failure appears to predispose to oral leukoplakia and there are associations between oral cancer and liver dysfunction. Iron deficiency in humans, as in the Patterson–Kelly (Plummer–Vinson) syndrome of sideropenia, achlorhydria and glossitis, appears to predispose to oral, pharyngeal and oesophageal carcinoma. Dietary factors such as vitamin A may be protective.

Habits

Pipe smoking

Pipe smoking may predispose to lip carcinoma.

Cigarette smoking

Smokers of more than 40 cigarettes per day appear to be about five times more likely to develop oral cancer than are non-smokers. Studies of those who abstain from smoking, for example, Mormons and Seventh Day Adventists, have shown a lower incidence of oral cancer. These persons may also abstain from alcohol use. Smoking and alcohol appear to have a synergistic effect in the aetiology of oral cancer.[28]

Reverse smoking

In reverse smoking, the lighted end of a cigarette is held in the mouth. Where this is practised, for example, in parts of India, oral cancer, particularly of the hard palate, may occur. This is an otherwise unusual site.

Cigar smoking

Some studies have shown an association with floor of mouth leukoplakia in women cigar smokers.

Bidi smoking

Bidi, made of tobacco rolled in a dried temburni leaf, is smoked in India and is associated with a high incidence of leukoplakia, particularly at the commissures, and oral cancer. Bidi emits larger amounts of potential carcinogens than do most Western cigarettes.

Tobacco chewing

Tobacco chewing predisposes to oral cancer. In parts of Asia, tobacco is chewed or held in the mouth for long periods, along with a variety of ingredients in a 'betel quid' which often also contains betel vine leaf, betel nut, catachu and slaked lime. This habit appears to predispose to oral cancer. Betel chewing together with smoking increases the risk of oral cancer by about 25 times.

Snuff dipping

The placing of snuff in the buccal sulcus predisposes to gingival and alveolar carcinoma. Currently there is concern that the use of smokeless tobacco may predispose to similar lesions.

Mouthwashes

There have been suggestions, that the frequent use of proprietary alcohol-containing mouthwashes over prolonged periods predisposes to oral cancer, but only in those patients who neither smoke nor drink alcohol.

Alcohol

Several studies have shown an association between high alcohol consumption and oral cancer. Many alcoholic drinks contain cogeners and some local brews may contain cogeners that are carcinogens responsible for oral cancer. For example, in Brittany there is a close relationship between the consumption of Calvados (a pot-stilled apple spirit) and cancer of the oesophagus and mouth. Indeed, Brittany has the highest incidence of oral cancer in Western Europe.

It should be noted that many patients who may drink alcohol heavily may have liver dysfunction and may also smoke heavily.

Oral sepsis

Some oral carcinomas develop in sites closely related to a denture flange or to a sharp or carious tooth. There is no study that unequivocally demonstrates that these dental factors are aetiological. However, oral cancer is uncommon in a well-cared-for mouth. Patients who have a low interest in oral hygiene and oral care[31] are likely to be high consumers of tobacco and alcohol. It is possible that the oral cancers develop as a response to these factors rather than to the poor oral hygiene.

Infections

Syphilis

Although early studies showed positive syphilis serology in a small minority of patients with oral carcinoma, they failed to point out that the incidence was no higher than in control patients without oral cancer. Many patients with tertiary syphilis (now rare) were also heavy smokers and drinkers, factors equally likely to be incriminated in the aetiology of oral cancer. Arsenicals or other agents used in the treatment of syphilis may have been implicated.

Candida albicans

Some leukoplakias, especially commissural and speckled leukoplakias which are the more premalignant forms, may be infected with *C. albicans*. This seems not to be simply a secondary infection of a damaged, already displastic, epithelium. *C. albicans* can produce nitrosamines, and these may induce the dysplasia.

Viral infections

There is a weak association between herpes simplex virus and labial carcinoma. Papillomaviruses have been detected in some leukoplakias and some oral cancers, but they are also found in other non-malignant lesions, and their role, if any, in the oncogenesis of oral cancer is unclear. Other potentially oncogenic viruses such as adenoviruses and Epstein–Barr virus have been proved not to be associated with oral cancer.

Actinic radiation

There is a higher incidence of lip cancer in outdoor workers than in office workers, indicating a relationship with exposure to sunlight (and ultraviolet irradiation). There is also a particular predisposition of fair-skinned people living in sunny climates to develop lip cancer, as well as skin cancer and melanoma. The fact that lip cancer commonly involves the more exposed lower lip rather than the upper lip also supports a relationship with actinic radiation.

Occupational factors

The relationships between buccal cancer and snuff dipping, and between lip cancer and exposure to sunlight in outdoor workers are discussed above. Some workers in the textile industry are at risk from oral cancer, apparently related to exposure to dust from carding raw cotton and wool.

Racial and geographic factors

Racial factors appear to influence the development of oral cancer, though this may be as much due to different habits and environmental factors such as diet, as to genetic factors.

Premalignant lesions

White lesions

The most common cause of oral white lesions is keratosis due to smoking, trauma, or other causes (Fig. 4.7). Most keratoses are benign and some, particularly stomatitis nicotinia, regress if smoking is stopped. However, there is a premalignant potential in some, especially in keratoses in the floor of the mouth and ventrum of the tongue (sublingual keratosis – see Figure 4.8). This potential is particularly marked when the keratosis is warty in appearance (verrucous or nodular), has a speckled white and red surface (speckled), or is histologically associated with *Candida* species (candidal leukoplakia).

Biopsy is often required in order to exclude dysplasia. Predisposing factors such as smoking should be stopped and, if they do not regress, some keratoses will need to be removed surgically.

Medical treatment of keratoses with vitamin A derivatives, or cytotoxics such as bleomycin, is still in its infancy but shows promise.

Red and pigmented lesions

Red oral lesions are often inflammatory in origin and benign, but they can be premalignant or even malignant. Isolated, red velvety lesions in the elderly (erythroplasia) can exhibit severe cellular dysplasia in up to 85% of cases. Biopsy and excision are indicated.

Examination

Carcinoma is seen most commonly on the lower lip, the lateral margin of the tongue and the floor of the mouth. The clinical appearance is highly variable: most are red or white lesions, lumps, or ulcers, often with rolled edges (Figs 4.9, 4.10). Spread is predominantly local and to anterior cervical lymph nodes. Dissemination to the lungs, liver or bone is seen only in advanced disease. As always, the whole mucosa should be examined because there may be widespread dysplastic mucosa ('field change'), or even a second neoplasm, which is not uncommon in the head and neck, lung or oesophagus. Lymph node examination is of paramount importance in the detection of metastasis.

Any chronic oral lesions should be regarded with suspicion. Features which particularly suggest malignancy include the following:

- The presence of erythroplasia
- A granular appearance or an ulcer with fissuring or raised exophytic margins

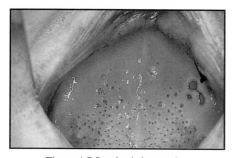

Figure 4.7 Smoker's keratosis

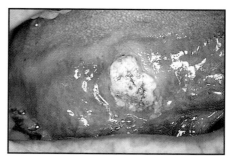

Figure 4.9 Oral squamous cell carcinoma. Note the rolled edges

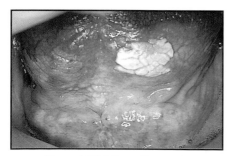

Figure 4.8 Sublingual keratosis

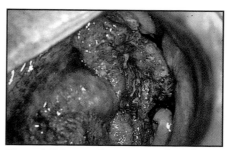

Figure 4.10 Late oral squamous cell carcinoma

- The presence of abnormal blood vessels supplying a lump
- Induration beneath a lesion, that is to say, a firm infiltration beneath the mucosa
- Fixation of the lesion (or node) to deeper tissues or to overlying skin or mucosa
- Cervical lymph node enlargement, especially if nodes are hard or fixed to deeper tissues.

Pain is only a late feature in malignancy. Any suspicious lesion, including any ulcer that does not heal within 2–3 weeks, must be biopsied and a specialist opinion should be sought at an early stage.

Other causes of mouth ulcers

Most mouth ulcers in the elderly are traumatic, often related to an overextended denture flange[32] (Fig. 4.11). Aphthae are uncommon in the elderly, but when they do appear for the first time, they often arise because the patient has stopped smoking, or has developed a haematinic deficiency or blood dyscrasia. It may be important to undertake blood tests, and should a haematinic deficiency be found, the cause should be sought and treated.

Treatment consists of replacement therapy for any deficiency state; and symptomatic relief, for example, with topical corticosteroids, of the aphthous ulcers.[33] This age-group also exhibits an increased incidence of vesiculobullous disorders. These cause multiple persistent ulcers. Dermatoses such as pemphigus, pemphigoid or lichen planus are usually responsible. These conditions tend to cause ulcers that persist for many weeks and

months, and the diagnosis can be established only by biopsy.

Lichen planus

The common oral lesions of lichen planus are white lesions without erosion or ulceration, though they may cause soreness (Fig. 4.12). A small number of patients suffer from atrophic or erosive forms of lichen planus which frequently affect the dorsum and lateral borders of the tongue, or the buccal mucosae on both sides. The erosions are often large, slightly depressed or raised with a yellow slough, and have an irregular outline. The surrounding mucosa is often erythematous and glazed in appearance, with loss of filiform papillae of the tongue, and pathognomonic whitish striae. Lichen planus may also produce a desquamative gingivitis and lesions elsewhere.

Biopsy is usually necessary to confirm the diagnosis and exclude keratosis, lupus erythematosus and other disorders. Some lichenoid lesions may be drug-induced, for example by non-steroidal anti-inflammatory agents, in which case it may be beneficial to change these. They may also be related to restorations and silver amalgam has been implicated. Topical corticosteroids are useful in controlling oral lichen planus.

In view of the slight possibility of premalignancy, especially in erosive lichen planus, a risk of the order of 1–4%, patients should be regularly reviewed.

Pemphigus

Pemphigus is a potentially lethal autoimmune bullous disease of the stratified squamous epithelium which almost exclusively affects late-middle aged or elderly adults. Serum autoanti-

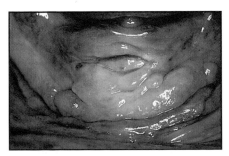

Figure 4.11 Denture-induced ulcer

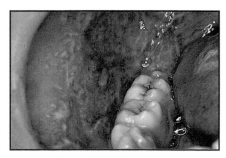

Figure 4.12 Lichen planus

bodies to intercellular substances of the supra-basal epithelium of skin and mucosa are found in most cases of pemphigus and are diagnostically helpful, especially where biopsy examination is difficult. The autoantibody titre is sometimes correlated with the severity of pemphigus. Direct immunofluorescence on biopsy demonstrates antibodies and complement components, bound to intercellular areas of epithelium.

The oral mucosa is almost invariably involved in pemphigus vulgaris and oral lesions are often the presenting feature (Fig. 4.13). Bullae appear on any part of the oral mucosa including the palate, but rapidly break down within hours to leave large, painful, irregular and persistent erosions. Other mucosae may be involved. Flaccid blisters eventually appear on the skin, especially in response to trauma – Nikolsky's sign.

Pemphigus is a life-threatening disorder. Untreated, patients inevitably die, usually from staphylococcal septicaemia. In view of the seriousness of a diagnosis of pemphigus, it is important to biopsy a lesion for conventional histology and immunostaining. Smears for cytology are of little practical value.

Systemic corticosteroids or immunosuppressants are invariably required in the management of pemphigus.

Pemphigoid

Pemphigoid is a bullous disorder with a less serious prognosis than pemphigus, though it may affect the eyes. Pemphigus is probably an autoimmune disease. Serum autoantibodies directed against basement membranes of stratified squamous epithelia may be found, with tissue immune deposits at the epithelial basement membrane zone.

The bullae in pemphigoid are subepithelial and tend to persist for longer than those of pemphigus (Fig. 4.14). The usual lesion is a desquamative gingivitis characterized by erythematous, glazed, sore gingiva. Bullous lesions are also usual, particularly on the soft palate, and may rupture to form erosions. The bullae may be filled with blood or serous fluid. The skin is rarely involved in mucous membrane pemphigoid but if it is tense, blisters form. Involvement of the eyes, and occasionally the larynx, is serious because there may be scarring.

A biopsy is necessary. Subepithelial bullae are diagnostic and there are deposits of complement components and immunoglobulin at the epithelial basement membrane zone. An ophthalmological opinion should be sought. Systemic corticosteroids may occasionally be required; topical steroids will help if the lesions are restricted to the oral mucosa.

Angina bullosa haemorrhagica (localized oral purpura)

This is the term given to a benign condition of unknown aetiology that usually presents in the elderly with blood blisters in the palate that rupture to leave ulcers. The patients appear well otherwise, with no immunological disease or disorder of haemostasis. Only symptomatic care is available.

Dry mouth

The number of people who complain of dry mouth increases with age and up to 40% of the elderly may be affected. Generally, it has been believed that dry mouth or decreasing

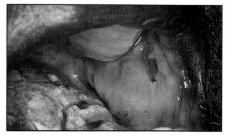

Figure 4.13 Pemphigus vulgaris (and leukoedema): extensive superficial oral ulceration of the tongue and buccal mucosa. The yellow discoloration is caused by amphotericin

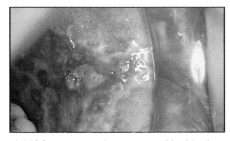

Figure 4.14 Mucous membrane pemphigoid: here the ulceration is deeper than in pemphigus vulgaris, and re-epithelialization is occurring

salivary function is caused by increasing age. The saliva of old people probably contains less total protein, and has qualitative protein and electrolyte differences, with a decreased pH and buffering capacity, than does that of younger individuals. However, more recent research has shown that diminished salivary output is not an ageing phenomenon but is caused by drugs, or disorders like Sjögren's syndrome that manifest with increasing age.[34–37] The commonest causes of dry mouth are listed in Table 4.4.

Drugs with an anticholinergic activity or with a parasympathomimetic activity are the main cause of xerostomia–tricyclic antidepressants being a classic example (see Table 4.9). Patients who have been irradiated for tumours around the head and neck frequently suffer quite severe salivary gland hypofunction. The severity of salivary gland destruction in irradiated subjects will depend upon the radiation dose. It may not become fully manifest until some time after the cessation of treatment, and is usually permanent in nature. Some of the cytotoxic drugs can cause similar problems.

Diseases that cause xerostomia include Sjögren's syndrome, sarcoidosis and diabetes mellitus. The combination of dry mouth with dry eyes is called primary Sjögren's (sicca) syndrome, and is associated with autoantibodies and a generalized exocrine gland hypofunction.[35] The triad of xerostomia, xerophthalmia and one of a number of connective tissue disorders (classically rheumatoid arthritis) is termed secondary Sjögren's syndrome. Sjögren's syndrome predisposes to lymphoma of the major salivary glands.

Xerostomia can give rise to problems with denture retention, increase the risk of dental caries, and infection, and cause problems during mastication and swallowing (Fig. 4.15).[20]

Table 4.4 Causes of dry mouth

Iatrogenic	
Anticholinergics	Propantheline bromide
	Atropine
	Benzhexol hydrochloride
Systemic antihistamines	Chlorpheniramine maleate
(H_1 Blockers)	Diphenhydramine hydrochloride
	Promethazine hydrochloride
Antidepressants	Amitriptyline
	Imipramine
	Despiramide
Antipsychotics	Chlorpromazine
	Prochlorperazine
	Haloperidol
Systemic bronchodilators	Terbutaline
	Theophylline
	Aminophylline
CNS stimulants	Amphetamines
Antineoplastic agents	
Diuretics	Thiazide diuretics
	Loop diuretics
	Potassium sparing diuretics
Antihypertensives	Clonidine
	Beta-adrenoceptor blockers
	Methyldopa
	Captopril
Radiotherapy to the salivary glands	
Graft versus host disease	
Disease	
Sjögren's syndrome	
Sarcoidosis	
Diabetes mellitus	
HIV disease	
Others	

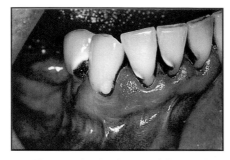

Figure 4.15 Xerostomia: the dryness of the mouth and soft tissues is also associated with root surface caries

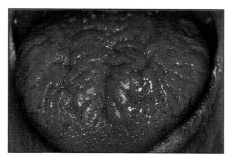

Figure 4.16 Sjögren's syndrome: lobulation of the tongue. Note the dryness of the lingual mucosa

The oral mucosae of patient's with dry mouth are often delicate and can be more sensitive to chemical stimuli. In addition, ascending sialadenitis and candidosis are more common, and sometimes there is a characteristic lobulation of the tongue (Fig. 4.16).

Many other old people complain of a dry mouth, often with an absence of clinical signs and, in these cases, depression may be a cause.

Management of xerostomia

[with Crispian Scully, Robin Seymour, Edwina Kidd and Angus Walls]

In order to prevent and treat the sequelae that may result from the dryness and to prevent further hyposalivation, aggravating factors such as smoking, drugs with anticholinergic activity, and alcohol should be avoided.

Management strategies for the xerostomic patient fall into two groups, first for patient's who have some residual function for whom alteration in drug regimens or salivary stimulation will be a benefit, and second, for those who have minimal function where salivary substitution is the key to success.

Patient's with some residual salivary function

Drug-induced xerostomia is often reversible when the patient's medication is changed. This must be done only in consultation with the subject's medical practitioner. There seems to be some variation in the ability of specific medicines within a pharmacological group to induce dry mouth.[38] Changing an individual's medication to an agent with a lesser xerostomic effect may be of some benefit. Equally, an alteration in the pattern of drug delivery may be helpful. For example, tricyclic antidepressants are often given as a single bolus dose last thing at night. As a result, maximum levels of salivary depression, which correspond to peak blood levels, occur during the night when ambient secretory levels are already low. A better option might be to take the drug dose first thing in the morning. Although the levels of salivary suppression would be the same, the patient would have the opportunity to take steps to mitigate the effects of the induced xerostomia.

Stimulation of salivary flow can be achieved using both gustatory and pharmacological approaches.

Gustatory stimuli

Gustatory stimuli can take the form of acids (citric and malic), although these may cause both dietary erosion and/or induce caries with prolonged use. Diabetic sweets and sugar-free chewing gum may be preferable.[39] Sorbitol-containing products are best avoided in dry mouths. There is some evidence that in dry mouths oral micro-organisms may metabolize sorbitol to acid.

Pharmacological stimuli

Pharmacological stimulation can be achieved using cholinergic agonists,[40] for example, bethanechol chloride, pilocarpine, pyridostigmine, and Sialor, and with nicotinamide. Many of the pharmacological stimulants have potential side effects, particularly within the gastrointestinal tract. The long-term use of pilocarpine may have an adverse effect upon the cardiovascular or central nervous systems.

Patients with minimal salivary function

Such patients will require the provision of salivary substitutes.

Salivary substitution

Salivary substitution can take two forms, either the use of a low viscosity fluid which will simply provide temporary oral wetness and symptomatic relief, or the use of a high viscosity liquid which is designed to remain within the mouth for some time. This latter approach attempts salivary substitution rather than palliation.

Low viscosity liquids that have been used include water, saline, sodium bicarbonate solution and milk of magnesia. These will all provide transient symptomatic relief and are used as required. High viscosity liquids contain a bulking agent such as glycerine, polyethylene oxide, liquid paraffin, sodium carboxymethylcellulose, carmellose sodium and sterile pig gastric mucin. Some preparations also contain a salivary stimulant, which is usually acidic, for example glycerine and lemon mouthwash. These should not be used in dentate subjects.

Most saliva substitutes are available in a bottle. Glandosane,[a] Luborant[b] and Saliva Orthana[c] are put out in aerosol form with the advantage that they can be carried with ease in a pocket or bag and are readily available for use. Their pH is somewhat higher than other artificial salivas. Both Saliva Orthana and Luborant have been shown to have a remineralizing action on carious lesions.[41] Saliva Orthana uses pig gastric mucin as its bulking agent and should not be prescribed for people with religious objections to porcine products or for vegetarians.

The problems of xerostomia are particularly profound in full denture wearers. Techniques have been described to incorporate a reservoir within the structure of an upper prosthesis to permit sustained release of an appropriate substitute for long-term use.[42]

Artificial salivas seldom relieve symptoms for more than an hour or two, and by no means all patients derive benefit greater than that afforded by frequent sips of water. Further development of saliva substitutes and improved methods of delivery are needed.[43]

Prevention

Dentate patients who have profound reduction in salivary flow should also be placed on a rigorous preventative regimen to limit the development of carious lesions. This would include the use of both professionally applied and topical fluorides, a fluoride-containing dentifrice, supersaturated calcium phosphate remineralizing solutions and chlorhexidine gluconate applications as gels or mouthrinses.[44,45,46] Obviously, appropriate control of both oral hygiene and diet will be necessary, and antifungal treatment may be required on a relatively frequent basis.

Facial pain

The incidence of facial pain increases with age. Facial pains have been considered in Chapter 2 under the headings of their cause.

Burning tongue syndrome

Burning mouth (glossopyrosis; glossodynia; oral dysaesthesia) is, for the patient who suffers it, a very real pain. The condition usually affects middle-aged and elderly females. The tongue is most frequently involved. There is usually bilateral discomfort which is often relieved by eating and drinking, in contrast to the pain associated with inflammatory lesions which is made worse by food.

Oral examination shows no abnormalities. Laboratory screening for anaemia, diabetes, a deficiency state or candidosis should be undertaken, but anxiety, depression or a cancerophobia is frequently the underlying cause. Reassurance and occasionally psychiatric care are indicated.

[a] Glandosane: Fresenius, Manor Road, Runcorn, Cheshire, WA7 1ST
[b] Luborant: Antigen Europe, Ellesfield Avenue, Bracknell, Berkshire, RG12 4YS
[c] Saliva Orthana: Nycomed (UK) Ltd, Coventry Road, Sheldon, Birmingham, B26 3EA

References

1 Hill M.W., The influence of aging on skin and oral mucosa, *Gerodontology 1984*; 3: 35–45

2 Heeneman H., Brown D.H., Senescent changes in and about the oral cavity and pharynx, *J. Otolaryngol. 1986*; 15: 214–16

3 MacEntee M.I., Silver J.G., Gibson G., Weiss R., Oral health in a long-term care institution with a dental service, *Commun. Dent. Oral. Epidemiol. 1985*; 13: 260–3

4 Scott J., Cheah S.B., The prevalence of oral mucosal lesions in the elderly in a surgical biopsy population: a retrospective analysis of 4042 cases, *Gerodontology 1989*; 8: 83

5 Skinner R.L., Weir J.C., Histologic diagnoses of oral lesions in geriatric dental patients, *Gerodontics 1987*; 3: 198–200

6 Axell T., A prevalence study of oral mucosal lesions in an adult Swedish population, *Odontol. Revy 1976*; 27: suppl. 36

7 Ambjornsen E., An analytic epidemiologic study of denture stomatitis in a group of Norwegian old-age pensioners, *Gerodontics 1985*; 1: 207–12

8 Grabowski M., Bertram U., Oral health status and need of dental treatment in the elderly Danish population, *Commun. Dent. Oral Epidemiol. 1975*; 3: 108–14

9 Hand J.S., Whitehill J.M., The prevalence of oral mucosal lesions in an elderly population, *JADA 1986*; 112: 273–6

10 Hoad-Reddick G., Oral pathology and prostheses – are they related? Investigations in an elderly population, *J. Oral Rehabil. 1989*; 16: 75–87

11 Kandelman D., Bordeur J.M., Simard P., Lepage Y., Dental needs of the elderly: a comparison between some European and North American Surveys, *Comm. Dentl Health 1986*; 3: 19–39

12 MacEntee M.I., The prevalence of edentulism and diseases related to dentures – a literature review, *J. Oral Rehabil. 1985*; 12: 195–207

13 MacEntee M.I., Scully C., Oral disorders and treatment implications in people over 75 years, *Commun. Dent. Oral Epidemiol. 1988*; 16: 271–3

14 Makila E., Oral health among the inmates of old people's homes. IV. Soft tissue pathology, *Proc. Finn. Dent. Soc. 1977*; 73: 173–8

15 Manderson R.D., Ettinger L., Dental status of the institutionalised elderly population of Edinburgh, *Commun. Dent. Oral Epidemiol. 1975*; 3: 100–7

16 Osterberg T., Ohman A., Heyden G *et al.*, The condition of the oral mucosa at age 70: a population study, *Gerodontology 1985*; 4: 71–5

17 Rise J., Heloe L.A., Oral conditions and need for dental treatment in an elderly population in Northern Norway, *Commun. Dent. Oral Epidemiol. 1978*; 6: 6–11

18 Smith J.M., Sheiham A., Dental treatment needs and demands of an elderly population in England, *Commun. Dent. Oral Epidemiol. 1980*; 8: 360–4

19 Vigild M., Oral mucosal lesions among institutionalised elderly in Denmark, *Commun. Dent. Oral Epidemiol. 1987*; 15: 309–13

20 Diu S., Gelbier S., Oral health screening in elderly people attending a community care centre, *Commun. Dent. Oral Epidemiol. 1989*; 17: 212–5

21 Cook R.J., Response of the oral mucosa to denture wearing, *J. Dent. 1991*; 19: 135–47

22 Jorge J., Almeida O.P., Bozzo L., Scully C., Graner E., Oral mucosal health and disease in institutionalised elderly in Brazil, *Commun. Dent. Oral Epidemiol. 1991*; 19: 173–5

23 Budtz-Jorgensen E., Oral mucosal lesions associated with the wearing of removable dentures, *J. Oral Pathol. 1981*; 10: 65–80

24 Scully C., Chronic atrophic candidosis, Leading article, *Lancet 1986*; ii: 437–8

25 Harding S.M., Wilson M., Dickinson C., Howlett J., Hobkirk J., The cultivable microflora of denture plaque from patients with denture-induced stomatitis, *Microbial Ecology 1991*; 4: 149–57

26 Walker D.M, Stafford G.D., Huggett R.M, Newcombe R.G., The treatment of denture-induced stomatitis, *Br. Dent. J. 1981*; 151: 416–19

27 Scully C., Prime S.S., Boyle P., Oral cancer, *Lancet 1989*; 2: 311–12

28 Boyle P., Zheng T., MacFarlane G.J., McGinn R., Maisonneuve P., La Veechia C., Scully C., Recent advances in etiology and epidemiology of head and neck cancer, *Current Opinion in Oncology 1990*; 2: 539–45

29 Ed. N.W. Johnson, *Risk markers for oral disease: 2 oral cancer*, Cambridge University Press, Cambridge 1991

30 Scully C., Boyle P., Tedesco B., The recognition and diagnosis of cancer arising in the mouth, *Postgraduate Doctor 1992*; 15: 134–41

31 Zheng T., Boyle P., Hu H.F., Duan J., Jiang PJ., Ma DQ, Shui L.P., Niu S., Scully C., MacMahon B., Dentition, oral hygiene and risk of oral cancer: a case-control study in Beijing, People's Republic of China, *Cancer Causes and Control 1990*; 1: 235–42

32 Gratton C.E.H., Scully C., Oral ulceration: a diagnostic problem, *Br. Med. J. 1986*; 292: 1093–4

33 Scully C., Porter S.R., Recurrent aphthous stomatitis: current concepts of aetiology, pathogenesis and management, *J. Oral Pathol. Med. 1989*; 18: 21–7

34 Scully C., Xerostomia and its management (Leading article), *Lancet 1989*; i: 884

35 Scully C., Sjögren's syndrome: clinical and laboratory features, immunopathogenesis and management, *Oral Surg. 1986*; 62: 510–23

36 Epstein J.B., Scully C., The role of saliva in oral health and the causes and effects of xerostomia, *J. Canad. Dent. Assoc. 1992*; 58: 217–21

37 Epstein J.B., Stevenson-Moore P., Scully C., Management of xerostomia, *J. Canad. Dent. Assoc. 1992*; 58: 140–3

38 Gilman A.G., Goodman L.S., Gilman A., in, *The pharmacological basis of therapeutics*, Macmillan Publishers, New York 1980; pp. 403, 423

39 Jensen M.F., Wefel J.S., Human plaque pH response to meals and the effects of chewing gum, *Brit. Dent. J. 1989*; 167: 204–8

40 Greenspan D., Daniels T.E., Effectiveness of pilocarpine in postradiation cancer, *Cancer 1987*; 59: 1123–5

41 Joyston-Bechal S., Kidd E.A.M., The effectiveness of three commercially available saliva substitutes on enamel in vitro, *Brit. Dent. J. 1987*; 163: 187–90

42 Vissink A., 's-Gravenmade E.J., Panders A.K., Oltof A., Visch L.L., Artificial saliva reservoirs, *J. Prosthet. Dent. 1984*; 52: 701–15

43 Duxbury A.J., Thakker N.S., Wardell D.G., A double-blind crossover trial of a mucin containing artificial saliva, *Brit. Dent. J. 1989*; 166: 115–20

44 Billings R.J., Brown L.R., Kasten A.G., Contemporary treatment strategies for root surface dental caries, *Gerodontics 1985*; 1: 20–7

45 Katz S., The use of fluoride and chlorhexidine for the prevention of radiation caries, *J. Am. Dent. Assoc. 1982*; 104: 164–70

46 Johansen E., Papas A., Fong W., Olsen T.O., Remineralisation of carious lesions in elderly patients, *Gerodontics 1987*; 3: 47–50

5

Dental pharmacology problems for the elderly

Robin Seymour

In the healthy elderly patient, drugs frequently used in dental practice are unlikely to cause any problems, since age is not a specific contraindication to the usage of these drugs. However, old people do have a reduced tolerance to drugs, many of which are prescribed in combination. The dentist must be aware of the hazards of prescribing drugs to old people, of the possible side effects, of possible drug interactions, and of the effect that drugs may have, both on the dental condition and the delivery of dental care.

Introduction

It has been estimated that 40% of the elderly need at least one drug per day for them to pursue the normal activities of daily living. Furthermore, 80% of people over the age of 75 are on regular drug treatment.[1] It is therefore essential that the dental surgeon takes a detailed drug history from all his patients and is aware of the special problems that exist in the elderly patient. We shall consider three aspects of pharmacological problems in the aged.

- The physiological changes that accompany the ageing process and which may affect the pharmacokinetics and pharmacodynamics of many drugs.
- Adverse drug reactions which have a higher incidence in the elderly. These reactions may manifest themselves in the mouth and related structures.
- The increased risk of drug interaction between a patient's day-to-day medication and drugs prescribed by the dental surgeon.

Pharmacokinetic changes and the aged

Pharmacokinetics may be defined as the study of the time-course of absorption, distribution, metabolism and excretion of drugs, and the corresponding pharmacological response. Many of the body's systems are involved in these processes, and most are affected by age changes.

After oral administration, a drug diffuses through the intestinal mucosa and enters the portal venous system, where several processes commence almost simultaneously. The drug is bound in a reversible fashion to plasma protein. During the first-pass through the liver, drug extraction and metabolism occur. The amount of first-pass metabolism varies markedly from drug to drug. After passing through the liver, drugs enter the systemic circulation and are available to enter the tissues and exert a therapeutic effect. Many drugs are eliminated from the body by excretion, either through the kidney in the urine, or through the liver in the bile, and thence in the faeces, or by metabolism in the liver.

Drug absorption

There are well-recognized age changes which occur in the gastrointestinal tract which, theoretically, could have an effect on drug absorption. These changes include an increase in gastric pH, which may alter drug solubility,[2] a reduction in gastric emptying, gastric motility, and intestinal and splanchnic blood flow.[3] The latter changes may impair drug absorption if absorption is dependent upon gastrointestinal activity. However, most drugs are absorbed by simple diffusion and the rate of absorption appears to be unaffected by age changes in the gastrointestinal tract.

Drug binding and distribution

Drugs are transported in the plasma in two forms, namely, 'unbound' and 'bound'. Unbound drug is that fraction which is available to diffuse into the tissues (it is sometimes referred to as 'active drug'). Bound drug is that which is attached to plasma protein (usually albumin) and acts as a mobile reservoir from which drug is released. Serum albumin concentrations decrease with age,[4] hence there will be a reduction in the number of drug binding sites and a higher level of unbound drug in the plasma. We shall see later that the changes in plasma protein binding with age become very significant in drug interactions.

The distribution of drugs to the tissues is dependent upon cardiac output, blood flow to the tissues and the volume of distribution (Vd). The latter is defined as the volume of fluid into which the drug appears to distribute with a concentration equal to that in the plasma. With increasing age, the proportion of body water, of intracellular water and of lean body mass decrease, whereas the proportion of body fat increases.[5] Drugs which are distributed in body water or lean body mass, such as paracetamol, may be predicted to have a decreased Vd and therefore a higher plasma concentration in the elderly. Conversely, the opposite applies to lipid soluble drug (e.g. diazepam). Alterations in a drug's Vd and hence plasma concentration, may, in theory, have an effect on the therapeutics of the drug, or increase its toxicity. In dentistry this may be particularly applicable to the benzodiazepines where dose reductions are required in the elderly to reduce the risk of confusion.

Cardiac output declines by approximately 1% per year between the ages of 50 and 86 years.[2] Blood flow to the heart and brain remains constant, but blood flow to the liver, kidneys and gastrointestinal tract reduces with age. These differences in blood flow may affect the behaviour of all pharmacokinetic parameters of a drug. This can result in delayed drug metabolism and excretion.

Drug elimination

The pharmacological action of a drug is terminated either by its elimination from the body in unchanged form or by its biotransformation into pharmacologically inactive or less active metabolites, which are subsequently excreted. Biotransformation occurs predominantly in the liver.

Hepatic biotransformation of drugs and ageing

Certain liver changes occur with age which may influence the biotransformation of a drug. These include a reduction in hepatic mass, a decrease in hepatic blood flow and a decline in hepatic drug metabolizing enzymes.[6,7] Drugs such as paracetamol, which are metabolized in the liver, will show slower metabolism in the elderly. Also, the liver changes described, also account for the 10% decrease in serum albumin which occurs between the ages of 40 and 80 years. The clinical significance of age-related liver changes remains to be determined. Interindividual variation in liver metabolism for specific drugs may be more important than age-related changes.

Renal excretion

Many drugs are excreted through the kidney either by glomerular filtration, or tubular excretion or reabsorption. Renal function reduces with age, so that by the age of 80 years, function is 40% less than in a young healthy adult. Age changes include, a reduction in the number of functioning nephrons, and decreases in renal blood flow, glomerular filtration rate and tubular secretory function. As a consequence of these changes, there is an increase in the plasma half-life of those drugs excreted through the kidney.

Pharmacodynamic changes with age

The term pharmacodynamics refers to the interaction of a drug at its receptor site. Certain age changes can affect a drug's pharmacodynamics. The elderly are more sensitive to drugs which act on the central nervous system, for example hypnotics and anxiolytics. This may be due to altered drug pharmacokinetics or alteration in receptor binding or both. The autonomic nervous system shows age changes which can alter the response to drugs. For example, elderly patients who use beta-blocking drugs such as propranolol and atenolol are more susceptible than the young to their cardiac action. This increased susceptibility is due to the increased ratio of drug to receptor, because there are a decreased number of receptors available for binding.

Further special considerations in the elderly

Compliance with prescribed medications is a major problem for all age-groups. In the elderly, it has been estimated that one-third to one-half of patients fail to comply with their drug regimens.[7]

Adverse drug reactions

These reactions occur when a drug is administered to a patient and subsequently causes a troublesome or potentially harmful effect. A reaction can be classified as type A or type B.[8]

Type A reactions are the result of an exaggerated, but otherwise normal, pharmacological action of a drug given in the usual therapeutic doses. These reactions are more likely to develop in individuals lying at the extreme of the dose response curves for pharmacological effect. Type A reactions are largely predictable on the basis of a drug's known pharmacology, and examples include xerostomia with anticholinergic drugs, an increase in bleeding time with aspirin and drowsiness from the benzodiazepines. These reactions are usually dose-dependent and although their incidence and morbidity in the population is high, their mortality is low.

Type B reactions are totally aberrant effects that are not to be expected from the known pharmacological actions of the drug, when given in the usual therapeutic doses to a patient whose body handles the drug in the normal way. Examples of type B reactions include malignant hyperpyrexia from general anaesthetic agents, acute porphyria from barbiturates, and many immunological reactions.

Elderly patients are particularly susceptible to adverse drug reactions,[9] the manifestations of which can affect the mouth and associated structures. Reactions that are of particular concern in the elderly include oral ulceration, lichenoid eruptions, discoloration of the oral mucosa, drug-induced infections, xerostomia, pain and swelling of the salivary glands, disturbances of taste and extrapyramidal syndromes.

Oral ulceration

Drug-induced oral ulceration can arise from local application of the drug or systemic usage. Those drugs, implicated as aetiological agents in oral ulceration which are particularly relevant to the elderly, are listed in Table 5.1. All cases of oral ulceration, especially in the elderly, should be investigated. Persistent lesions should be biopsied. Patients should have a full haematological screening, because many drug-induced lesions are secondary to blood dyscrasias. In many cases of locally produced oral ulceration, it is often a matter simply of identifying the cause, for example, an aspirin burn, and of preventing the lesion from becoming secondarily infected. Chlorhexidine mouthwash 0.2% is particularly useful for this purpose. If the oral ulceration is the result of systemic medication, then the patient's physician must be informed and hopefully, the medication changed.

Drugs which are commonly implicated as the cause of local ulceration include aspirin, potassium chloride and isoprenaline. Aspirin is a weak organic acid and some patients may attempt to relieve their toothache by placing an aspirin tablet against the offending tooth. The corrosive action of the acidic aspirin may

Table 5.1 Drugs implicated in causing oral ulceration

Local irritants		
Aspirin		
Isoprenaline		
Potassium salts		
Toothache solutions		
Hydrogen peroxide		
Other agents acting systemically	The ulcerations occur primarily or secondary to a leucopenia	
Antineoplastic drugs	methotrexate	
	fluorouracil	
	actinomycin D	
	doxorubicin	
	bleomycin	
	carbamazepine	
	sulphonylureas	
	penicillamine	
	proguanil hydrochloride	
	thiazides	
	gold salts	

result in a fairly large area of ulceration. There is no evidence that this practice has any benefit in the management of toothache. Aspirin has also been incorporated into chewing gum and this has similarly been associated with oral ulceration.[10]

Potassium salts are frequently used in the management of certain cardiovascular conditions and many elderly patients may be on potassium supplements. Potassium chloride can cause ulceration of the oral mucosa, especially if the tablets are sucked. Slow release preparations reduce this problem, and patients should be advised to swallow the tablet.[11]

Isoprenaline tablets are often placed sublingually to relieve bronchospasm. It has been reported that such an application can lead to ulceration of the floor of the mouth and undersurface of the tongue.[12]

Oral ulceration, either primary or secondary to leucopenia, may be caused by antineoplastic drugs such as methotrexate, fluorouracil, actinomycin D, doxorubicin and bleomycin.[13] Similarly, non-steroidal anti-inflammatory drugs, such as naproxen and ibuprofen have been implicated in causing oral ulceration secondary to a severe neutropenia.[14,15]

Stevens–Johnson syndrome, erythema multiforme and lupus erythematosus are severe mucocutaneous disorders which can be drug-induced. Lists of drugs which have been im-plicated as aetiological factors in these conditions are given in Table 5.2.

Lichenoid eruptions

The term 'lichenoid drug eruption' can be used in two senses; first, lichenoid drug eruptions that are similar to or identical with lichen planus, and second, drug eruptions which do not necessarily appear like lichen planus, but have histological features very like this condition. Beta-adrenoreceptor blocking drugs, for example propranolol and atenolol, are examples of drugs which cause lichenoid eruptions of the latter category. Other drugs which have been suggested as causative agents for this condition are listed in Table 5.3. The mechanism for drug-induced lichenoid eruptions is uncertain, but they may be the oral manifestations of a hypersensitivity type reaction.

Disorders of the oral mucosa which result in breakdown of the oral epithelium are troublesome to any patient. However, in the elderly such lesions present further problems. They may impair eating which could have significant implications in a poorly nourished patient. Areas of ulceration may be slow to heal and will also prevent the wearing of dentures. The diagnosis and treatment of drug-induced lesions of the oral mucosa in the elderly is essential to prevent further discomfort to the patient.

Table 5.2 Drugs implicated in erythema multiforme (Stevens–Johnson syndrome) and lupus erythematosus

Erythema multiforme and Stevens–Johnson syndrome	Ampicillin	Phenylbutazone
	Barbiturates	Phenothiazines
	Benzodiazepines	Phenytoin
	Carbamazepine	Propranolol
	Chlorpropamide	Rifampicin
	Clindamycin	Salicylates
	Doxycycline	Sulphonamides
	Ethambutol	Theophylline
	Meprobamate	Minoxidil
	Penicillin	
Lupus erythematosus	Chlorpromazine	Primidone
	Isoniazid	Procainamide
	Hydralazine	Practolol
	Penicillamine	Sulphasalazine
	Phenytoin	Thiouracils

Table 5.3 Drugs implicated in lichenoid eruptions

Amiphenazole	NSAIDs
Beta-adrenoceptor blockers	Penicillamine
Captopril	Phenothiazines
Chlorpropamide	Quinine
Chloroquine	Quinidine
Lithium carbonate	Spironolactone
Methyldopa	Tetracyclines
Mepacrine	Thiazide diuretics

Discoloration of the oral mucosa

Some drugs can cause discoloration of the oral mucosa, either by direct contact or following absorption after systemic administration. In the past, staining of the oral mucosa was often due to treatment involving heavy metals such as silver, bismuth, gold, lead, mercury, zinc and copper. These treatments are rarely used now and the conditions are of historical interest. Of the systemic drugs that cause discoloration, the phenothiazines (especially chlorpromazine) are particularly relevant to the elderly. Chlorpromazine administration is reported to cause a bluish-grey discoloration of the oral mucosa. The incidence of this problem is less than 1%, and is probably caused by the accumulation of a metabolite in the tissues.[16]

Oral infections induced or aggravated by drugs

Many types of systemic drug therapy can alter the oral flora and therefore predispose the mouth to infection. Drugs which have been implicated in this problem and relevant to the elderly include corticosteroids, antimicrobials, antimetabolites and immunosuppressive drugs. The most common drug-induced oral infection is candidiasis.

Corticosteroids inhibit the inflammatory response and are immunosuppressive. These drugs are often used as aerosols in the treatment of asthma, where the incidence of oropharyngeal candidiasis associated with such usage is approximately 13%.[17]

Antimetabolites are used extensively in the treatment of cancer. Their use has been associated with the activation of herpes labialis.[18] It is suggested that this infection occurs as a consequence of the inflammatory reaction induced by the drug.

Patients who have had organ transplants are invariably taking immunosuppressive drugs, such as azathioprine, prednisone and cyclosporin. As their name suggests, these drugs suppress various components of the immune system and therefore render the patient more susceptible to infection. These infections are usually bacterial or fungal in origin, but fatal herpes simplex has been reported in an immunosuppresed patient.[19]

Elderly patients may be more susceptible to infections, because of diet, alteration in their immune response, some concomitant illness, or to the drugs mentioned above. The main infections in these patients are candidiasis and herpes. Thus, the dental surgeon should be aware of these high risk patients and treat or advise the treatment of infection when the need arises.

Salivary gland disorders

The salivary glands are under control of the autonomic nervous system, mainly the parasympathetic division. Because of this innervation, salivary gland function can be affected by a variety of drugs. In addition, certain types of systemic drug therapy can produce pain and swelling of the salivary glands.

Xerostomia

Xerostomia can be very troubling and may have a number of causes, including drugs (see Table 5.4).[20,21] The causes, problems and treatment of dry mouth have been considered in the preceding chapter.

Pain and swelling of the salivary glands

Salivary gland swelling is associated with a number of drugs (see Table 5.5). Swelling usually subsides when the offending drug is discontinued. The mechanism of drug-induced salivary swelling is uncertain. In the case of phenylbutazone it may be a hypersensitivity reaction.

Iodine compounds, which are used extensively in radiographic contrast media, may cause painful swelling of the parotid and submandibular gland. The salivary glands can

Table 5.5 Drugs implicated in pain and swelling of the salivary glands

Bethanidine	Methyldopa
Bretylium	Nitrofurantoin
Chlorhexidine	Oxyphenbutazone
Clonidine	Phenylbutazone
Iodides	Warfarin sodium

concentrate iodide up to 100 times the plasma levels and this high concentration may cause inflammation of the gland and oedema of the duct mucosa. This in turn obstructs the flow of saliva which causes the gland to swell.

Disturbances of taste

Taste acuity diminishes with age, but many drugs (see Table 5.6) induce abnormalities of

Table 5.6 Drugs which have been associated with disturbances of taste

Aspirin	Imipramine
Carbimazole	Lithium carbonate
Chlorhexidine	Lincomycin
Clofibrate	Levodopa
Ethionamide	Metformin
Ethambutol	Metronidazole
Griseofulvin	Penicillamine
Gold salts	Phenindione

Table 5.4 Drugs which frequently cause xerostomia

Anticholinergics	Propantheline bromide
	Atropine
	Benzhexol hydrochloride
Systemic antihistamines	Chlorpheniramine maleate
(H₁ blockers)	Diphenhydramine hydrochloride
	Promethazine hydrochloride
Antidepressants	Amitriptyline
	Imipramine
	Despiramide
Antipsychotics	Chlorpromazine
	Prochlorperazine
	Haloperidol
Systemic bronchodilators	Terbutaline
	Theophylline
	Aminophylline
CNS stimulants	Amphetamines
Antineoplastic agents	
Diuretics	Thiazide diuretics
	Loop diuretics
	Potassium sparing diuretics
Antihypertensives	Clonidine
	Beta-adrenoceptor blockers
	Methyldopa
	Captopril

taste. The mechanism for this change is poorly understood. The alteration in taste may be a blunting or decreased sensitivity in taste perception (hypogeusia), a total loss of the ability to taste (ageusia), or a distortion in the perception of the correct taste of a substance, i.e. sour for sweet (dysgeusia).

Drug-induced taste disturbances may be mediated by their action on trace metal ions such as nickel, zinc and copper. These mechanisms modulate the interaction of tastants with the membrane proteins of the taste pores.[21]

Drug-induced oral dyskinesias

Oral dyskinesias are movement disorders (sometimes referred to as extrapyramidal reactions), characterized by severe dystonia, involuntary movements of the facial, oral and cervical musculature. The tongue, lips and jaws are particularly involved. Oral dyskinesias are common in the aged and can be drug-induced. Drugs which have been implicated are predominantly the antipsychotic drugs, e.g. phenothiazines and butyrophenones. Other drugs that have produced oral dyskinesias include metoclopramide, tricyclic antidepressants, anticonvulsants, diazoxide, levodopa and reserpine.

Drug interactions

Drug interactions have a high incidence in the elderly simply because they are taking more drugs than any other group of the population. Dental surgeons must know what drugs their patients are taking and the possible interactions that can occur with the drugs they may prescribe to the patient. There are several drug interactions which can occur with drugs used in dental practice, but those of particular relevance to the aged are detailed in Table 5.7.

Table 5.7 Drug interactions in dentistry which are especially applicable to the elderly

Drug prescribed or recommended by dentist	Patient's medication	Possible outcome of interaction
Aspirin	Warfarin	Increase in anticoagulant effect NSAIDs due to displacement of warfarin from plasma binding site. Aspirin also inhibits platelet aggregation which causes a prolongation of bleeding time. The interaction can result in a disastrous haemostasis problem
Aspirin	Heparin	Heparin prolongs bleeding time and potentiates aspirin-induced prolongation in bleeding time
Aspirin	Insulin	Aspirin at doses of 3–4 g/day has a hypoglycaemic action and can potentiate the hypoglycaemic action of insulin
Aspirin	Chlorpropamide	Aspirin displaces chlorpropamide from protein binding sites. Hence a prolonged hypoglycaemic effect can result which is potentiated by the hypoglycaemic actions of aspirin
Aspirin	Captopril	Aspirin reduces the hypotensive actions of catropril
Aspirin	Ethyl alcohol	Both drugs have an adverse effect on the gastric mucosa, there is therefore an increased risk of gastrointestinal damage
Aspirin	Sodium valproate	Aspirin displaces sodium valproate from plasma binding sites and there is an increased risk of haemostatic problems
Aspirin	Corticosteroids	Both drugs have an adverse effect on the gastrointestinal tract and increase the risk of peptic ulceration
Aspirin	Spironolactone (aldosterone antagonist)	Salicylates interfere with the tubular secretion of canerone, the active metabolite of spironolactone; this decreases the effectiveness of the parent drug
Aspirin	Acetazolamide	An increase in CNS toxicity of acetazolamide, leading to increased drowsiness and paraesthesia
Ibuprofen	Digoxin	Increase in serum concentration of digoxin
Ibuprofen	Phenytoin	Increase in plasma levels of phenytoin

Table 5.7 (*cont.*)

Drug prescribed or recommended by dentist	Patient's medication	Possible outcome of interaction
Ibuprofen	Lithium	Ibuprofen and other NSAIDs can facilitate renal proximal resorption of lithium and therefore increase plasma concentration of the drug
Ibuprofen and NSAIDs	Digoxin	Increase digoxin plasma levels and other exacerbation of heart failure
Ibuprofen and other NSAIDs	Cyclosporin	Both drugs are associated with nephrotoxicity. When used in combination there is an increased risk of renal damage
Benzodiazepines	Levodopa	Can produce a Parkinsonism-like syndrome and an increased incidence of extrapyramidal side effects
Diazepam	Cimetidine	Impaired elimination of diazepam and therefore an increase in sedative actions
Diazepam	Ethyl alcohol	Enhanced disruption of psychomotor performance and an increase in CNS depression
Carbamazepine	Mono-amine oxidase inhibitors (MAOIs)	Carbamazepine enhances drug metabolizing enzymes and increases the risk of toxicity from MAOIs
Carbamazepine	Sodium valproate	A lowering of the concentration of sodium valproate and an increase in plasma concentration of carbamazepine, leading to increased drowsiness
Carbamazepine	Erythromycin, cemetidine, diltiazem, verapamil	All of these drugs impair the hepatic metabolism of carbamazepine leading to an increase in plasma concentration and more drowsiness
Carbamazepine	Barbiturates, butyrophenones, clonazepam, coumarin anticoagulants, oral hypoglycaemics, phenytoin, corticosteroids, theophylline, thyroid hormone	Carbamazepine stimulates hepatic drug metabolizing enzymes. The metabolism of drugs in this list will all be enhanced by carbamazepine, leading to reduced plasma levels and an impaired therapeutic effect
Carbamazepine	Lithium	Increases CNS toxicity of lithium
Morphine	Cimetidine	Serious CNS unwanted effects, i.e. apnoea, confusion, disorientation and respiratory depression
Pethidine	Mono-amine oxidase inhibitors	Severe hypotension, hyperpyrexia and convulsions
Corticosteroids (systemic)	Cardiac-glycosides, diuretics, antihypertensives	Corticosteroids have a marked mineralo-cortiacoid action which can affect electrolyte balance and oedema formation. These actions can result in a hypokalaemia, can cause fluid retention, and exacerbate any type of heart failure
Corticosteroids	Chlorpropamide/insulin	Corticosteroids are hypoglycaemic and may enhance the hypoglycaemic action of chlorpropamide and insulin
Doxycycline	Coumarin anticoagulants	Potentiation of anticoagulant effect
Tetracyclines	Antacids	Tetracyclines chelate with calcium, aluminium and magnesium ions. The subsequent chelate is poorly absorbed
Tetracyclines	Digoxin	Increased risk of digoxin toxicity.
Tetracyclines	Lithium carbonate	Increase in serum concentrations of lithium and therefore increase in toxicity
Tetracyclines	Colestipol, cholestyramine	These lipid lowering drugs will bind to tetracyclines in the gut and result in impaired absorption
Erythromycin	Carbamazepine	Impaired metabolism of carbamazepine in the liver
Erythromycin	Warfarin	Potentiation of warfarin-induced hypoprothrombinaemia
Erythromycin	Digoxin	Potentiates the effect of digoxin, probably by enzyme inhibition
Erythromycin	Theophylline	Inhibition of theophylline metabolism by erythromycin results in high and potentially toxic concentrations of the drug
Erythromycin	Disopyramide	Increased risk of ventricular arrhythmias
Metronidazole	Ethyl alcohol	Impaired metabolism of alcohol, which results in an accumulation of acetaldehyde
Metronidazole	Coumarin anticoagulants	Metronidazole inhibits hepatic drug metabolizing enzymes, thus there is impaired metabolism of warfarin and hence a potentiation of the anticoagulant effect

Table 5.7 (*cont.*)

Drug prescribed or recommended by dentist	Patient's medication	Possible outcome of interaction
Metronidazole	Lithium	Possible renal damage
Metronidazole	Cimetidine	Cimetidine inhibits the P450 hepatic enzymes which metabolize metronidazole. Thus increase in plasma concentration
Metronidazole	Phenytoin	Increase phenytoin levels due to impaired metabolism
Co-trimoxazole	Warfarin	Potentiation of hypoprothrombinaemic effect
Co-trimoxazole	Oral hypoglycaemic drugs	Enhancement of hypoglycaemic action
Co-trimoxazole	Diuretics	Increased risk of thrombocytopenia, especially in the elderly with heart failure
Ephedrine	MAOIs	Provokes release of noradrenaline from sympathetic nerve endings and potentiates its pressor effects

References

1 Davison W., Principles of geriatric therapeutics, ed, J.C. Brocklehurst, *Geriatric pharmacology and therapeutics*, Blackwell, Oxford 1984: 27–40

2 Bender A.D., Effect of age on intestinal absorption: implications for drug absorption in the elderly, *J. Am. Geriatr. Soc. 1968*; 16: 1331–9

3 Montgomerie R., Heaney M.R., Ross I.N., The ageing gut: a study of intestinal absorption in relation to nutrients in the elderly, *Quart. J. Med. 1978*; 47: 197–211

4 Bender A.D., Post A., Meier J.P, Higson J.E., Reichard G., Plasma protein binding as a function of age in adult human subjects, *J. Pharm. Sci. 1975*; 65: 1711–13

5 Vestal R.E., Drug use in the elderly: a review of problems and special considerations, *Drugs 1978*; 16: 358–82

6 Farah F., Taylor W., Rawlins M.D., James O., Hepatic drug acetylation and oxidation: effects on ageing in man, *Br. Med. J. 1977*; 2: 255–6

7 Ouslander J.G., Drug therapy in the elderly, *Ann. Intern. Med. 1981*; 95: 711–22

8 Rawlins M.D, Thompson J.W., Pathogenesis of adverse drug reactions, in, *Textbook of adverse drug reactions*, ed, D.M. Davies, Oxford University Press, Oxford 1977; 44

9 Hurwitz N., Admission to hospital due to drugs, *Br. Med. J. 1969*; 1: 539–40

10 Claman H.N., Mouth ulcers associated with prolonged chewing of gum containing aspirin, *J. Am. Med. Assoc. 1967*; 202: 651–2

11 McAvoy B.R., Mouth ulceration and slow release potassium tablets, *Br. Med. J. 1974*; 4: 164–5

12 Brown R.D., Bolas G., Isoprenaline ulceration of the tongue: a case report, *Br. Dent. J. 1973*; 134: 336–7

13 Bottomley W.K., Perlin E., Ross G.R., Antineoplastic agents and their oral manifestations, *Oral Surg. 1977*; 44: 527–34

14 Guggenheimer J., Ismail Y.H., Oral ulceration associated with indomethacin therapy: report of 3 cases, *J. Am. Dent. Assoc. 1975*; 90: 632–4

15 Kaziro G.S., Oral ulceration and neutropenia associated with naproxen, *Aust. Dent. J. 1980*; 25: 833–4

16 Vogel R.I., Deasy M.J., Extrinsic discoloration of the oral mucosa, *J. Oral Med. 1977*; 32: 14–16

17 McAllen M.K., Kochanowski S.J., Shaw K.M., Steroid aerosols in asthma: an assessment of betamethasone valerate and a 12 month study of patients on maintenance treatment, *Br. Med. J. 1974*; 1: 171–5

18 Burnett J.W., Further observations of two unusual complications of topical fluorouracil therapy, *Arch. Dermatol. 1982*; 118: 74–8

19 Montgomerie J.Z., Bedcroft D.M.O., Croxson M.C., Doak P.B., North J.D.K., Herpes simplex virus infection after renal transplantation, *Lancet 1969*; 2: 867

20 Ettinger R.L., Xerostomia – a complication of aging, *Aust. Dent. J. 1981*; 26: 365–71

21 Sreebny L.M., Swartz S.S., A reference guide to drugs and dry mouth, *Gerodontology 1986*; 3: 75–99

6

Management of the old patient

Ian Barnes, Robin Seymour, David Smith and Angus Walls

The management of the older patient is usually straightforward. It is based upon kindness, common sense, care, and on a foundation of knowledge.

Recently, one of the authors was told by a 92-year-old patient, at the end of an appointment for endodontic treatment, that it was a source of great pride to him that he had 'kept his teeth'. Despite their particular management needs, and the occasional clinical problem, the treatment of old people is usually a pleasure for the dentist, which is reciprocated by the warmth and gratitude of the patient. Old patients may welcome a trip to the dentist as a break from routine. Nevertheless, the various deteriorations that occur with age, discussed in earlier chapters, and the drug regimens that our patients may well be on, will affect our management of them. Old people require a special consideration.

It should not be assumed that older people are intellectually unable to cope with dental advice and instruction. Longitudinal studies reveal that most of adult life is characterized by little change in intellectual capacity.[1] Indeed, verbal and communication skills improve with increasing age. This would appear to be particularly true if the patient has been and remains intellectually stimulated. However, biological decline and health problems may adversely influence some intellectual functions. For example, the elderly perform psychomotor tasks requiring a high-speed response less efficiently. Also, learning,

through information processing into memory, is slower, especially when tasks are complex, or if the information is not meaningful or personally relevant.[2,3] It appears that in old age the memory is more susceptible to overload and 'interference' from stored previous experiences. In practical terms the learning should as far as possible be 'self-paced' (Fig. 6.1). The teacher must be patient, caring, and on occasions tactful. Sessions should be short, unhurried and stress free. Treatment plans should, wherever possible, be simple, and simply explained, without undue persuasion being exerted. It may be necessary to repeat instructions several times over, or to write them down. Old people may worry inordinately over quite small and, to the observer, inconsequential matters.[4]

For old people, as in the young, prevention is the very core of treatment and the effective delivery of information is important. The neurological implications have been alluded to above, but often little thought is given to other deteriorations that can impede learning. For example, visual accommodation deteriorates after 45 years (presbyopia), and distance and depth perception decline rapidly after 75 years. Sight and adaptation in low light is poor. On the other hand, elderly patients may be particularly susceptible to the glare from dental lights, which should be adjusted with care. One consequence is that the use of a hand mirror to demonstrate oral hygiene procedures may be of limited value as the subject may be unable to focus on the images in the

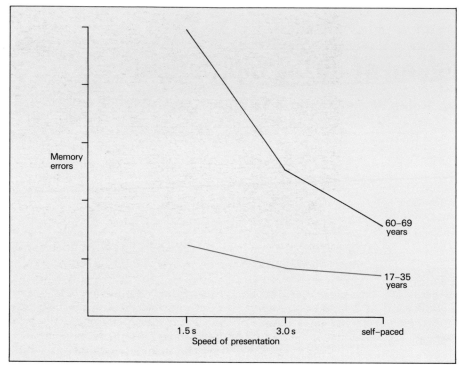

Figure 6.1 Learning errors in relation to age and speed of presentation. Older patients show marked improvement in learning when speed of presentation is reduced or self-paced

mirror. Greater reliance must be made on teaching the patient to detect plaque with their tongue.

Hearing loss (presbycusis) is a gradual change associated with ageing, although there will be variations in the severity of loss between individuals. There tends to be a loss of perception of higher frequency phonemes (f, s, sh, t, th, p, g). In addition there is a generalized increase in perception thresholds for other frequency levels (Fig. 6.2). Instructions and messages should be delivered slowly, and clearly enunciated (without being too deliberate!) whilst sitting close to and facing the patient. Talking from behind the chair is a bad enough practice in any event, but it is unsupportable when dealing with the elderly. Unnecessary, distracting, background noise in the surgery should be eliminated. The prevalence of tinnitus increases with age, as does 'acoustic recruitment'. Acoustic recruitment is responsible for the 'I can't hear you – don't shout' phenomenon. Often, when speaking to an older person, normal speech cannot be understood, but raising the voice results in the response 'there's no need to shout'. This is a product of acoustic recruit-

ment where the rate of loudness increase in sounds of gradually increasing intensity is greater than in a normal subject. Many older subjects depend on hearing aids and consequently have to contend with generalized sound amplification, including background noise. For ease of communication, background noise should be kept to a minimum. It may also be helpful to suggest that the hearing aid be turned off before the airotor is used.

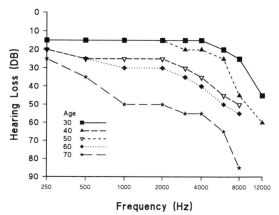

Figure 6.2 Probable maximum hearing loss due to the ageing process[6].

The heating aid should be switched back on before giving instructions, for example, in oral hygiene.

Dramatic life events and deterioration in personal roles, for example, retirement, the death of a spouse, or a loss of independence, may be expected to occur more frequently amongst the elderly. These events can have an adverse effect on self-concept and self-esteem, and may induce breakdown and depression, especially when combined with declining general health.[5]

Depression, like any other mental disorder, can impair the motivation to maintain oral hygiene, or to seek professional advice. The condition also reduces the capacity to comply with treatment. Such patients may be 'hard to reach'. They may forget clear instructions and find it difficult to make decisions about treatment. They may tire easily, and repeated short appointments may be desirable. In addition, antidepressant therapy may reduce salivary flow, and the patient may resort to sucking sweets to moisten the mouth. Some patients are prescribed ascorbic acid lozenges for the same reason. The outcome of this sequence of events is greater and more rapid plaque accumulation, which may lead to a deterioration in periodontal health and the development of root caries in susceptible individuals (Fig. 6.3).

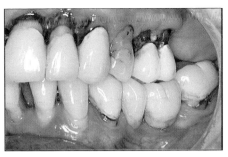

Figure 6.3 Sjögren's syndrome in a 68-year-old woman who struggled with plaque control around long clinical crowns and developed multiple lesions of root caries

In dealing with elderly patients with depression and other mental disorders it is wise to have a concerned, though low-key and flexible, attitude to treatment. Realistic objectives need to be set for treatment, recall schedules and domiciliary care. It is important to maintain contact with the patient, their family and friends, or institutional staff. Such patients are easily 'lost' to the system only to reappear after a year or so with a marked deterioration in their oral health.

Even though an old patient may not be overtly depressed, many will be helped by an approach that encourages self-esteem. They are of value to society. Their appearance is of importance (Fig. 6.4 a–d). There is no reason why they should settle for second best.

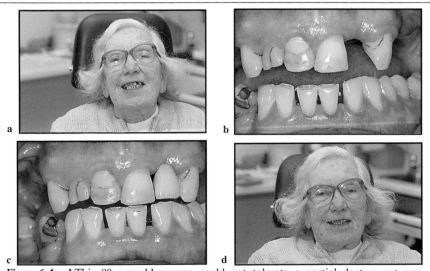

Figure 6.4a–d This 80-year-old woman could not tolerate a partial denture yet was unhappy to leave her house because of embarrassment about the missing upper lateral incisor teeth. The provision of a simple adhesive cantilever bridge worked well despite the lack of posterior support

It should not be forgotten that many old people will have had traumatic experiences of dentistry in the past, when for example, the provision of local anaesthesia for conservation was not the norm. They may not have overcome their fear.

The inadequacy of the carotid reflex has been mentioned earlier and if the patient is not to lose consciousness, the dental chair must be returned to the upright position slowly and the patient observed for a while before being escorted from the surgery. The old person will exhibit slow and incomplete physiological responses to both increases and decreases in blood pressure. They can react suddenly and dramatically both to small losses of blood, or slight increases in blood pressure caused, for example, by pain.

Most old people will tolerate the horizontal chair position, though many will welcome a small pillow to support the neck. However, those with lung conditions such as emphysema or congestive cardiac failure should be tilted at no more than forty-five degrees, or ten in severe cases. If in doubt, it can be helpful to ask the patient whether they can lie down to sleep, or if not, how many pillows they require. Even for the healthy old person, the cough reflex may be depressed and good nursing with efficient aspiration is essential at all times. The use of a rubber dam may sometimes be contraindicated for patients with breathing difficulties. Oxygen should always be to hand.

The avoidance of pain has been stressed. This means the provision of efficient local anaesthesia. A solution of 2% Lignocaine with 1:80 000 adrenaline is a safe drug in normal therapeutic dose for all, except those with severe myocardial insufficiency and hyperthyroidism. An aspirating technique is obligatory in order that the solution is not inadvertently injected into the venous system. If this precaution is taken, the risk from the injection of this concentration of adrenaline is probably less than if endogenous catecholamines were to be released in response to operative pain.

Intraligamentous injections are commonly assumed to be safe. However, Brannstrom has reported that the technique can be hazardous if used on the cardiac compromised patient, because the bulk of the solution is forced into cancellous bone where it may readily pass into patent venules and the venous return[7].

Though there does not seem to be documentary evidence, it may be unwise to use adrenaline impregnated gingival retraction cords (which contain therapeutically huge doses) during crown and bridgework on old people, particularly now that efficient styptics are available.

The prescription of drugs must be done with circumspection and in consultation with the patient's general medical practitioner.

The precautions discussed above should be taken for all patients. However, overt pathology will require particular management. Increasing numbers of patients with rheumatic heart disease, degenerative valvular disease and prosthetic heart valves are reaching old age. Appropriate antibiotic cover must be provided for blood-spilling or traumatic procedures such as scaling, root planing, periodontal surgery and the taking of impressions. Clear case-note entries and prescriptions should be made, especially if a dental hygienist is to carry out treatment. In this respect, medico-legally, it is very difficult to prove that a scaling did not lead to blood letting. Where possible, dental treatment should be avoided within six months of prosthetic heart valve replacement.

Cerebrovascular accidents are a frequent occurrence in the aged. Facial palsy reduces the overall cleaning of gross debris by the oral musculature, and paresis of limbs may cause considerable physical handicap to satisfactory plaque control. In these circumstances it is essential to involve family, friends or institutional staff in the oral hygiene motivation and instruction programme. Their commitment must be even greater if the patient has suffered a receptive dysphasia and is unable to be taught.

The incidence of Parkinson's disease and orofacial dyskinesias increases with age, and may be drug-induced. The unusual muscular activities of tremor, rigidity and tongue protrusion may make access for cleaning difficult for both the patient and the operator.

Muscle and joint disorders may make difficult attendance at or access to the clinic. Domiciliary care is considered in Chapter 20. However, most old people could readily be treated in practice were sufficient thought to be given to the design of the surgery. The absence of steep stairs, wide doorways, uncluttered space in the surgery, and an accessible lavatory with suitable handgrips are the most obvious essentials.

Management of the old patient relates largely to the general changes that accompany old age. *Treatment* attempts to deal with the deleterious local changes that may occur in the oral tissues as the patient ages, and this will be considered in the following chapters.

References

1 Schaie K.W., Translations in gerontology – from lab to life: intellectual functioning, *Am. Psychol. 1974*; 29: 802–7

2 Hoyer W.J., Plude D.J., Attentional and perceptual processes in the study of cognitive aging, in: L.W. Poon, ed., *Aging in the 1980s: Psychological issues*, American Psychological Association, Washington DC, 1980

3 Fozard J.L., The time for remembering, in: L.W. Poon, ed., *Aging in the 1980s: Psychological issues*, American Psychological Association, Washington DC, 1980

4 Canestrari R.E., Paced and self-paced learning in young and elderly adults, *J. Gerontol. 1963*; 18: 165–8

5 Gurland B.J., The comparative frequency of depression in various adult age groups, *J. Gerontol. 1976*; 31: 283–92

6 Hinchcliffe R., Correction of pure-tone audiograms for advancing age, *J. Lar. Otol. 1959*; 73: 830–832

7 Brännström M., Pashley D.H. and Gaberoglio R., Periodontal ligament anaesthesia: clinical experience and review of recent research, *Grafica* Editoriale; Asti, Italy: 1984

7

Periodontal disease and its treatment in the elderly

David Smith and Robin Seymour

The periodontium in dentate elderly patients invariably demonstrates the capacity to resist, overcome and repair the ravages of periodontal disease, despite age changes that may suggest increased vulnerability. Dentists often concern themselves with the amount of periodontal support that has been lost, rather than with the health of that which remains. In the elderly, periodontal health is still a prerequisite for successful restorative treatment. Effective and rewarding programmes of periodontal care are possible in the general practice, institutional and domiciliary settings. Perhaps the barriers to such care are to be found not principally with the patients, but in political and professional attitudes, and in understanding.

Active periodontal disease does not seem to play a major part in the dental management of old people. The consequences of earlier disease are, however increasingly apparent. The need for sound oral health measures is of paramount importance in the control of root surface caries.

Periodontal disease is a disease of the supporting structures of the teeth, namely, the gingival tissues, alveolar bone, cementum and periodontal ligament. The disease is a result of an interaction between the products from bacterial plaque and the resulting inflammatory and immunological responses within the periodontal tissues. Several types of periodontal disease can be identified, but these can be simply classified into gingivitis and periodontitis. In gingivitis, the inflammatory and immunological changes are confined to the gingival tissues. In periodontitis, these changes have spread to the deeper tissues of the periodontium. Periodontal disease is characterized clinically by inflammation of the gingival tissues, apical migration of the junctional epithelium, pocket formation and alveolar bone loss. If untreated, periodontal disease becomes a frequent cause of tooth loss in the adult population.

The pathogenesis of gingivitis is well documented and four distinct types of lesions have been described. These are, initial, early, established and advanced.[1] The lesions do not follow a well-defined chronological sequence. The early and established lesions may remain stable over prolonged periods of time. Furthermore, spontaneous or treatment-induced reversals may occur.

It is now recognized that, in cases of periodontal disease, activity appears to be episodic, with bursts of destruction followed by periods of quiescence.[2] Such bursts of activity may be randomized or asynchronized, and it is suggested that their incidence is considerably reduced in patients over the age of 40 years. In view of these findings on the pattern of periodontal destruction, periodontal disease may be a less significant problem in the elderly than was once believed. However, this does not lessen the difficulties experienced in trying to provide individual and community programmes of care for sufferers.

Epidemiology of periodontal disease in the elderly

One of the earliest epidemiological studies on the prevalence of periodontal disease and tooth loss in the adult population of the USA showed that periodontal disease was uncommon before the age of 18, and increased steadily with age.[3] After the age of 40, there was a rapid rise in edentulousness, and by the age of 60, 60% of the dentition was lost and 20% of the subjects were edentulous. This would suggest that periodontal destruction is age related. However, further studies have shown that this is not the case, but rather that each succeeding generation is less affected by periodontal disease.[4]

Cross-sectional studies have shown that the prevalence and severity of periodontal disease increase with age.[5,6,7] However, all studies report that only a small cohort of patients, irrespective of age, exhibited severe periodontal destruction. The size of this cohort appears to increase with age.

In the UK there is little meaningful information on the incidence and severity of periodontal disease in the elderly. This may be because of the high incidence of edentulism in the population aged 65 years and over, although there are regional variations. Findings from a survey carried out on 153 elderly subjects from the East Midlands showed an incidence of edentulism of 83%. Of the remaining subjects, the authors reported that their restorative, periodontal and surgical treatment needs were low.[8] A further problem when investigating the periodontal status of the elderly is in differentiating between the effects of the 'normal' ageing process on the periodontal tissues and the effects of disease. This particular problem arises when attachment loss is considered.

There have been several reports from Scandinavian countries on the dental state of the elderly. In Finland, 40% of the elderly aged 65 years and over retained some of their natural teeth, but only 2% of these had healthy periodontal tissues.[9] Of the dentate sample, 43% of the men and 27% of the women had severe periodontal disease with probing depths greater than 6 mm. Only 50% of the dentate men and 75% of the women brushed their teeth once a day. A similar figure for edentulism was found in a Norwegian study,

with 46% of subjects aged 67 years and older retaining some of their natural teeth.[10]

Other studies from Scandinavian countries have reported that periodontal treatment needs increase with age up to middle age. Thereafter, the periodontal health of most elderly people can be maintained by regular non-surgical management.[11,12,13]

Studies from the USA have shown that approximately 60% of the population aged 65 years and over are partially dentate,[14] with an average of 19 teeth remaining. Of the sample selected in this investigation, 90% needed periodontal treatment of some type such as oral hygiene instructions, scaling and root planing for pockets of 3–6 mm in depth. Only 1% of this cohort of patients had gingival bleeding and periodontal pockets greater than 6 mm. Another American study,[15] showed that age did not significantly correlate with the following parameters:

- The presence of gingival inflammation
- The accumulation of plaque and calculus
- Gingival recession
- The depth of periodontal pockets.

On the other hand, in a group of 65–74 year olds, a correlation was demonstrated between the number of remaining teeth and the periodontal status, as measured by the periodontal index. A high correlation was found with periodontal status and the standard of oral hygiene.[16] The number of retained teeth in the same age group also showed a positive correlation with the remaining alveolar bone height supporting the teeth.[17] This would indicate individual resistance to periodontal disease.

Other factors which may influence the retention of teeth in the elderly have been examined using multiple linear regression analysis.[18] Physical and medical variables are relatively unimportant factors for determining the proportion of retained teeth in the population sample. Significant correlations in this study were behavioural factors, especially tobacco consumption.

A recent 6-month longitudinal study[19] investigated risk indicators for clinical attachment loss. The findings show that baseline attachment levels and patients, age are major risk indicators for further attachment loss. Thus, patients with existing severe periodontal disease and those over the age of 60 years are at greatest risk from further attachment loss after treatment.

It may be inferred from these studies that the periodontal treatment needs of the elderly are few, comprising chiefly regular plaque control, dietary advice and professional tooth cleaning. This may not be as simple as first it might seem. Some elderly are cared for in long-term stay hospitals, or residential or nursing homes. One survey has shown that the dentate institutionalized elderly patient has poor plaque control and severe gingival inflammation.[20]

Patients who received 'assistance' with oral hygiene measures had more plaque and gingival bleeding than those who managed to clean their own teeth. The author concludes that both the elderly and the staff who care for them are in need of regular instructions in plaque control and mouth care. This subject is discussed further in the chapter on domiciliary care.

Effects of age on the periodontium

The periodontal tissues comprise the gingivae (epithelium and connective tissue), periodontal ligament, alveolar bone and cementum. These tissues are all affected by age changes. The clinical significance of such changes has yet to be determined in many instances.

Epithelium

The oral epithelium becomes thinner with age, less keratinized and there is an increase in cell density.[21,22] The interface between the epithelium and connective tissue also changes with age from a ridge-type interface to a papilla-type interface.[23] There is uncertainty about the effect of age on the mitotic activity of oral epithelium, with some studies reporting an increase with age, others reporting a constant rate of mitosis, and still others showing a decrease in activity.[24] These differences may be related to the level of inflammation present in the tissues prior to harvesting.

Connective tissue

It is now recognized that skin shows definite changes with age, for example, the appearance of wrinkles and the loss of elasticity. These features are largely caused by the loss of subcutaneous fat. Gingival tissue does not contain such fat and therefore such obvious changes do not occur. However, age changes are found in the gingival connective tissue, and include an alteration in texture from a fine to a more dense and coarsely textured tissue. The cellular component of connective tissues also decreases with age.

Periodontal ligament

The connective tissue component of the periodontal ligament also undergoes age changes. The fibre and cellular components decrease and the structure of the ligament becomes more irregular.[25] Other changes in this structure include a reduction in cell density and mitotic activity, a reduction in organic matrix production and a loss of acid mucopolysaccharide.

There are further conflicting findings concerning the effect of age on the width of the periodontal ligament. Some studies report an increase with age whilst others report a decrease.[24] However, it is now well established that the width of the ligament is related to the functional demands on the tooth. Differences in occlusal loading may account for these conflicting findings. Thus, fewer remaining teeth would take a greater proportion of the occlusal load. This may produce widening of the periodontal ligament and an increase in tooth mobility. In such circumstances, mobile teeth do not necessarily have a poor prognosis. It has also been reported that masticatory forces decrease with age, which may contribute to a reduction in the width of the periodontal ligament.[26]

Cementum

Cementum formation, mainly acellular, occurs continuously throughout life and the increase in width with age is most marked in the apical region of the tooth.[22] It has been suggested that the latter finding may be a response to passive eruption.[25] A slight increase in the remodelling of cementum also occurs with age and is characterized by areas of resorption and apposition,[28] which may account for the increased irregularity observed on cemental surfaces of older teeth.[29]

Alveolar bone

Alveolar bone shows changes with age that include an increase in the number of interstitial lamellae, producing a denser interdental septa, and a decrease in the number of cells in the osteogenic layer of the cribriform plate. With increasing age the periodontal surfaces of the alveolar bone become jagged, and collagen fibres show a less regular insertion into the bone.[25]

Ageing and attachment loss (see Fig. 7.1)

In health, the apical cell of the junctional epithelium is attached to the cemento-enamel junction. A feature of periodontal destruction is the apical migration of the junctional epithelium. There is controversy as to whether age also induces apical migration of this structure, as evidenced by the increase in periodontal breakdown with age. So, when examining an elderly patient with attachment loss, one might ask whether the attachment loss was due to periodontal disease, or part of the ageing process, or both.

Animal studies suggest that ageing is associated with a gradual, physiological recession of the gingival tissues, which occurs concomitantly with an apical migration of the junctional epithelium. This idea would support the theory of continuous passive eruption, which proposes that gingival recession occurs as a result of occlusal migration of the teeth in the presence of a stable gingival margin level. The migration compensates for occlusal wear (Fig. 7.1 b).

Subsequent studies have shown that occlusal movement of the teeth is not necessarily associated with apical migration of the junctional epithelium, provided that there is good gingival health.[30,31] It has been shown that the location of the mucogingival junction does not change with age,[32] and, in the absence of gingival recession, the width of the attached gingiva increases with age.[33] These reports point to the conclusion that the junctional epithelium remains at the cemento-enamel junction, and the width of the attached gingiva increases with age due to the eruption of the teeth or the dentoalveolar complex (Figs 7.1c, 7.2). These events only occur if the periodontal tissues are healthy. There is little evidence to support the physiological apical migration of the junctional epithelium with age.

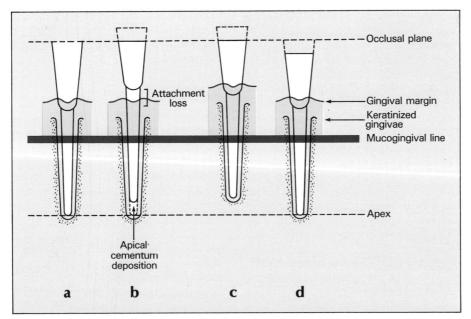

Figure 7.1 Attrition, attachment loss and attached gingiva. (a) 'Normal': no attrition, no periodontal disease. (b) 'Passive eruption': real attachment loss because of periodontal disease; attrition and compensatory eruption. (c) Dentoalveolar compensatory eruption: attrition, no periodontal disease and increased width of attached gingivae. (d) No compensatory eruption: presence or absence of periodontal disease; attrition producing reduced occlusal face height

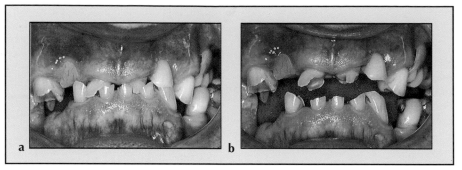

Figure 7.2 A 60-year-old man: (a) intercuspal position; (b) rest position – note no attachment loss; dentoalveolar eruption and wide zone of keratinized gingivae

Effects of age on plaque

Composition and formation

Various biochemical and microbiological changes occur in dental plaque with increasing age. The calcium and phosphorus levels increase, and this may relate to similar increases in salivary calcium and phosphorus levels.[34] The bacterial composition shows certain qualitative changes. Plaque from young patients contains more viable microorganisms per mg than plaque from the elderly.[35] The number of spirochaetes is reported to increase in plaque with increasing age.[36] Conversely, there is a fall in the number of streptococci.[35]

In the early stages of plaque formation (at 4 h) there are significantly fewer bacteria in the elderly patient. However, at 24 h, bacterial counts in both groups are similar. This may indicate a more rapid rate of plaque formation in the elderly.[37,38,39] This phenomenon may be caused by physiological changes in saliva; or by the greater surface area of roughened cementum surface that is exposed as a result of gingival recession; and the grooved, tilted, single-standing and less-accessible teeth that are found in the elderly (Fig. 7.3).[40] Softer diets, reduced oral activity and an increased incidence of xerostomia in the elderly may also contribute to gross accumulation of deposits.

Certain enzymic and immunological differences are apparent in the plaque from elderly patients. Levan hydrolase activity is markedly lower than in the young. This difference may be related to differences in the numbers of streptococci.[35]

The concentration of immune factors (IgA, IgM, C3, lactoferrin, lysozyme and lacto-

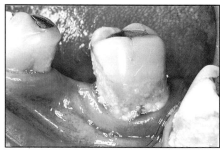

Figure 7.3 A 83-year-old woman, showing copious plaque around a single-standing ⌐7 with gingival recession

peroxidase) is reported to be higher in plaque obtained from older people. The clinical significance of this finding and whether such changes alter the pathogenicity of plaque with regard to periodontal breakdown have yet to be determined.

Response of the periodontal tissues

Various age-related alterations occur in the body's immune and inflammatory response and these may affect the resistance of the periodontium to bacterial plaque. A reduced immune response, as determined by the lymphocyte stimulation index, to plaque has been reported in the elderly.[41] Sensitization of peripheral blood leucocytes to lipopolysaccharides is a feature of experimental gingivitis in young adults. Such sensitization does not appear to occur in the elderly.[42] Also, an experimental model of gingivitis has shown that the rate of development of gingival inflammation (as assessed by gingival exudate and bleeding) increases with age.[40] This could be associated with a diminished immune response, but recent studies have shown that the susceptibility of an individual to periodontal disease is a more important determinant than age for the rate of development of periodontal inflammation.[43]

Musculo-skeletal system

Osteoarthritis, rheumatoid arthritis and other connective tissue disorders, such as polymyalgia rheumatica, can severely limit attempts at plaque control. Again, the assistance of a third party for daily cleaning may be crucial.

Drugs

The effects of certain drugs on the periodontium are seen increasingly in the elderly population. Epanutin (anticonvulsant), cyclosporin (immunosuppressant) and nifedipine (calcium channel blocker) can provoke gingival overgrowth in the susceptible individual (Fig. 7.4). A more rigorous three-monthly recall programme should be considered in such cases because the rate of overgrowth may be related to the degree of gingival inflammation. Some antihypertensives, for example methyldopa, may produce lichenoid reactions in the gingival tissues.

Patients taking anticoagulants may require adjustment of dose prior to surgery, although scaling and root planing can usually be carried out within the therapeutic range, that is to say, where the International Normalized Ratio (INR) does not exceed 2.5.

Immunosuppressants appear to have little effect on the progress of chronic inflammatory periodontal disease. However, oral ulceration and delayed healing may occur in the gingivae (Fig. 7.5).

Clinical aspects

Plaque and gingival inflammation appear to develop more rapidly in the elderly. Notwithstanding, successful therapeutic results can be obtained and maintained.

It is advisable to record and monitor simple plaque and bleeding indices, and pocket depths where possible. This is essential in the assessment of cleaning efficiency, patient compliance and disease progress. Furthermore, a visible record of performance can be just as powerful a motivational device for the elderly as for the young. We can commend a system of screening and monitoring based on the Community Periodontal Index of Treatment Need that has been recommended by the

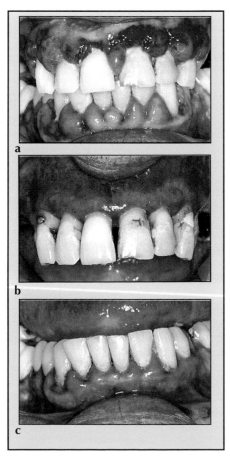

Figure 7.4 (a) Gingival overgrowth in a 60-year-old man taking nifedipine; (b) following gingivectomy 3|4; (c) following 3 months non-surgical management and discontinuation of nifedipine

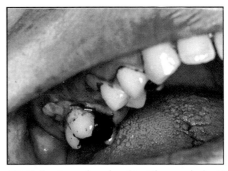

Figure 7.5 Refractory chronic ulcerative periodontitis in an elderly woman taking systemic steroids for rheumatoid arthritis

British Society of Periodontology for use in general practice in the UK.[44]

When plaque accumulates undisturbed, gingival inflammation appears to develop more rapidly in the older patient, but does not necessarily involve the deeper tissues (Fig. 7.6). It is generally true that the dentate individual who has survived to their seventh or eighth decade is less susceptible to destructive periodontitis. Indeed, some individuals have considerable resistance to periodontal disease. Frequently, a severely worn dentition is supported by a periodontium showing little signs of destruction. It is unusual therefore to see generalized advanced periodontitis, with many pockets deeper than 6 mm, in the elderly. More commonly, a spectrum of conditions is seen, ranging from early to moderate chronic periodontitis with varying degrees of gingival recession and localized advanced pocketing, especially where predisposing factors exist. In the older patient such factors may include radicular grooves, exposed furcations, split roots or impinging restorations (Figs 7.7, 7.8). These may partly account for the findings of a recent survey,[45] which indicated that untreated elderly patients between 60 and 79 years were more likely to experience sites of periodontal attachment loss greater than 2 mm annually, especially around molars. Furthermore, older patients with existing periodontitis developed more additional periodontal disease than younger subjects.

Periodontal inflammation is a stimulus to overeruption and subsequent drifting and tilting of teeth (Fig. 7.9). Loss of alveolar support and inflammation within the periodontium lead to increased tooth mobility, over and above that caused by excess functional loading. Such teeth may remain functional for many years, and may be crucial to a complex

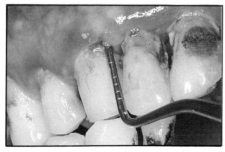

Figure 7.6 A 65-year-old man with very poor oral hygiene, but pocketing no greater than 3 mm

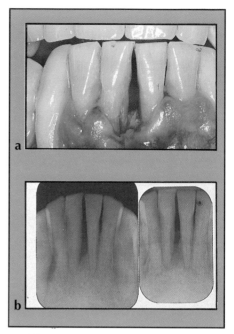

Figure 7.7 (a) Severe local pocketing on the deeply-grooved mesial aspect of $\overline{1|}$. (b) Radiograph showing extent of bone loss

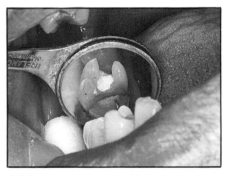

Figure 7.8 A severe, suppurating furcation involvement of $\overline{6|}$ in an elderly man was associated with a communicating root fracture

treatment plan, in which case it is essential in the first instance to establish periodontal health (Fig. 7.10).

Two conditions which were previously described as 'desquamative gingivitis' are also seen more frequently in the elderly, especially in women. These conditions are atrophic or erosive lichen planus (Fig. 7.11) and benign mucous membrane pemphigoid (Fig. 7.12). Owing to the thinness and fragility of the overlying epithelium, both conditions can give the appearance of severe gingival inflammation, which may in fact only be superficial.

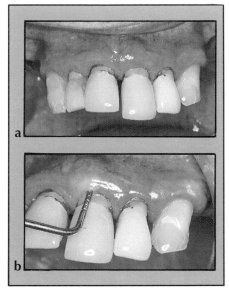

Figure 7.9 (a) Overeruption of ⌊12 in an 83-year-old woman associated with (b) moderate chronic periodontitis

Toothbrushing may produce discomfort and so discourage adequate plaque control. Persistence with an atraumatic brushing technique supported by chlorhexidine mouth rinses and professional tooth cleaning is usually sufficient to prevent deeper periodontal destruction. In more severe cases, topical or systemic steroid therapy is required.

Treatment

Treatment options for elderly patients depend upon many factors, for example, their attitudes and expectations, previous dental treatment, existing oral and dental health, medical complications, their mobility, and their domestic or institutional support. The choice of treatment is usually between three modalities.

- Minimum intervention so as to maintain the status quo. For example, occasional hygiene therapy, fillings and extractions as necessary.

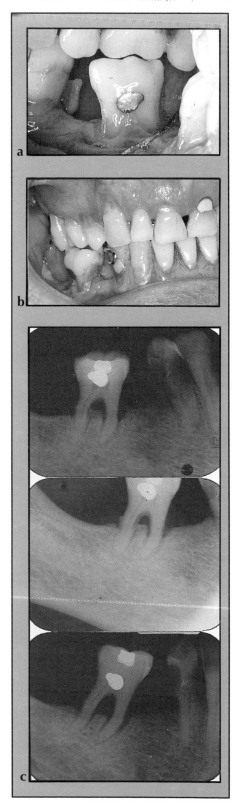

Figure 7.10 (a) A functional, furcation-involved 6⌉ with grade III mobility in a 66-year-old man. (b) After 5 years of non-surgical management and maintenance therapy, still mobile and functional. (c) Follow-up radiographs 6⌉ 1980 (top), 1982 and 1986

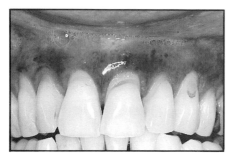

Figure 7.11 'Desquamative gingivitis' diagnosed as atrophic lichen planus in a woman in her mid-60s

- Multiple extractions and provision of dentures.
- More extensive periodontal and restorative treatment. This might include multiple root canal treatments and coronal restorations.

In the UK, elderly patients have traditionally been offered the first two options only, usually on the grounds of limited life expectancy, cost and poor periodontal or dental prognosis. However, with respect to the latter, longitudinal studies have shown that in older patients suffering from advanced periodontitis, successful therapeutic results can be obtained and maintained for many years, provided that optimal plaque control is achieved.[46]

Plaque control

The demand and requirement for good instruction, demonstration and motivation is just as great for the old as for the young, and is within the gift of every dental practitioner (Fig. 7.13). The problems of management of and communication with the old patient, discussed in Chapter 6, are of particular relevance here. The following recommendations should improve communication with the older patient:

- Structure the plaque control message in a chronological step-by-step manner, for example, the stages of a brushing routine.
- Avoid giving too much information at one time. No patient, and certainly not an elderly person, can be expected to absorb instructions for disclosing, brushing, flossing, and so on, in a single session.
- Allow time for explanation and clarification of terms. Use slower and clearer speech, but avoid shouting and overexaggeration, which can so easily cause offence. During instruction, the simple expedients of facing the patient, sitting closer, and avoiding background noise are appreciated by patients with poor hearing.
- Listen for, and encourage, feedback – if necessary by direct enquiry. Also listen to the overtly, or covertly, expressed needs

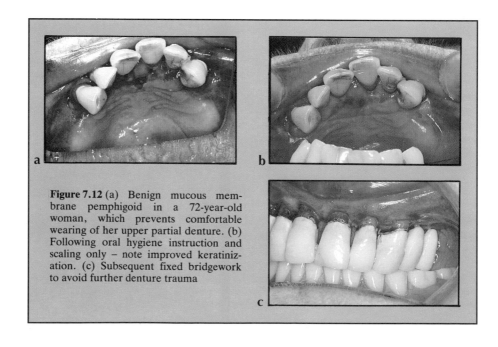

Figure 7.12 (a) Benign mucous membrane pemphigoid in a 72-year-old woman, which prevents comfortable wearing of her upper partial denture. (b) Following oral hygiene instruction and scaling only – note improved keratinization. (c) Subsequent fixed bridgework to avoid further denture trauma

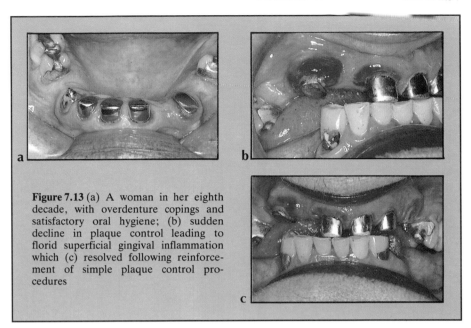

Figure 7.13 (a) A woman in her eighth decade, with overdenture copings and satisfactory oral hygiene; (b) sudden decline in plaque control leading to florid superficial gingival inflammation which (c) resolved following reinforcement of simple plaque control procedures

of the patient with regard to appearance, function, transport and home support. Good rapport is more likely to result in compliance and return visits.

- Use several modes of communication to support the same message. Wherever possible, let the patient see and feel the presence of plaque, calculus and inflammation for themselves. The 'tell, show and feel' of correct toothbrushing can be supported by written advice. The written message should be simple, pithy and printed in large, bold characters with contrasting colours.
- Set realistic objectives. Crevicular and interproximal brushing is desirable and achievable for patients of all ages if they have reasonable manual dexterity. For the less able, a simple scrub technique supplemented by a once or twice daily rinsing with 0.2% chlorhexidine gluconate is more appropriate. For infirm patients, it is necessary to involve the family, or institutional staff, in a similar simple and regular regimen, augmented by professional tooth cleaning every 3–6 months.
- Modified toothbrush handles for improved grip and access can be purchased or easily made (Fig. 7.14). A good range is now available of handle-mounted interproximal brushes. These are essential for cleaning of the wider interdental spaces and open

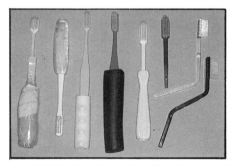

Figure 7.14 Modified toothbrush handles. Simple padding, acrylic, bicycle handle grips, etc., can be used to thicken the handle and improve grip

furcations often present in the aged dentition. Contra-angled, single-tufted brushes are invaluable for reaching single-standing posterior teeth and those with long clinical crowns (Fig. 7.15). A double-headed

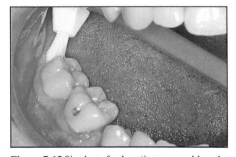

Figure 7.15 Single-tufted or 'interspace' brush

toothbrush designed for simultaneous cleaning of two tooth surfaces may find application in the physically handicapped elderly patient (Fig. 7.16). Automatic toothbrushes, preferably of the rechargeable type and having an elliptical head movement (Fig. 7.17), confer the real benefits of being less tiring and less painful for some elderly patients. In situations where finger and wrist or arm movements are limited, a pulsed-jet water irrigator can be used once daily to deliver 400 ml of a 0.02% solution of chlorhexidine gluconate (Fig. 7.18). Floss holders also relieve less mobile fingers of complex manipulations (Fig. 7.19). A plaque control programme and scaling is often all that is required in cases of early or moderate chronic periodontitis.

Surgery?

Age does not contraindicate periodontal surgery. However, recent longitudinal studies[47] have shown that in patients with moderately advanced periodontal disease, where adequate plaque control was achieved, there was no significant difference between sites treated surgically and those treated non-surgically by

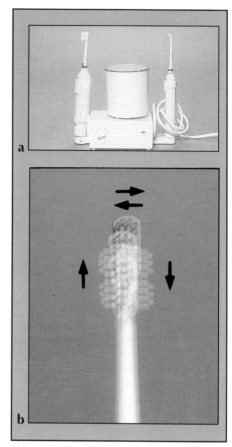

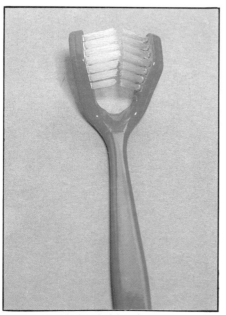

Figure 7.16 A double-headed brush which can clean two surfaces simultaneously and facilitate location of bristles at the gingival margin

Figure 7.17 (a) Automatic toothbrush with (b) both arcuate and horizontal movement

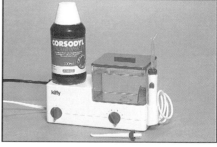

Figure 7.18 Pulsed-jet irrigator with 400 ml of a 0.02% solution of chlorhexidine gluconate in the reservoir

OHI, scaling and root planing. Although surgery produced a greater reduction in depth of severe pockets, both treatment modalities were capable of arresting periodontal destruction. Thus, for most elderly patients, especially those with medical complications or inadequate home care, a non-surgical approach is advisable. When root planing, it

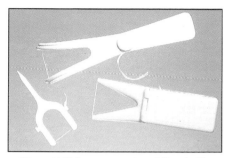

Figure 7.19 Some examples of floss holders

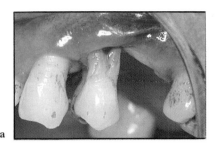

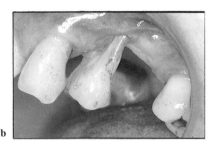

Figure 7.21 (a) A 65-year-old woman with a grade III furcation involvement of the two buccal roots of ⌐4. (b) 15 months after root filling and mesio-buccal root amputation. Residual 3 mm pocketing

should be noted that repeated and excessive removal of cementum is unnecessary and may lead to dentinal hypersensitivity.

Gingivectomy (see Fig. 7.4), flap surgery (Fig. 7.20) and root amputation (Fig. 7.21) are probably the most useful surgical techniques for the older patient. These procedures facilitate visual and mechanical access to the root surface for cleaning by the patient or by the clinician. Although teeth with furcation involvements were once thought to have poor prognosis, long-term surveys indicate a high survival rate into old age when managed surgically or non-surgically.[48]

Response to surgery

In both animal and human studies, wound healing is reported to be adversely affected by age. Factors include the rate of healing, and the strength of the healed tissues. This may be a reflection of altered fibroblastic function and slower revascularization in the elderly. However, it appears that age is not a clinically significant factor with regard to healing of the periodontal tissues. It has been reported that healing after gingivectomy is not affected by age.[49] More recent evidence suggests that the amount of periodontal breakdown, and hence susceptibility to periodontal disease, is of greater import in determining healing following periodontal surgery than age.[50]

It is apparent that an older dentate patient with the same degree of periodontal breakdown as a younger person may be regarded as being more resistant to the disease process.

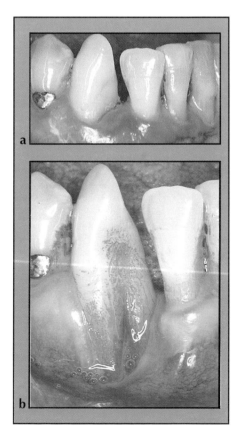

Figure 7.20 (a) A refractory 10 mm pocket on the mesial of ̄3⌐. (b) Two years after a replaced flap that had a vertical relieving incision over the buccal root of ̄3⌐, 3 mm residual pocketing. Note mesial groove and 'inadequate' plaque control

Furthermore, such resistant individuals have been succesfully treated surgically and nonsurgically even with a less-than-ideal standard of plaque control.[51] It should be emphasized that surgery performed on any patient with poor oral hygiene may constitute 'over-treatment', and may result in even greater damage being done to the periodontium.[52]

Splinting

Mobile teeth with no active periodontal disease may remain functional and in a stable position for many years. Splinting should not be undertaken lightly because it often encourages plaque accumulation and inhibits its removal. However, splinting is indicated when the mobility of a tooth is increasing, or is so great that exfoliation is threatened, or when it causes discomfort. When treatment planning, mobile teeth are more suitably used as abutments for fixed bridgework than for removable prostheses because the distribution forces can be better controlled.[53]

References

1 Page R.C., Schroeder H.E., Pathogenesis of inflammatory periodontal disease, *Lab. Invest. 1976*; 33: 235–49

2 Sockransky S.S., Haffajee A.D., Goodson J M., Lindhe J., New concepts of destructive periodontal disease, *J. Clin. Periodontol. 1984*; 11: 21–32

3 Marshall-Day C., Stephens R., Quickley L., Periodontol disease: prevalence and incidence, *J. Periodontol. 1955*; 26: 185–203

4 Miller A., Brunelle J., Carlos J., Oral health of the United States, *National Institutes of Health Publication 1987*; 87

5 Yoneyama T., Okamoto H., Lindhe J., Socransky S.S., Haffajee A.D., Probing depth, attachment loss and gingival recession. Findings from a clinical examination in Ushiku, Japan, *J. Clin. Periodontol. 1988*; 15: 581–91

6 Papapanou P.N., Wennstrom J.L., Grondahl K., Periodontal status in relation to age and tooth type. A cross-sectional radiographical study, *J. Clin. Periodontol. 1988*; 15: 469–78

7 Baelum V., Fejerskov O., Manji F., Periodontal diseases in adult Kenyans, *J. Clin. Periodontol. 1988*; 15: 445–52

8 Taylor C.M., King J.M., Sheiham A., A comparison of the dental needs of physically handicapped and non-handicapped elderly people living at home in Grimsby, England, *Gerodontics 1986*; 2: 80–82

9 Lappalainen R., Widstrom E., Markkanen H., Periodontal condition, remaining teeth and dental health habits of the aged in Finland, *Gerodontics 1988*; 4: 277–9

10 Rise J., Heloe L.A., Oral conditions and need for dental treatment in an elderly population in Northern Norway, *Community Dent. Oral Epidemiol. 1987*; 15: 134–6

11 Hugoson A., Jordan T., Frequency distribution of individuals aged 20–70 years according to severity of periodontal disease, *Community Dent. Oral Epidemiol. 1982*; 10: 187–92

12 Markkanen H., Rajala M., Paunio K., Periodontal treatment needs of the Finnish population aged 30 years and over, *Community Dent. Oral Epidemiol. 1983*; 11: 25–32

13 Plasschaert A.J.M., Folmer T., Van den Heuvel J.L.M., Jansen J., Opijnen L., Wouters S.L.J., An epidemiological survey of periodontal disease in Dutch adults, *Community Dent. Oral Epidemiol. 1978*; 6: 65–70

14 Hunt R.J., Beck J.D., Lemke J.H., Kahout F.J., Wallace R.B., Edentulism and oral health problems among elderly rural Iowans: The Iowa 65+ Rural Health Study, *Am. J. Public Health 1985*; 75: 1177–81

15 Roper R.E., Knerr G.W., Gocka E.F., Stahl S.S., Periodontal disease in aged individuals, *J. Periodontol. 1972*; 43: 304–10

16 Burt B.A., Ismail A.I., Eklund S.A., Periodontal disease, tooth loss and oral hygiene among older Americans, *Community Dent. Oral Epidemiol. 1985*; 13: 93–6

17 Palmqvist S., Sjodin B., Alveolar bone levels in a geriatric Swedish population, *J. Clin. Periodontol. 1987*; 14: 100–4

18 Levy S.M., Heckert D.A., Beck J.D., Kahout J., Multivariate correlates of periodontally healthy teeth in an elderly population, *Gerodontics 1987*; 3: 85–8

19 Grbic J.T, Lamster I.B., Gelenti R.S., Fine J.B., Risk indicators for future clinical attachment loss in adult periodontitis. Patient variables, *J. Periodontol. 1991*; 62: 322–9

20 Vigild M., Oral hygiene and periodontal conditions among 201 dentate institutionalised elderly, *Gerodontics 1988*; 4: 140–5

21 Shklar G., The effects of aging upon oral mucosa, *J. Invest. Dermatol. 1966*; 47: 115–20

22 Ryan E.J., Toto P.D., Gargiulo A.W., Aging in human attached gingival epithelium, *J. Dent. Res. 1974*; 53: 74–6

23 Löe H., Karring T., The three-dimensional morphology of the epithelium-connective tissue interface of the gingiva as related to age and sex, *Scand. J. Dent. Res. 1972*; 79: 315–26

24 Van der Velden U., Effect of age on the periodontium, *J. Clin. Periodontol. 1984*; 11: 281–94

25 Severson J.A., Moffett B.C., Kokich V., Selipsky H.,

A histological study of age changes in the adult human periodontal joint (ligament), *J. Periodontol. 1978*; 49: 189–200

26 Helkimo E., Carlsson G.E., Helkimo M., Bite force and state of dentition, *Acta Odont. Scand. 1977*; 35: 297–303

27 Zander H.A., Hurzeler B., Continuous cementum apposition, *J. Dent. Res. 1958*; 37: 1035–44

28 Henry J.L., Weinmann J.P., The pattern of resorption and repair of human cementum, *J. Am. Dent. Assoc. 1951*; 42: 270–90

29 Grant D., Bernick S., The periodontium of aging humans, *J. Periodontol. 1972*; 43: 660–7

30 Manson J.D., Passive eruption, *Dent. Practice 1963*; 14: 2–9

31 Anneroth G., Ericsson S.G., An experimental histological study of monkey teeth without antagonist, *Odont. Rev. 1967*; 18: 345–59

32 Ainamo A., Influence of age on the location of the maxillary mucogingival junction, *J. Periodont. Res. 1978*; 13: 189–93

33 Ainamo A., Ainamo J., Poikkens R., Continuous widening of the band of attached gingiva from 23 to 65 years of age, *J. Periodont. Res. 1961*; 16: 595–9

34 Kleinberg I., Goldenberg D.J., Kaufmann H.W., Plaque formation and the effect of age, *J. Periodontol. 1971*; 42: 497–507

35 Holm-Pedersen P., Folke L.E.A., Gawronski T.H., Composition and metabolic activity of dental plaque from healthy young and elderly individuals, *J. Dent. Res. 1980*; 59: 771–6

36 Socransky S.S., Gibbons R.J., Dale A.C., Bortnick L., Rosenthal E., MacDonald J.B., The microbiota of the gingival crevice area of man: 1 Total microscopic and viable counts of specific organisms, *Arch. Oral Biol. 1963*; 8: 275–9

37 Brecx M., Holm-Pedersen P., Theilade J., Early plaque formation in young and elderly individuals, *Gerodontics 1985*; 1: 8–13

38 Holm-Pedersen P., Dolbe L.E.A., Gawronski T.H., Composition and metabolic activity of dental plaque from healthy young and elderly individuals, *J. Dent. Res. 1980*; 59: 771–6

39 Holm-Pedersen P., Agerbaek N., Theilade E., Experimental gingivitis in young and elderly individuals, *J. Clin. Periodontol. 1975*; 2: 14–24

40 Holm-Pedersen P., Agerbaek N., Theilade E., Experimental gingivitis in young and elderly individuals, *J. Clin. Periodontol. 1975*; 2: 14–24

41 Church H., Dolby A.E., The effect of age on the cellular immune response to dento-gingival plaque extract, *J. Periodontol. Res. 1978*; 13: 120–6

42 Holm-Pedersen P., Gaumer H.R., Folke L.E.A., Aberrant blastogenic response to LPS in experimental gingivitis of elderly subjects, *Scand. J. Dent. Res. 1979*; 87: 431–4

43 Van der Velden U., Abbas F., Experimental gingivitis in relation to age, *IADR, NOF Meeting 1982* abs. no. 60

44 A system of periodontal screening for general dental practice in the UK, British Society of Periodontology.

45 Lindhe J., Okamoto H., Yoneyama T., Haffajee A., Sockransky S.S., Longitudinal changes in periodontal disease in untreated subjects, *J. Clin. Periodontol. 1989*; 16: 662–70

46 Lindhe J., Nyman S., The effect of plaque control and surgical pocket elimination on the establishment and the maintenance of periodontal health. A longitudinal study of periodontal therapy in cases of advanced disease, *J. Clin. Periodontol. 1975*; 2: 67–79

47 Pihlstrom B.L., McHugh R.B., Oliphant T.H., Otiz-Campos C., Comparison of surgical and non-surgical treatment of periodontal disease. A review of current studies and additional results after 6 1/2 years, *J. Clin. Periodontol. 1983*; 10: 524–41

48 Ross I., Thompson A., A long term study of root retention in the treatment of maxillary molars with furcation involvement, *J. Periodontol. 1978*; 49: 238–44

49 Stahl S.S., Witkin G.J., Cantor M., Brown R., Gingival healing. II, Clinical and histological repair sequences following gingivectomy, *J. Periodontol. 1968*; 39: 109–18

50 Abbas F., Van der Velden U., Wound healing after periodontal surgery in relation to age, *IADR, NOF Meeting 1982* abs. no. 11

51 Van der Velden U., Regeneration of the interdental soft tissues following denudation procedures, *J. Clin. Periodontol. 1982*; 9: 455–9

52 Nyman S., Lindhe J., Rosling B., Periodontal surgery in plaque-infested dentitions, *J. Clin. Periodontol. 1977*; 4: 240–9

53 Ed: J. Lindhe, *Textbook of Clinical Periodontology*, Munksgaard, Copenhagen 1983; Ch. 21, 22, 24

8

Root caries

Edwina Kidd

Dental decay often develops on the roots of older patients' teeth. Such root surface caries can be difficult to control and treat. In the light of the greater proportion of old people who are retaining their natural dentition, it may well become the major caries problem of the future.

Introduction

Dental decay has generally been considered a disease of childhood or early adulthood. However, the problem of dental caries is increasingly being met during the treatment of the older patient who has retained his or her teeth. These carious lesions are found mainly on the roots of the teeth rather than the crowns. Such lesions may become more prevalent with a greater retention of the natural dentition in adults and an upward shift in the mean age of the population.

Local factors leading to the development of root surface caries include an increasing exposure of root surfaces to the oral environment as a result of periodontal disease. There is now a considerable interest in this pattern of decay among practitioners and researchers, and it is thought that this will become the major caries problem, certainly of the near future.[1] However, despite the interest in, and the importance of, the subject there remain many gaps in our understanding of the disease.

Clinical features of root surface caries

Carious lesions may occur on all exposed root surfaces but are predominantly found on the approximal and buccal aspects. In its early stages the lesion appears as one or more well-defined, discoloured areas predominantly located along the cement–enamel junction.[2] Clinically, both active and inactive (arrested) lesions can be distinguished (Figs 8.1, 8.2).[3]

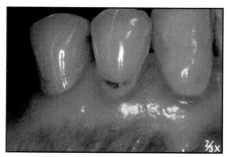

Figure 8.1 Active root caries

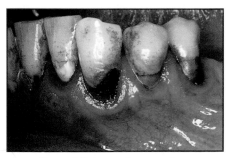

Figure 8.2 Arrested root caries

The consistency of the demineralized tissue appears to be the most relevant factor in judging its activity. Active lesions are soft or leathery, whereas inactive lesions are hard and shiny. Whilst colour has been considered to be of diagnostic relevance, dark lesions being regarded as inactive,[4,5] recent work has shown that colour may be no certain guide in making a diagnosis of active or inactive.[6]

Active lesions tend to spread laterally and coalesce, and may eventually encircle the tooth. They less often spread apically as the gingival margin recedes as a consequence of periodontal breakdown. Thus, a passive lesion can be located at the cement–enamel junction, apparently left abandoned by the receding gingiva. However, new lesions may develop later at the level of the repositioned gingival crest. Active lesions are usually found close to the gingival margin.[6]

Cavitation is commonly seen in active lesions, and thick yellow or white plaque often fills the defect. Pulpal involvement, with pain, is not a common complaint.

Epidemiology of root surface caries

The problem of root caries is not a recent phenomenon.[7] Skulls and mandibles from anthropological studies of ancient populations show that dental caries was a minor problem overall, but most of the lesions that had developed were on root surfaces.

In modern times most epidemiological investigations of dental caries have been confined to coronal carious lesions, particularly in school children who are easily accessible for surveys. In contrast, representative populations of adults and elderly people are difficult to gather. For this reason the prevalence of root surface caries has been described in certain specific communities[2] such as patients from a mental hospital, insurance company employees, patients at a dental school, military personnel, groups with periodontal diseases and institutionalized old persons. These data are difficult to compare, because they represent extreme diversities of age, sex, cultural backgrounds and socio-economic characteristics.

Studies of root caries in the USA,[8] and Scandinavia[9] have shown that root caries prevalence increases with age. Studies on older dentate people living in the community[5,10,11] have demonstrated 56.8%–69.7% of subjects to have 'active' root caries. In a UK population[6] most of the subjects (84.4%) showed evidence of root caries, but the disease was only judged to be active in 31.5% of these cases.

Another problem is that different methods have been used to assess root caries. A standardized method was described in 1980 by Katz.[8] However, this method does not include the use of bitewing radiographs, and arrested caries does not count towards the 'score'. These are important omissions.[12]

Whilst data on the prevalence of root caries is limited, data on rate of progression is virtually non-existent. This presents enormous problems for those involved in clinical trials of agents proposed to prevent or manage the disease, because there is little indication as to how long such a trial should last. Our ignorance of the natural history of the disease also poses great problems to practitioners, who have to manage it.

Microbiology of root surface caries

The microbiology of enamel caries has been extensively investigated, and *Streptococcus mutans* and Lactobaccillus species have been strongly implicated. In contrast, relatively little information is available concerning the microbiological aspects of root caries. Actinomyces or *S. mutans* have both been implicated as causative pathogens in animal models. However, whilst Actinomyces have been found to be present in large numbers in the human carious root surface, they do not appear to be related to 'active decay'.[13] Both *S. mutans* and lactobacilli have been found in higher proportions in dental plaque samples taken from subjects with root caries compared with subjects having exposed root surfaces but no root caries.[14]

Whilst it is tempting to search for a specific organism responsible for caries it is possible that this may be an oversimplification of the complex microbial shifts that take place over the developing lesion. In future, microbiologists may define 'carogenic communities' rather than using the presence of a single organism as an indicator of risk.[15] This information may well prove to be of practical importance and not just of academic interest. A knowledge of the microbiology of the disease may make possible specific microbiological screening tests to predict root caries risk. In addition, it may encourage chemical plaque control as a method of managing the disease.

Diagnosis of root caries

The diagnosis of caries requires sharp eyes, but blunt probes and high-quality bitewing radiographs.[16] The visual signs of arrested and active root surface lesions have already been described, but if these are not to be missed the teeth must be examined clean and dry. This may well necessitate scaling, prophylaxis and oral hygiene instruction prior to any attempt at definitive diagnosis.

Some authors advocate the use of sharp probes in the diagnosis of root caries,[17] suggesting that the defects should be penetrated by a sharp explorer which is then removed to see whether the lesion is sticky. Although the consistency of the lesion is important in the diagnosis of active disease, this approach seems unwise, because it is likely to make a hole in the lesion which will subsequently fill with plaque thus encouraging progression rather than arrest of the carious process. Such an approach may well have been justified when lesions were automatically managed operatively. However, operative measures alone will not prevent recurrence and nowadays the treatment of choice is early diagnosis and preventive efforts to arrest the disease. Perhaps a better way of assessing the texture of a lesion is the judicious application of the edge of a sharp excavator.

Interproximal areas are often difficult to see directly and therefore bitewing radiographs are of importance (Fig. 8.3). Such films must be carefully taken so that the rays pass tangentially to the surface of the lesion without overlap of the image of the adjacent tooth. Figures 8.4a, b illustrate how differences in angulation of the tube can affect what is seen on the resultant radiograph. A film holder that will facilitate reproducible radiographs is a distinct advantage (Figs 8.5, 8.6). It can be difficult to distinguish between the cervical radiolucency and root caries. When in

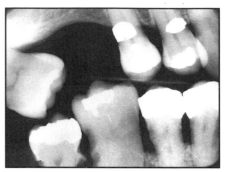

Figure 8.3 Bitewing radiograph showing root caries

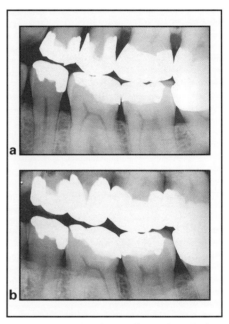

Figure 8.4a, b Two bitewing radiographs of the same patient. Note how the change in angulation confuses the picture

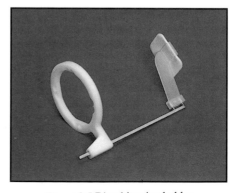

Figure 8.5 Rinn bitewing holder

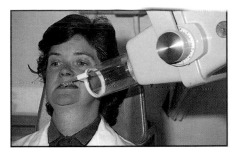

Figure 8.6 Rinn bitewing holder in use

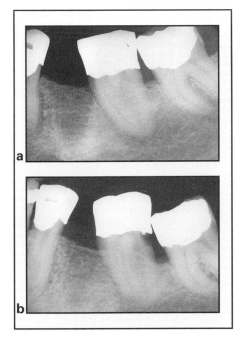

Figure 8.7a, b Radiographs of a retired dentist. The recall interval of one year between these two pictures was too long

doubt, radiographic data must be supplemented by visual examination and *gentle* probing to feel for cavitation.

In recent years there has been considerable discussion on the appropriate intervals between dental examinations.[18,19] Some workers have suggested that the time-honoured six-month recall is an outdated concept which should be replaced with an annual examination. Others suggest that longer intervals are appropriate for older people because dental caries is a disease of the young. This argument does not pertain to root caries, which is chiefly a disease of the elderly. Very little scientific information is available on the speed of progression of root caries in a susceptible patient, and the frequency of recall appointments currently relates to clinical judgement based upon experience. The wise practitioner will seek to extend the diagnostic net to try to predict individuals who are at risk to disease and examine these patients more frequently than those who are not caries-prone. However, matters are not as simple as at first they might seem. Figures 8.7a, b show radiographs of a retired dentist taken a year apart. The progress of the lesion has been unexpectedly rapid, despite the knowledge of caries control that the patient might have been expected to have, and the reduced caries incidence which could have been hoped for. In this case an interval of a year between examinations was evidently too long.

Factors which predispose to root caries

Several factors are known to predispose towards root caries. They may usually be identified in a particular patient by means of a careful history and clinical examination.

Diet

The Vipeholm Dental Caries Study[20] showed that increases in enamel and cemental caries incidence coincided with an increased daily intake of sugar, especially when taken between meals. Thus, diet analysis may assist in the diagnosis of caries risk. It is helpful to ask the patient to keep a diet sheet on which all food and drink consumed, together with the time of eating, is recorded over a 3–4 day period (Fig. 8.8). At present, there is a lack of specific information on the importance of dietary factors in root caries. It is intriguing to note that ancient man appeared to suffer from the disease despite very little sucrose in the diet. This might be thought to implicate starch as a cause of the condition. However, until further research work has been carried out, it is difficult to know whether or not frequent starch intake constitutes a risk in modern man.

	THURSDAY	
	Time	Item
BEFORE BREAKFAST	6.50	Lucozade
	7.12	Grapefruit juice
	7.30	Lucozade
Breakfast	9.30	Cereal, milk, glucose, toast, marmalade, Coffee with glucose
MORNING	10.15	Tablets Lithium Valium
	11.05	Lemon drink
	12.20	Guiness
	1.00	Tablets Lithium
Mid-day Meal	1.45	Macaroni cheese Tomato Shortbread Biscuits Water
AFTERNOON	2.40	Lemon drink, sugar & lemon juice
	3.40	Water
	4.35	Tea and glucose Lemon drink
Evening Meal	6.45	Omelete, potato Biscuits, raisins, water
EVENING & NIGHT	8.10	Water
	8.45	Lime juice
	9.45	Peanuts: water
	9.55	Glacé cherry
	10.05	Tablets Lithium Valium Largactil
	1.10	Lucozade
	3.30	Lucozade
	5.30	Lucozade

Figure 8.8 One day from a diet sheet of a patient who was thirsty because of her medication

Oral flora

Because it has been demonstrated that *Streptococcus mutans* and lactobacilli are associated with root caries, salivary counts of these organisms may be useful in predicting caries risk. It is possible that in the future microbiological testing will become a routine diagnostic test. Commercial kits[a] are already available for the estimations of salivary bacterial counts. Large-scale clinical trials on the predictive value of such tests for root caries have yet to be undertaken. However, the number of lactobacilli in saliva was found to be a useful assessment of caries risk in patients treated for advanced periodontal disease.[21]

[a]Dentocult LB; Dentocult SM; LIC Dental, Smidgesvagen 1, S-171 83 Solna, Sweden. (Available from Rexodent Ltd, Middlesex and Vivacare, Ivoclar/Vivadent, 2 Meridian South, Leicester, LE3 2WY)

Periodontal disease

Exposure of the cementum or dentine to the oral environment is a prerequisite for the development of root surface caries. One epidemiological study has found approximately twice as many decayed and filled root surfaces in patients with untreated as opposed to treated periodontitis.[22] Another study, which sought to identify predictors of root caries in the elderly, noted that patients with poor oral hygiene, calculus and few remaining teeth were particularly susceptible[23] and male denture wearers were at risk in another study.[6] However, a group of 31 patients successfully treated for periodontal disease whose oral hygiene was good were not immune from root caries.[21] In follow-up examinations over four years, approximately two-thirds of the patients developed lesions although the total increment was low, being present on less than 5% of exposed root surfaces. In this study previous root caries experience, high lactobacillus counts, increasing age and low salivary secretion rate were found to be the best predictors of caries risk.

Xerostomia

Xerostomia or dry mouth is an important factor that predisposes to root caries.[24] Causation and management is discussed in Chapter 4.

Age

Epidemiological studies have shown an increase in root caries experience with advancing age. This is hardly surprising because old people are likely to have gingival recession and may well be taking one of the medicaments that have a xerostomic effect. Patients with drug-induced xerostomia may frequently be consuming drinks, sucking sweets or using a sugar-containing chewing gum and these dietary changes favour caries. Even in the absence of xerostomia, detrimental changes in the diet will often occur, simply as a consequence of the general disabilities of ageing. Retirement, bereavement or ill health can all result in an increase in the amount and frequency with which sugar-rich snacks and convenience foods are consumed. Finally, old people often find it more difficult to carry out effective oral hygiene regimens.

Management of root caries

Ideally, the management of root caries should be preventive in nature. Prevention depends upon the assessment of caries risk, early diagnosis and efforts to arrest the disease at an early stage.

Operative intervention may be required to restore the integrity of the tooth surface in deeply cavitated lesions, to aid plaque control, to prevent pulpal involvement or to improve appearance in the anterior part of the mouth.

Assessment of caries risk

An attempt should be made to assess the risk of root caries in all patients with exposed root surfaces. The important factors, which have already been discussed, include advancing age, *a history of high caries experience*, partial dentures, xerostomia, poor oral hygiene, a cariogenic diet and high salivary counts of *Streptococcus mutans* and lactobacilli. Assessment must include a decision as to whether lesions appear active or whether they are arrested, because the latter only require regular monitoring.

Preventive treatment of root caries

As with coronal caries, preventive efforts should be directed towards dietary advice, effective plaque removal and fluoride therapy. There appear to be no studies available on the effect of dietary advice alone in the management of the disease. It would seem logical to attempt to reduce the frequency of intake of cariogenic food and drinks.

Mechanical plaque control is important, not only because it disturbs the causative organisms, but also because the use of a fluoride-containing dentifrice results in regular topical application of the fluoride ion, in low concentration, at the site of acid attack. A clinical trial has shown the cariostatic effect of a fluoridated dentifrice on root caries.[25] Because some patients may be using toothpastes which do not contain fluoride, it is important to check the brand of toothpaste used. Oral hygiene instruction should be specific to the sites of the lesions, stressing the need for scrupulous cleanliness in those areas. The patient needs to be aware of how plaque control can help arrest the condition. Where

necessary, toothbrushes should be modified and interdental brushes provided to allow the patient to clean the lesions. Oral hygiene instruction must be carried out in the patient's mouth. Models are not very helpful in this site-specific problem.

Disclosing agents are essential to help patient and dentist see the plaque. A disposable mouth mirror and a supply of disclosing tablets will be needed for home use. It has been shown that, within 2–6 months, active lesions with soft, greasy and yellowish surfaces can be converted to leathery or hard, darkly discoloured tissues using such a regimen.[26]

Professional plaque control, perhaps every two months, may have a role to play in managing the disease, although this hypothesis has yet to be tested in a clinical trial. Meticulous home care may be an impracticable objective to set for a confused or infirm old person. In such cases chemical plaque control using chlorhexidine might be considered.[27] One clinical trial carried out on a group of radiotherapy patients has demonstrated the beneficial effect of combinations of chlorhexidine and topical fluoride.[28] A suitable chlorhexidine regimen would be the use of chlorhexidine gel (Corsodyl, ICI) applied to the teeth in custom-made applicator trays. This may either be carried out by the patient or professionally. Where the patient is to apply the gel, daily five-minute applications for two weeks have been shown to reduce salivary levels of *S. mutans* but, since the organism recolonizes, this treatment should probably be repeated every three months. An alternative regimen, which may be chosen where patient compliance is in doubt, is for the patient to have professional chlorhexidine applications on two consecutive days. On the first day, four five-minute applications are given with a water rinse in between applications, whilst on the second day, three such treatments are done. Again, the applications should be repeated at three-monthly intervals.

Several clinical studies and reports on the management of root caries have used fluoride in some form. The optimum fluoride regimen has yet to be determined and the practitioner must therefore select a regimen based on the severity of the disease and the degree of patient compliance that is expected.

The use of a fluoride-containing dentifrice[25] and various combinations of fluoride mouthwash (0.05% sodium fluoride), topical fluoride gel application,[29] and daily self-application of 1.0% gel in custom-fitted trays[17] have all been described. The use of gel has been advocated in cases of severe xerostomia such as may be found in patients who have had radiotherapy in the region of the salivary glands. However, there is a potential toxicity problem in the long-term home use, of fluoride-containing gels. Preliminary studies[30] show injury to the gastric mucosa of healthy adults after ingestion of as little as 20 mg of fluoride. For this reason, home use of fluoride mouthwashes together with professional gel application may be a safer approach.

Patients with severe xerostomia benefit from the use of an artificial saliva[31,32] which may be based upon either carboxymethyl cellulose or mucin. Laboratory studies[33] have shown that both formulations are capable of promoting remineralization of early caries-like lesions, provided the preparation contains fluoride. A mucin-based product (Saliva Orthana[b]) and a methyl cellulose preparation (Luborant[c]) are both available.

Operative management

Incipient lesions, where there is no obvious surface defect, can often be treated by preventive measures alone, the aim being to transform active lesions to arrested lesions. One study[26] has used this approach to good effect on slightly cavitated lesions. Other workers have suggested that shallow cavitated lesions benefit from recontouring and smoothing, together with topical fluoride application.[17] Conventional finishing and polishing materials are used, such as mounted abrasive points and flexible polishing discs. Interdentally, a special handpiece with a reciprocating action (the Eva[d] system) can aid access.[29] When shallow lesions are smoothed, it is neither necessary nor desirable to remove all stained dentine. To do so would result in an unacceptable surface defect which would require restoration. The purpose of the recontouring and smoothing is to eliminate the soft

tissue, leaving a smooth and easily cleansable root surface.[17]

Recent histological studies have shown that arrested lesions frequently exhibit signs of considerable surface wear.[34] It may be, therefore, that recontouring and smoothing by the dentist only hastens what will happen naturally if further carious destruction is prevented.

In vitro studies of recontouring techniques have shown that infected dentine is not completely removed following the smoothing of lesions. Histological analysis of smoothed sites demonstrated that microbial invasion extends up to 1 mm into clinically 'sound' dentine. Coccoid and filamentous organisms were seen at the depth of the lesion. However, such lesions can be treated successfully by a combination of smoothing and the application of topical fluorides.

Cavities, which cannot be made cleansable by recontouring, or of such depth that the pulp is endangered, require restorative intervention. A glass ionomer cement, which is chemically adhesive to dentine, is the material of choice for restoring root surface dental caries. It was first described in the dental literature in 1972[35] and since that time the physical properties and potential uses for the material have been extensively reported.[36] No adverse or irreversible pulpal responses have been noted to the restorative versions of these materials, as a result of *in vitro* biological evaluations. However, deep cavities, especially those where there is freshly cut dentine at the base, should be lined with a proprietary cement containing calcium hydroxide. Glass ionomer cements contain fluoride, and the release of this material exerts a cariostatic effect upon the surrounding tooth tissue. Gingival tissues respond well to the material. The second- and third-generation materials have solved some of the earlier problems such as a long setting time and poor aesthetics. Some of the new systems are encapsulated and when triturated produce a homogeneous and consistent mix. Placement is straightforward but technique-sensitive.[36] Salivary contamination of the cleaned and dried tooth surface must be avoided because this will interfere with bonding. Once the material is placed it must continue to be protected from moisture contamination until the initial set is complete. When the matrix is removed, a light-cured bonding resin should be applied to

[b]Saliva Orthana, Nycomed (UK) Ltd, Coventry Road, Sheldon, Birmingham
[c]Luborant: Antigen Europe, Ellesfield Avenue, Bracknell, Berkshire RG12 4YS
[d]EVA system, Dentatus, Sweden

the exposed surface of the cement to prevent dehydration and crazing of the material. Initial finishing should be minimal, and sharp hand instruments are preferable to rotary instruments. When it is essential to use fine diamond or multi-bladed tungsten carbide finishing burs, or abrasive discs, these should be lubricated with petroleum jelly.

Conventional glass ionomer cements are radiolucent, and this can make difficult the radiographic detection of interproximal recurrent caries. In these situations the use of radio-opaque Cermet is advisable. Such materials have silver particles incorporated within the glass element of the powder.[36]

An important development in clinical technique is the bonding of resin-based filling materials to glass ionomer cements, either by means of etching the surface of the set glass ionomer cement,[37] or preferably by the use of a dentine bonding agent. In this technique, the glass ionomer has been likened to replacement dentine, the composite resin as an 'enamel substitute'. The technique may be used for the restoration of root caries in the anterior part of the mouth where the appearance and surface finish of a composite resin is thought to be more desirable, particularly if the lesion extends into the enamel.

Although the advent of the glass ionomer cements has greatly simplified the restorative management of root caries, treatment of the condition is far from easy. Access to approximal lesions can present great difficulty, particularly if they lie deep within the trifurcation or bifurcation of a posterior tooth. In the absence of an existing coronal restoration, access from the buccal is often the most convenient approach. However, if the root caries has developed at the cervical margin of an existing restoration, access may more simply be gained by removing the filling. Vision is often difficult as the operator is peering down a long dark tunnel. The margin of the cavity may lie well subgingivally and in such cases periodontal surgery may be required before a definitive restoration can be placed, especially if a glass ionomer cement is to be used to restore the carious surface. Access to lingual lesions in the lower arch is often difficult and made worse by the presence of the tongue and floor of the mouth. The placement of rubber dam can occasionally be of help in gaining access.

References

1 Katz R.V., Root caries: is it the caries problem of the future? *J. Can. Dent. Assoc. 1985*; 51: 511–14

2 Nyvad B., Fejerskov O., Root surface caries: clinical, histopathological and microbiological features and clinical implications, *Int. Dent. J. 1982*; 32: 312–26

3 Miller W.A., Massler M., Permeability and staining of active and arrested lesions in dentine, *Br. Dent. J. 1962*; 112: 187–97

4 Miller A.J., Brunelle J.A., Carlos J.P., Brown L.J., Löe H., Oral Health of United States Adults. Mass USA: *National Institute for Dental Research, 1987* (Pubn 87/2868)

5 Locker D., Slade G.D., Leake J.L., Prevalence of and factors associated with root decay in older adults in Canada, *J. Dent. Res. 1989*; 68: 768–72

6 Hellyer P.H., Beighton B., Heath M.R., Lynch, E.J.R., Root caries in older people attending a general dental practice in East Sussex, *Br. Dent. J. 1990*; 169: 201–6

7 Banting D.W., Ellen R.P., Carious lesions on the roots of teeth: a review for the general practitioner, *J. Can. Dent. Assoc. 1976*; 42: 496–504

8 Katz R.V., Assessing root caries in populations: the evolution of the root caries index, *J. Publ. Health Dent. 1980*; 40: 7–16

9 Vehkalahti M., Occurrence of root caries and factors relating to it, *Proc. Finn. Dent. Soc. 1987*; 83: Suppl iv–v, pp. 1–99.

10 Beck J.D., Hunt R.J., Hand J.S., Field H.M., Prevalence of root and coronal caries in a non-institutionalised older population, *J. Am. Dent. Assoc. 1985*; 111: 964–7

11 Wallace M.C., Retief D.H., Bradley E.L., Prevalence of root caries in a population of older adults, *Gerodontics 1988*; 4: 84–9

12 Fejerskov O., Luan Wen Min., Nyvad B., Gadegaard P., Holm-Pedersen P., Budtz-Jorgensen E., Root surface caries in a population of elderly Danes, *J. Dent. Res. 1985*; 64: 187 abs. 116

13 Keltjens H.M.A.M., Schaeken M.J.M., van der Hoeven J.S., Hendricks J.M.C., Microflora of plaque from sound and carious root surfaces, *Caries Res. 1987*; 21: 193–9

14 Fure S., Romanier M., Emilson C.G., Krasse B., Proportions of *Streptococcus mutans*, lactobacilli and Actinomyces spp in root surface plaque, *Scand. J. Dent. Res. 1987*; 95: 119–23

15 Bowden G., Which bacteria are cariogenic in humans?, in: risk markers for oral diseases, vol. *1 Dental Caries*, ed.: Johnson N.W., Cambridge University Press, Cambridge, 1991

16 Kidd E.A.M., The diagnosis and management of the 'early' carious lesion in permanent teeth, *Dent. Update 1984*; 11: 69–81

17 Billings R.J., Restoration of carious lesions of the root, *Gerodontology 1986*; 5: 43–9

18 Elderton R.J., Six-monthly examinations for dental

caries, *Br. Dent. J. 1985*; 158: 370–4

19 Anon., Routine six-monthly checks for dental disease? *Drug Ther. Bull. 1985*; 23: 69–72

20 Gustafsson B.E., Quensel C-E., Lanke L.S., Lundqvist C., Grahnen H., Bonow B.E., Krasse B., The Vipeholm dental caries study. The effect of different levels of carbohydrate intake on caries activity in 436 individuals observed for five years (Sweden), *Acta Odontol. Scand. 1954*; 11: 232–364

21 Ravald N., Hamp S-E., Prediction of root surface caries in patients treated for advanced periodontal disease, *J. Clin. Periodontol. 1981*; 8: 400–414

22 Hix J.O., O'Leary T.J., The relationship between cemental caries, oral hygiene status and fermentable carbohydrate intake, *J. Periodontol. 1976*; 47: 398–404

23 Kitamura M., Asuman N., Kiyak H., Mulligan K., Predictors of root caries in the elderly, *Community Dent. Oral Epidemiol. 1986*; 14: 34–8

24 Kidd E.A.M., Joyston-Bechal S., Saliva and caries, in: *Essentials of dental caries: the disease and its management*, John Wright, Bristol, 1987; 58–67

25 Jensen M.E., Kahout F., The effect of a fluoridated dentifrice on root and coronal caries in an older adult population, *J. Am. Dent. Assoc. 1988*; 117: 829–32

26 Nyvad B., Fejerskov O., Active root surface caries converted into inactive caries as a response to oral hygiene, *Scand. J. Dent. Res. 1986*; 94: 281–4

27 Kidd E.A.M., The role of chlorhexidine in the management of dental caries, *Int. Dent. J. 1991*; 41: 279–86

28 Katz S., The use of fluoride and chlorhexidine for the prevention of radiation caries, *J. Am. Dent. Assoc. 1982*; 104: 164–70

29 Nicholls C.B., Root caries: a rationale for treatment, *Dent. Update 1987*; 14: 145–53

30 Spak C-J., Sjostedt S., Eleborg L., Veress B., Perbeck L., Ekstrand J., The tissue reaction of human gastric mucosa after fluoride ingestion, *Caries Res. 1989*; 23: 100

31 Shannon I.L., McCrary B.R., Starke E.N., A saliva substitute for use by xerostomic patients undergoing radiotherapy to the head and neck, *Oral Surg. 1977*; 44: 656–61

32 Vissink A., S-Gravenmade E.J., Panders A.K., Vermey A., Petersen J.K., Visch L.L., Schaub R.M.H., A clinical comparison between commercially available mucin – and CMC – containing saliva substitutes, *Int. J. Oral Surg. 1983*; 12: 232–8

33 Joyston-Bechal S., Kidd E.A.M., The effect of three commercially available saliva substitutes on enamel in vitro, *Br. Dent. J. 1987*; 163: 187–90

34 Fejerskov O., Nyvad B., Active or inactive root surface caries – clinical and histological entities? *Caries Res. 1988*; 22: 91

35 Wilson A.D., Kent B.E., A new translucent cement for dentistry: the glass ionomer cement, *Brit. Dent. J. 1972*; 132: 133–5

36 Wilson A.D., McLean J.W., *Glass ionomer cement*, Quintessence Publishing, Chicago 1988

37 McLean J.W., Prosser H.J., Wilson A.D., The use of glass ionomer cements in bonding composite resins to dentine, *Brit. Dent. J. 1985*; 158: 410–14

9

Toothwear: Aetiology and diagnosis

Bernard Smith

In the light of the constant use to which they are put it is surprising that the teeth and supporting oral structures last so well. Nevertheless, wear does take place as the patient ages. A small degree of wear must be considered as normal. Increasingly, however, cases of extreme wear are being seen by dentists, and their treatment poses problems. This chapter considers the causes of toothwear and discusses the diagnosis, prognosis and possible avenues for treatment.

The use of the term 'toothwear' has been increasing in the last few years and is to be encouraged. A general term such as this does not prejudge the aetiology of the condition, as does the casual use of one of the terms erosion, attrition or abrasion, which are sometimes used, usually before a proper diagnosis has been made.

Toothwear, particularly in the elderly, is often the result of a complex combination of causes. In such instances, it can be difficult to attribute the aetiology to a single factor, and it is thus wrong to use a specific term which implies cause and effect. Use of such terminology could lead to both inappropriate management and treatment. The simple term 'toothwear' is readily understood by patients, and so helps good communication between the patient and dentist. This is necessary in order to determine the aetiology of the toothwear, the means of preventing further wear and the management of the condition. The term 'tooth surface loss' has also been proposed, based on the idea that the wear is occurring at the surface of the tooth rather than in the sub-surface layer, as with enamel caries. This subtle distinction is of no particular help in diagnosing or managing the condition, and by suggesting that only the surface of the tooth is lost, the term tends to devalue a condition which can be of major significance to the dentition (Fig. 9.1).

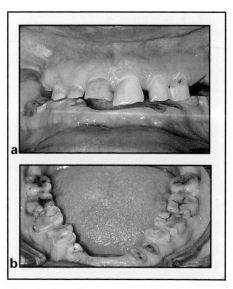

Figure 9.1 a, b Extensive toothwear which has contributed significantly to the collapse of this dentition

Erosion, attrition and abrasion

It is legitimate to use the terms erosion, abrasion and attrition only when there is a clear indication of the specific aetiology in the case under investigation.

Erosion

Erosion is the loss of enamel and dentine resulting primarily from chemical attack (usually acids), other than those chemicals produced intra-orally by bacteria. If dietary or other acids are applied to the surface of an extracted tooth, etching occurs, much as with the preparation of a tooth for an acid-etched retained restoration, and the surface becomes frosty and white. The decalcified surface produced does not look the same as clinical 'erosion', which is smooth and polished. Clinical erosion probably does not occur alone, and some minor physical wear is necessary to rub away the softened, decalcified surface. The erosive component is, however, of prime importance. Strictly speaking, therefore, these lesions should always be attributed to erosion/abrasion or erosion/attrition. However, when the principal aetiology is chemical rather than physical it is common practice to use the term 'erosion' on its own.

Attrition

Attrition is the physical wear of one tooth surface against another, with tooth tissue loss occurring on the contacting surfaces. Slight wear occurs at the contact points but the principle loss occurs occlusally and incisally. Such wear can be particularly marked in people with 'primitive' diets. Attrition may occur alone but is commonly accelerated by an erosive factor. The clinical appearance is similar whether the wear is purely physical, or partly physical and partly chemical. This similarity leads to considerable difficulty in diagnosis which will be discussed later.

Abrasion

Abrasion is defined as physical wear by objects other than another tooth. It may occur, for example, as a result of biting sewing thread or a fishing line, or chewing a pipe stem. However, the commonest abrasion lesions are thought to result from over-vigorous tooth brushing with abrasive toothpastes or brushing dentine exposed on the labial or buccal surfaces of the tooth following gingival recession. Again, it is likely that a full explanation of these lesions is not as simple as it first seems. The presence of 'abrasion' lesions on instanding teeth, and on some teeth in an arch and not others, and on teeth where standards of oral hygiene are poor, suggests that other factors, such as erosion, or the softening of tooth substance through decay, are also at work.

Typical lesions of erosion, attrition and abrasion are shown in Figure 9.2a, b, c. Those illustrated in Figure 9.2d and e are combined lesions. However, the extracted lower canine tooth in Figure 9.3 not only has a buccal lesion that would traditionally be described as 'toothbrush abrasion' but also a similar lingual lesion, which could hardly be the result of excessive tooth brushing. The cause is unclear.

Aetiology of toothwear in the elderly

Dental hard tissues have the capacity, within the oral environment, for some repair and change. This is seen in the remineralization of early carious lesions, and the deposition of peritubular dentine. However, they are not replaced in the way that hair, skin and most other tissues of the body are. It is not surprising, therefore, that all patients show some degree of toothwear by the time they are elderly. It is remarkable, with life expectancy increasing and with more people keeping a natural dentition into old age, that there are not more complaints about dentitions wearing out.

The effects of toothwear are cumulative throughout life, and so it is more difficult to assess the aetiology in old patients than it is in the young. The rate at which toothwear occurs may vary during different periods of life. Thus, although the net cumulative effect of wear is seen in old age, the period when the condition progressed most rapidly may have been decades earlier. For example, a woman who has suffered from morning sickness during several pregnancies may well have suffered regurgitation erosion affecting the

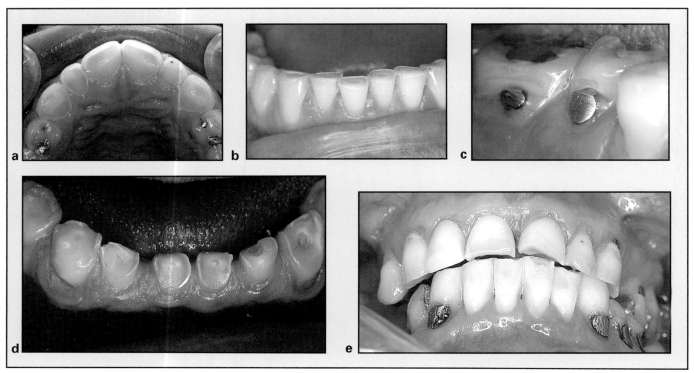

Figure 9.2 Examples of toothwear. (a) Typical dental erosion arising from regurgitation of stomach acid. Enamel has been eroded away from the palatal surfaces of all the upper anterior teeth, and the incisal edges show typical cupping-out which is associated with erosion. (b) Typical attrition with flat wear facets with no cupping-out. The wear facets have sharp edges and can be brought into close contact with the opposing teeth. Both arches wear at approximately the same rate when attrition is the main cause of the wear. (c) Typical abrasion with both tooth tissue and amalgam restorations being worn away. The second premolar tooth is instanding in the arch and yet, strangely, the abrasion is worse than in the first premolar tooth. The dentine is being worn more than the amalgam, but the amalgam shows horizontal abrasion marks. (d) Combined erosion and attrition. There is a degree of cupping-out but not so much as with erosion alone. The patient gave a history of regurgitating and was also aware of bruxing. (e) Gross toothwear where the aetiology is unclear but is likely to be a combination of all three main causes: erosion, attrition and abrasion

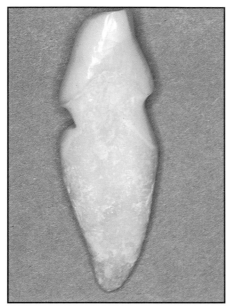

Figure 9.3 An extracted lower canine tooth showing a labial cervical notch lesion which would commonly be attributed to toothbrush abrasion. However, there is a similar lesion on the lingual side which is almost as deep. The incisal edge is also very worn. It would be a remarkable coincidence if these three lesions do not have some common factor as part of their aetiology

palatal surfaces of her upper teeth, of which she was unaware at the time. Only much later, when the thin incisal edges begin to wear down and chip does she become aware of the problem. Also, patients may have experienced toothwear of different aetiologies at different times in their life. However, it is also possible that the rate of progress of toothwear accelerates in older patients. The following paragraphs list some possible explanations for this.

Regurgitation and dietary erosion

Erosion is almost always caused by acid from one of three sources: hydrochloric acid from the stomach, acids within the diet, or acid present in the atmosphere of an individual's workplace. The elderly patient is unlikely to be currently exposed to an acidic industrial environment, so only the first two need to be considered as a cause for a currently progressive erosion, which requires attention.

Regurgitation

Regurgitation erosion may increase in older patients as a result of various digestive dis-

turbances which vary in severity between acute peptic ulcers, to low-grade non-specific grumbling indigestion. Figure 9.4 shows the result of regurgitation erosion in a patient in his late sixties whose peptic ulcer was treated surgically two years prior to this photograph. Following treatment of the ulcer, there has been no further deterioration of the worn tooth surfaces. Regurgitation erosion can occur in the absence of frank vomiting. Mild indigestion which the patient attempts to control with proprietary antacid preparations can cause damage. Patients may be aware only of occasional indigestion pains or heartburn, or they may suffer a chronic condition such as an hiatus hernia. It has been reported that the incidence of toothwear in diabetics is increased, possibly as a result of regurgitation.[1]

Alcoholism, too, must be considered. Alcoholism is not uncommon amongst older people, and has many serious side effects, including chronic gastritis. Most alcoholics do not vomit regularly, nevertheless regurgitation does occur though they may be unaware of this. The accumulative effects of erosion may be noticeable in the old person, particularly if he or she has been an alcoholic for many years. The popular image of the elderly alcoholic is of a derelict, sleeping rough in the streets. This is only part of the picture, especially as these patients rarely seek dental treatment other than for acute emergencies. The discreet, often secretive, middle-class alcoholic is far more likely to seek dental treatment, and it is usually difficult or impossible to obtain a reliable history.

The incidence and/or rate of dietary erosion may increase in some older patients as a result

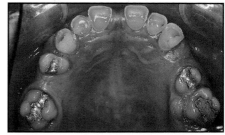

Figure 9.4 A patient in his late sixties who had a peptic ulcer treated surgically two years before this photograph was taken. Monitoring with models since then has shown that no further deterioration has taken place. Although the wear is primarily on the incisal edges, the aetiology is clearly erosion more than attrition

of a change in diet. Food fads are not a prerogative of the young, and many old people take to drinking lemon tea, chewing vitamin C tablets, or sucking acid drops.

Saliva and dry mouth

It is a common clinical observation that older patients suffer from dry mouths. The numerous reasons for this have been discussed in Chapters 3, 4 and 5. The profoundly dry mouth that follows surgical excision of one or more salivary glands or radiotherapy, produces both rapid caries development and dental erosion. Dental erosion may increase in such patients because acids are less well buffered and diluted by saliva. Thus, a patient who has always eaten a couple of items of fruit per day with no ill-effect may suffer erosion in old age as the saliva dries up, or salivary buffering capacity is altered.

Attrition

It has been assumed for many years that loss of posterior teeth accelerates the rate of wear of anterior teeth. Many older patients are left with only their anterior teeth, and perhaps poorly supported dentures replacing the lost posterior teeth. This scenario is commonly offered as an explanation for the accelerated anterior toothwear that may be seen in old people. However, this assumption has seldom been tested and may be a gross over-simplification. There is no reliable evidence to show that a patient who loses his or her posterior teeth increases the number of chewing strokes on the anterior teeth in proportion. A review of the literature[2] and a recent study[3] found no evidence of a relationship between the number of missing teeth and wear of the remaining teeth. The incidence and force of bruxism appear to decline in older patients. Chewing habits are often maintained, but the powerful, destructive grinding habits of young and middle-aged patients are reduced. This may be a consequence of reduced muscle power, accommodation to the occlusal arrangement which may have been improved by the wearing away of interferences, or simply a coming-to-terms with life in general. Against this may be set the increase in the abrasivity of food and opposing teeth in a mouth that is poorly lubricated with saliva. Despite this, it is likely that attrition will play a decreasing rather than an increasing role in toothwear as the patient becomes older.

Abrasion

Life-long habits such as pipe smoking or aberrant toothbrushing techniques will show their accumulated effect in old age. It is more difficult to alter these habits in old people than in the young and so this aetiological factor may persist.

Diagnosis of toothwear

Diagnosing that the teeth are worn is easy; deciding whether they are worn pathologically or whether the wear is within physiological limits is less so. Identifying the aetiology can also often be very difficult.

A limited degree of toothwear must be accepted as a 'normal' age-related change in older patients. If, on examining a patient, it seems likely that the toothwear is progressive and has occurred at the same rate for some time, then it is possible to estimate the effect of continued wear at the same rate in ten or twenty years time. If this projection suggests that the patient will be left with a dentition that remains functional, symptomless and of a reasonable appearance, then the wear may be considered to be physiological, or within acceptable limits.

If, on the other hand, the wear has already produced an unsatisfactory appearance, sensitivity, or mechanical problems such as a reduction in occlusal vertical dimension or very thin teeth, then the toothwear is pathological. If the rate of wear projected into the future is likely to give rise to one or more of these conditions before the patient is likely to die, then again the rate of wear must be considered to be pathological.

Such estimates are difficult enough when an assumption is made that the wear is progressing at a steady rate. However, this is often not the case and it is important to determine if the major event producing wear was in the past and the current rate is slow, or if the rate is accelerating. Thus, a period of monitoring is necessary in order to decide the appropriate management.

A complete, relevant history can be very difficult to obtain. It is necessary to go back to adolescence in taking the dietary and the medical history in relation to regurgitation. Similarly, it is necessary to ask about stress and associated bruxism, and tooth cleaning and other habits which may have given rise to abrasion throughout life. It is unreasonable to expect a patient to recall all the possible details that may have a bearing on the diagnosis, but major events such as pregnancies, living in tropical climates and drinking large quantities of carbonated drinks or other similar events may be recalled. The current medical, drug and dietary history are easier to obtain and may, or may not, be relevant. The clinical examination will give a clue as to the probable aetiology but, even so, care must be taken not to jump to conclusions. For example, wear of the incisal edges or occlusal surfaces may well be partly due to erosion as well as attrition (see Fig. 9.4). Many patients are seen with wear of both the occlusal and buccal surfaces. It is possible that, by coincidence, they are suffering simultaneously from unrelated attrition and abrasion, but although coincidences do sometimes occur, it is much more likely that the two observations have a common cause and that erosion is a primary aetiological factor, with attrition and abrasion as secondary factors.

Epidemiology of toothwear

There have been few epidemiological studies of toothwear. Most indices of toothwear have been designed in order to study selected groups, for example patients suffering from industrial acid erosion. A Toothwear Index (TWI)[4] has recently been developed to record levels of toothwear, irrespective of the cause, and to take account of the normal progression of toothwear throughout life. This index has been used in a limited number of studies. The prevalence of unacceptable levels of toothwear in the 'normal' population has not yet been clearly established but in one study, of 100 consecutive referred patients with pathological levels of toothwear, the commonest cause by far was erosion, of which regurgitation erosion accounted for the most extensive cases.[5] Interestingly, no definitive diagnosis

could be reached for 31 of these patients, emphasizing the need for a general term 'toothwear' so as to avoid the need to guess an aetiology.

The management of toothwear – general principles

In many cases, toothwear is a progressive, lifelong, problem, and it is wise to take a long-term view of its management. Active interventive treatment is required only if the patient is actually suffering a problem as a result of the toothwear. Such problems may include sensitivity of teeth, an alteration in appearance that the patient is no longer willing to accept, reduced occlusal vertical dimension, or teeth which are progressively wearing and becoming unrestorable. In the absence of one of these conditions, patient management should be aimed at prevention and control, rather than premature treatment, which may not be necessary and which, in some cases, may give rise to more trouble than the condition itself. Most patients who have survived into old age with a slowly progressing toothwear problem will be happy to continue with the condition, provided it is not accelerating. Some, however, decide at a certain point in life, perhaps retirement, that although the condition is only progressing slowly, the time has come to improve their appearance as they intend to keep their teeth for the remainder of their life, which may be several decades.

Monitoring

It will be clear that in order to make the proper decisions about both diagnosis and management, a reliable system of monitoring the progression of toothwear is essential. Several methods are used including photographic records, various measurements, and the Toothwear Index referred to earlier. However, for the individual patient, rather than for epidemiological studies, study casts are the most reliable method. Figure 9.5 shows two study casts of the same patient taken six years apart. This patient was sixty-two when the first cast was made. She suffers from achlorhydria. Prior to the first cast she was taking liquid hydrochloric acid by mouth

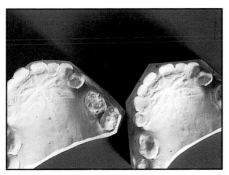

Figure 9.5 Study casts taken six years apart showing that no further erosion occurred in this patient with achlorhydria once the method of administration of the medicinal hydrochloric acid was changed to the encapsulated form. No treatment was necessary

and this was causing dental erosion. Just before the cast was made the method of administration was changed to encapsulated hydrochloric acid so that the acid did not contact the teeth. The second study cast taken six years later shows no change in the extent of the erosion. Had the patient been younger these thin, weak teeth would probably have needed crowning in order to protect them from the risk of breaking. However, in this delicate lady with no sporting or other vigorous pastimes, and who had learned to eat in a gentle manner avoiding undue force on these teeth, the provision of crowns was not necessary. The patient was happily in control of the situation.

Figure 9.6 shows a progressive condition where the aetiology of the toothwear is unclear and general preventive advice has not been successful. In this situation, active treatment is required.

Prevention

The aetiology of the toothwear must be clearly understood before preventive measures can be effective. For example, if the aetiology is erosion but a false assumption is made that it is attrition, and an acrylic bite plane is constructed to prevent attrition, the erosion will worsen because acids will be trapped between the appliance and the teeth.

Regurgitation erosion is difficult to prevent because most of the chronic causes are not amenable to simple treatment. Some patients should be referred to their general medical practitioner or to a gastro-enterologist, but in

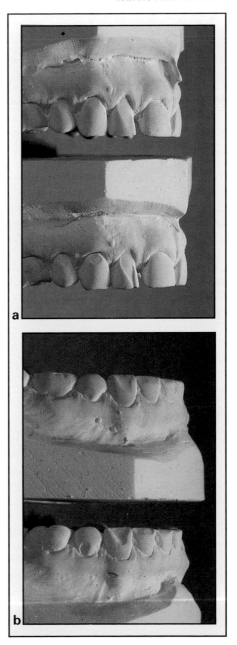

Figure 9.6 Casts of a patient taken three years apart. (a) The upper casts showing that toothwear is continuing. A marked change has occurred with the upper right lateral incisor and the cervical lesion on the canine tooth is also worse. (b) The lower casts of the same patient again showing deterioration of the lower canine and first premolar. The aetiology in this case has not been determined although the clinical appearance is one of erosion. As the condition is continuing, the patient is concerned about appearance and a preventive approach has been unsuccessful, the upper right lateral incisor and the lower right canine will be crowned now and the other teeth reviewed at regular intervals

the milder chronic cases most patients are controlling the condition as far as possible by self-medication and dietary control.

Dietary erosion can be prevented if a single item of food or drink which the patient is taking to excess can be identified, and if they are willing to forgo this. If dietary or regurgitation erosion is being exacerbated by a reduction in salivary flow, this should be investigated further, and if possible reversed. It may be possible for the medical practitioner to find alternative drugs that produce a less dry mouth; or a salivary stimulant may be prescribed. Unfortunately, many of the artificial saliva substitutes themselves have a low pH and may contribute to dental erosion rather than prevent it (Chapter 4).

A hard acrylic bite plane may be made to prevent attrition. However, it should first be used as a diagnostic appliance to confirm that bruxism is contributing significantly to the aetiology. The bite plane is fitted and adjusted in the mouth and an impression taken of it. Three months later the cast of this impression may be compared with the occlusal surface of the bite plane. If no wear has taken place, attrition is not a major part of the aetiology. If the acrylic has worn, the patient should continue to wear the bite plane to prevent further wear. Hard acrylic is softer than the dental tissues and wears away in preference to them. The appliance is replaced periodically and this will slow down wear resulting from attrition. Soft plastic appliances should not be used as they wear too rapidly.

The abrasive effects of aggressive toothbrushing habits can be reduced, but it is often difficult to wean patients off their favourite toothpaste and brush after a lifetime of using them. Other habits can also be changed, though often with difficulty.

The effectiveness of all these preventive measures must be monitored over a period of time, whether or not other active treatment is undertaken. Only if the teeth are to be extracted or crowned can it be assumed that toothwear will be arrested. In some cases the teeth that are not being treated must also be monitored.

Desensitization

If the teeth are sensitive, fluoride-containing varnishes, such as Duraphat, can be applied, or the patient may be prescribed a fluoride mouth rinse. Dentine adhesive systems are now being investigated for the purpose. However, it is unusual for the teeth to be sensitive in older patients who have slowly progressive toothwear, and if this is the case it is likely either that the condition has started to progress rapidly or that a pulpitis has developed.

Restorations

Intracoronal restorations will not prevent toothwear. Figure 9.7 shows a typical picture of an amalgam standing proud from a tooth surface which has eroded away around it. Similarly, composite or glass ionomer restorations placed in cervical erosion/abrasion lesions do not prevent the condition recurring around the margins, and in some cases the tooth is in a worse condition a few years after being restored than it would have been had it not been filled (Fig. 9.8).

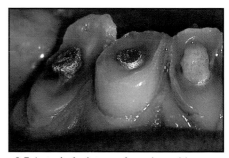

Figure 9.7 A typical picture of erosion with an amalgam restoration standing proud of the tooth surface. The restoration has had no effect in preventing further toothwear

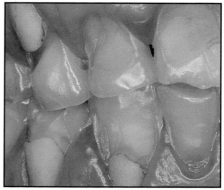

Figure 9.8 When the cause of cervical abrasion/erosion lesions has not been prevented, simply restoring the surface does little to prevent further wear of the surrounding enamel and dentine

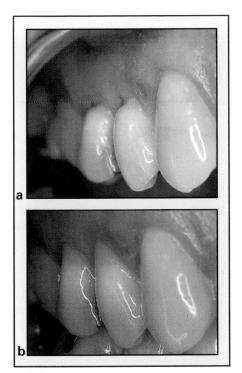

Figure 9.9 Toothwear requiring restoration. (a) Cervical erosion/abrasion lesions in the premolar teeth. These were sensitive and the patient was concerned about their appearance. (b) Glass ionomer and composite layered restorations were used

On occasions, the provision of intracoronal restorations may be necessary, if only as a temporary or semi-permanent measure; for example, when the defect is aesthetically unacceptable, in some cases of sensitivity, as a holding measure where large numbers of teeth require treatment, or in older patients who are having difficulty with oral hygiene pro-

cedures and accumulate plaque in the defects. In these cases dentine-bonded and acid-etch retained composite, glass ionomer or amalgam restorations may be used as appropriate (Fig. 9.9).

Endodontic treatment

In most cases secondary dentine is laid down at a sufficient rate to prevent pulp exposure from toothwear. However, pulp exposure or death of the pulp sometimes occurs, necessitating endodontic treatment. Intractable sensitivity which cannot be controlled by more conservative means may sometimes be more readily, reliably and permanently dealt with by endodontic treatment than with crowns or other restorations.

References

1 Robb N.D., Smith B.G.N.,Walls A.W.G., Presentation of pathological toothwear in patients with typical diabetes mellitus, *J. Dent. Res. 1990*; 69 (special issue): 304 abs. 304

2 Käyser A.F., Witter D.J., Oral functional needs and its consequences for dentulous older people, *Community Dent. Health 1985*; 2: 285–91

3 Robb N.D., Smith B.G.N., The influence of missing posterior teeth on anterior toothwear in dental attenders *J. Dent. Res. 1992*; 71: 625 abs. 881

4 Smith B.G.N., Knight J.K., An index for measuring the wear of teeth, *Br. Dent. J. 1984*: 156: 435–8

5 Smith B.G.N., Knight J.K., A comparison of patterns of toothwear with aetiological factors, *Br. Dent. J. 1984*; 157: 16–19

10

Toothwear: Treatment of the worn dentition

Richard Ibbetson and Derrick Setchell

A person should not be denied the benefits of restorative treatment because they are old. Most treatment will be as straightforward to do as for a younger patient. However, factors such as toothwear will sometimes make matters problematical.

The treatment of toothwear may involve either fixed or removable restorations or a combination of both. There must be a good indication for the provision of complex fixed work, and a decision to proceed with this should not be made, simply or solely because the patient has expressed a wish to avoid a removable prosthesis. Also, where the replacement of missing teeth is indicated, it should be remembered that the slavish provision of twenty-eight occlusal surfaces is not a requirement if the existing dentition is acceptable in function and appearance.[1] Overdentures, or a combination of abutment crowns with a removable partial denture, may be more manageable than fixed bridgework in the long term, especially when only a limited number of sound abutments are available. The provision of anterior crowns on weak roots in the hope that occlusal support and stability can be gained by the provision of a partial denture is not sensible. Heroics, that may ultimately threaten the preservation of what sound teeth remain, should be avoided.

Where laboratory-constructed restorations are to be used, metal castings are generally required to restore function and to protect the remaining tooth structure. Porcelain should be confined to a veneering role, in areas where appearance is critical. There is seldom sufficient space for all-porcelain crowns and often, particularly in wear cases, the full occlusal coverage of ceramo-metal crowns with porcelain will be impracticable because of the lack of space. In such situations the patient may have to accept some compromise in the appearance. Experience suggests that all-metal restorations, sadly unfashionable these days, are very durable. They are relatively easy to make, and require limited tooth reduction. If cemented having a sandblasted occlusal surface they are simple to adjust; the articulating paper clearly marking the matt surface. Cast metal surfaces provide predictable occlusal contacts against opposing natural tooth structure or metal surfaces. Porcelain, especially when it has been adjusted and not reglazed, is abrasive and can damage antagonists, except other porcelain surfaces.

There have been substantial improvements in resins intended for crown and bridge purposes. To date they remain interim materials, for use in non-occluding areas. Few cases are seen where the small economies accompanying their selection can be justified in relation to the overall costs of the fixed work.

Considerations in planning restorative care

The considerations that must be made when planning restorative care can be divided into those that relate to the whole mouth, particularly the occlusion and those that relate to the individual tooth.

Decisions relating to the whole mouth

The occlusion – conformative or reorganized?

The practitioner who thinks only with the turbine in his or her hand is unlikely to address one of the most fundamental planning decisions that has to be made when treating a case of toothwear. Namely, should the restorations adapt to a conformative or a reorganized occlusion?

Conformative

Restorations that are constructed to be conformative will fit in with the patient's existing intercuspal position (ICP), that is to say the simply assessed, obvious 'bite'. Most simple restorative dentistry is done this way, when many teeth are present but few are being treated. When the dentition is extensively worn there is a risk, if this approach is adopted, that what is being conformed to will be inappropriate.

Although in the younger dentition an occlusion may 'wear in', there seems little doubt that an occlusion can also 'wear out'. The risk in adopting a conformative approach, particularly if the treatment is done piecemeal, is that we begin by making one or two restorations to suit a heavily worn occlusion, only to find that, later, several more become necessary. Subsequently, many of the increasing difficulties that are met, in terms of space, contour and appearance, could with forethought have been avoided. Fewer problems may be encountered if a planned change is made to the occlusion, so that a new jaw relationship will result when the restorative work is completed.

In summary, a conformative approach is justified where:

- A full examination of the occlusion has been made
- It can be predicted with confidence that few teeth are likely to require cast restorations within the foreseeable future
- Sufficient teeth remain to provide an acceptable occlusion

- Wear is not severe and space considerations permit acceptable restorations to be made.

An exception to these guidelines occurs when the anterior teeth are heavily worn and there is a 'close bite'. In such circumstances it is not sensible to provide anterior crowns as a localized procedure, unless the posterior occlusion is stable (Fig. 10.1a, b).

Neither does the decision to take a conformative approach exclude the possibility of making localized corrections to increase the space available for a given restoration or to improve its relationship with the opposing teeth. Such modifications will usually be relatively minor and can be accomplished by local tooth movement or adjustment (see Chapter 11).

The reorganized approach

Many problems may be overcome if a planned change is made to the occlusion, so that a new jaw relationship results when the restorative work has been completed. This is a 'reorganized' approach, and is seen in a simple way whenever an onlay partial denture is made (Fig. 10.2). There is more to this procedure than simply 'raising the vertical dimension', a potentially hazardous procedure that can produce spectacular failures in removable prosthetic work.

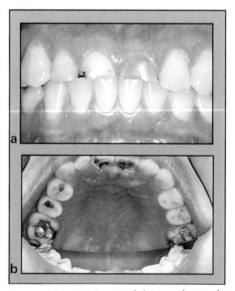

Figure 10.1a, b Localized wear of the anterior teeth and a 'close bite'

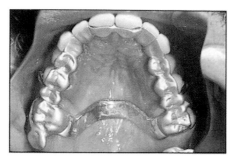

Figure 10.2 Occlusion restored at an increased vertical dimension by a removable chrome–cobalt onlay appliance

Dentists are sometimes reluctant to take up the benefits that can be gained by adopting a well-applied reorganized approach when undertaking fixed restorative work. They may fear that an older person will not be able to tolerate a changed occlusion, or be concerned about the clinical problems of managing such a change. In practice, the magnitude of change that can be successfully made in the natural dentition is limited by factors such as anterior tooth length and position. The authors have never seen a patient who could not tolerate a sensible change where the result provided the three characteristics of a satisfactory occlusion described by Wise:[2]

- **Multiple, even posterior tooth contacts in closure** The existing 'intercuspal position' cannot exist when the teeth are no longer in contact or have been prepared. Thus, a convenient guide to a jaw relationship in which multiple, even posterior tooth contacts can be achieved is the **retruded axis position**, or centric jaw relationship.
- **Acceptable anterior guidance** In jaw movements away from the reorganized intercuspal position, tooth surfaces near the front of the arch should prevent the posterior cusps from clashing.
- **Non-working side disclusion** If possible, posterior teeth on the side away from which the lower jaw is moving, the non-working side, should not contact and so obstruct the guidance established by the anterior teeth.

These are simple concepts. No dentist should be deterred from attempting to achieve them because of the esoteric jargon which sometimes surrounds the hallowed, albeit important, subject of occlusion. These concepts should be simply tested in each practical case by providing either a simple occlusal splint or temporary restorations before making the commitment to definitive restorations. This is not done to test the patient's toleration of the change but so that the operator can perceive the requirements for the finished work. The laboratory can then produce a diagnostic wax-up that 'rehearses' the final contours. Without this forward planning it is difficult or impossible to determine the various necessary stages of treatment. Also, the patient is able to see what is proposed, and can understand any limitations that there may be. A diagnostic wax-up is for fixed work what a wax try-in is for dentures.

Diagnostic waxing requires the study casts to be mounted in a semi-adjustable articulator, a procedure that is within the scope of general practice. The various types of highly sophisticated and often very complicated fully adjustable articulators are simply ways of achieving a desired result, not the means of restorative dentistry.

The reorganized approach is likely to be appropriate when wear is present to a marked extent and the criterion of an acceptable occlusion cannot be met by means of local adjustments. Such cases will usually exhibit many missing teeth, compensatory over-eruption, drifting, or repeated fracture of teeth and restorations. There may be symptoms of an occlusal functional disturbance. However, reorganization should not be undertaken simply to impose order on disorder, nor as the first line of treatment for dysfunction. Reorganization may be selected mainly or even exclusively for the convenience that it affords in carrying out treatment, in that it allows the use of a reference position–the retruded axis position (RAP)–that will remain relatively constant during treatment even when many teeth have been prepared, and from which movements may be arranged in a controlled way. It may also allow the disengagement of occluding surfaces so as to make sufficient space available to allow restorative treatment. This release of space will require less reduction to be made of already short teeth, and an improved contour and appearance of the restorations. It will also permit the restored surfaces to be related to each other in such a way that further wear is minimized.

Reorganization may require the adjustment of some teeth and the restoration of others. In many 'wear cases' a large number of occlusal surfaces will require to be restored. Provided that the new occlusion is adequately supported by periodontal ligament, it seems to us to matter little whether the new surfaces are removable onlays, conventional cemented crowns or 'adhesive' cast restorations.

When undertaking a reformative rehabilitation there is little likelihood of achieving a satisfactory result simply by inspired guesswork. The fundamental principle must be first to determine the correct occlusal relationship, then to restore to it. This may be done in stages, if that is easier. A wise preliminary is the construction of a full-coverage occlusal splint on the unprepared teeth (Figs 10.3, 10.4). This will require an increase in vertical dimension, which may be used to verify its acceptability. However, the chief effect of such a splint is to relax the masticatory musculature so as to allow the mandible to be guided into the RAP. A permanent increase in vertical dimension may prove not to be necessary once this has been achieved (Figs 10.5, 10.6).

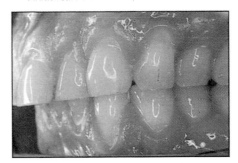

Figure 10.5 Intercuspal position

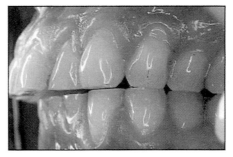

Figure 10.6 Retruded axis position. This patient displays a large horizontal and smaller vertical discrepancy between RAP and ICP

Practical aspects of reorganized occlusion

General principles have been discussed. It may now be helpful to consider the practical procedures involved in the treatment of two clinical situations that are commonly met with in the elderly dentition. These are, first, relatively severe wear of the anterior teeth where the posterior dentition is not so badly affected and second, relatively severe wear of both the anterior and posterior teeth.

Wear of the anterior teeth where the posterior dentition is less damaged

Excessive wear of the anterior teeth, the posterior teeth being less affected, is found when the tooth tissue has been lost as a result of localized erosion, parafunctional activity, or a combination of both. Analysis of the aetiological factors will have been made, initial measures instituted to control the causes, and any immediate problems dealt with, as described in Chapter 9.

Wear of the functional surfaces of anterior

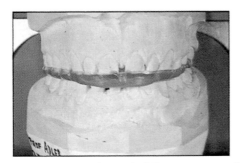

Figure 10.3 Anterior view of full-coverage maxillary occlusal splint

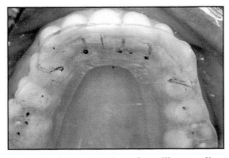

Figure 10.4 Occlusal view of maxillary appliance

teeth without compensatory eruption of the antagonists is uncommon. It is probable that there will be insufficient space to allow the placement of aesthetic anterior crowns. Casts should be mounted in the RAP, and the tooth contact on closure observed. If the casts are then 'slid' into the intercuspal position, it can be noted how far the mandible has had to close in order to reach this position. This distance comprises the **vertical component** of the slide. It can also be seen by how much the mandible has had to move forward, the **horizontal component** of the slide. The size of each of these components is important and will have a significant bearing on the way in which the worn anterior teeth should best be restored.

Where the vertical component is large and the horizontal component small, adjustment of the posterior teeth to provide even contacts in RAP at the patient's normal vertical dimension will not move the mandible very far posteriorly. When the horizontal component of the discrepancy between RAP and ICP is large, adjustment to make all the posterior teeth meet evenly in the retruded position will create a new ICP which is placed some distance posterior to the position of the patient's previous habitual closure. This concept will perhaps be made clearer by Figure 10.7. In the latter instance, if there is a large horizontal component, the adjustment to create a new intercuspal position at RAP may make sufficient room anteriorly for crowns to be placed on the worn anterior teeth. The adjustment should first be carried out on a second set of mounted study casts to see whether the expected result can be achieved. An unrehearsed occlusal adjustment should never be performed upon a patient. The casts can also be used to assess the stability of the occlusion, according to the criteria mentioned earlier. Occlusal interferences and discrepancies in the occlusal plane are easier to see on mounted casts than in the mouth.

Another way of obtaining the extra space necessary for the provision of anterior crowns is to move the teeth axially by means of a Dahl appliance[3] (see Chapter 11).

Diagnostic waxing

The adjustment of the casts made either before occlusal adjustment, or after tooth de-

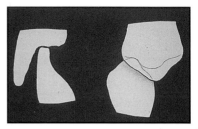

Figure 10.7a Worn palatal aspects of upper anterior teeth with patient in ICP

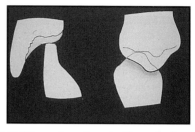

Figure 10.7b Where there is a significant horizontal component of slide between RAP and ICP the inclined planes of the posterior teeth (mesial upper, distal lower) may be adjusted to give occlusal stability in a more posterior position. Space is thereby created for anterior restorations (courtesy Mr R. Wassell)

pression by means of the Dahl appliance, is followed by trial waxing of the anterior teeth that require crowns. This is done in order to see whether sufficient space has been gained to achieve form and function of the crowns that are to be placed, and whether sufficient tooth height remains to allow retentive preparations to be cut.

The completed wax-up can be discussed with the patient so that he or she may have an idea of the finished result, and what will be involved in producing it. The diagnostic wax-up can also be used to construct matrices in either silicone putty or vacuum-formed acetate sheet. These act as guides for tooth preparation and are used for the construction of temporary restorations (Figs 10.8–10.12).

The occlusal adjustment is then performed on the patient's teeth to create the new intercuspal position, thereby making the space for the anterior crowns. When this has been done the anterior teeth are prepared and the temporaries made using a matrix from the diagnostic wax-up.

High-quality temporary coverage is the key to success in this type of treatment. Where worn anterior teeth are to be restored, the

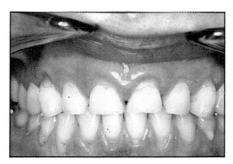

Figure 10.8 Worn anterior teeth (courtesy Mr Lloyd Searson)

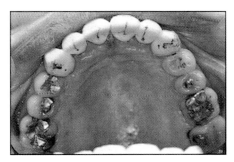

Figure 10.12 Palatal view of temporary restorations constructed in acrylic resin using matrix (courtesy Mr Lloyd Searson)

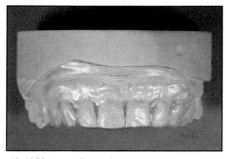

Figure 10.9 Diagnostic wax-up of upper anterior teeth (courtesy Mr Lloyd Searson)

functional form required for the final crowns is always a matter for educated guesswork. The intelligent use of temporary restorations made from the diagnostic wax-up removes the need for chairside clairvoyance. The temporaries must be constructed from a durable material because they will have to remain in place until the patient is happy with the appearance and the dentist is satisfied with their functional aspects. Anterior guidance, sufficient to prevent interferences posteriorly on mandibular movement, should be established on the temporary restorations.

The temporary crowns must be aesthetically and phonetically acceptable to the patient. The criteria used to assess occlusal success are three-fold. The temporaries must remain cemented, they must not fracture, and the teeth should not show signs of progressively increasing mobility. If any of these problems is seen, it is a sign that the functional form of the temporary crowns is incorrect. If so, they should be adjusted and left in place for a further period of assessment. This may take some time, hence the need for durability.

When the temporary crowns are stable, working impressions, a face-bow transfer and a jaw registration are made to allow construction of the final crowns.

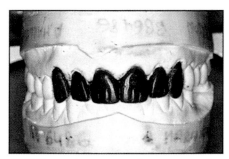

Figure 10.10 Vacuum-formed matrix on stone cast made from diagnostic wax-up (courtesy Mr Lloyd Searson)

Transfer of information to the laboratory

The technician should be provided with as much information as possible, and it is helpful if they can be involved in colour matching. It is also important that the information gained from the careful adjustment of the temporaries is not lost. Thus, an alginate impression should be made of the temporaries in the

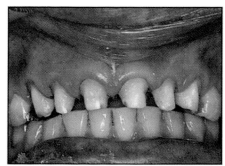

Figure 10.11 Anterior tooth preparations (courtesy Mr Lloyd Searson)

mouth so that the technician can use the cast to copy their form in the final restorations. This may be done with matrices or by making a custom anterior guide-table on the articulator (Fig. 10.13a, b).

Try-in and adjustment of the final crowns

The crowns are tried-in prior to final glazing in order to define the occlusal contacts and axial contour. However, if the temporaries have been copied accurately, a correct jaw registration has been made, and the temporaries have remained stable in the mouth, little adjustment should be needed. It is sensible to temporarily cement the crowns with

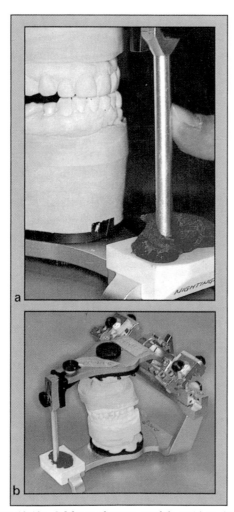

Figure 10.13a, b Mounted stone models used to form a custom anterior guide-table on the articulator (courtesy Mr Lloyd Searson)

a zinc-oxide/eugenol soft cement. This will allow a further period for assessment of both appearance and function. When the patient is happy and the occlusion stable, using the same criteria as used for the temporaries, the crowns can be cemented finally.

Wear of anterior and posterior teeth

Toothwear is often associated with derangements of the posterior occlusion. When the condition is advanced, restoration of nearly all the teeth may be necessary. Such treatment uses many of the principles that have been outlined already.

Full arch reconstruction is not easy, and is really best undertaken only when the practitioner has gained experience from the successful completion of several cases involving multiple crowns in localized areas of the mouth.

Where all the teeth are to be restored, for whatever reason, there is seldom an indication for the use of the conformative approach to the occlusal scheme. To do so will make treatment more difficult, because the crowns will have to be provided in a series of small stages in order to prevent the existing inter-cuspal position from being lost. This approach is generally inappropriate when the teeth are worn, because few corrections of the occlusion are possible. Rather, a reorganized approach to the occlusion is indicated, with the new crowns being made so that they furnish multiple even contacts in the retruded axis position.

In discussing the treatment options we will again assume that the diagnostic procedures discussed in the previous chapter have been undertaken.

Initial treatment

Initial treatment must include the management of any acute problems, including preliminary endodontics, caries control and the extraction of unsalvageable or useless teeth.

Preliminary diagnostic measures

Study casts are mounted in a semi-adjustable articulator using a face-bow transfer and an inter-occlusal record made in the retruded axis position. These casts will complement the clinical examination in an analysis of the occlusion. The information which will be gained includes the following:

- The nature and extent of the RAP–ICP discrepancy
- Discrepancies in the occlusal plane
- The degree of wear of the teeth
- The size and extent of any edentulous areas
- The amount of clinical crown height available for preparation
- The relationship of the upper and lower anterior teeth (i.e. the prospects for anterior guidance)
- The relationship of the teeth both statically and on excursive movements of the mandible.

Preparation of the mouth

The subsequent stages of initial treatment comprise the detailed investigation of individual teeth. Existing restorations are removed and cores placed where necessary. Any necessary endodontic treatment is carried out.

When the assessment of the individual teeth has been done, a maxillary occlusal splint is provided for the patient. This is worn and adjusted until a stable jaw relationship is achieved. Fresh study casts are remounted in the articulator in this stable relationship, and the treatment plan is reassessed.

At this stage, means of achieving sufficient space for the restorations can be considered. This will be influenced by the amount of crown height available, the morphology of the teeth, and the anatomical features of their roots, such as furcations and root grooves.

The effect of a possible increase in the vertical dimension is examined. In particular, the relationship of the anterior teeth is assessed. It is important that contacts between the restored anterior teeth be maintained so as to provide anterior guidance and stability. However, as the vertical dimension is increased, so will the overjet increase anteriorly because the mandible moves posteriorly as it opens.

These factors have all to be considered when determining the methodology for achieving the necessary clearance to allow retentive crowns with accessible margins to be made and fitted, and to allow corrections in

tooth position and occlusal form. This will usually be done by increasing the vertical dimension, by crown lengthening, or commonly a combination of both. Crown lengthening, when necessary, is carried out at this stage, and the tissues are allowed to heal. The clinical procedure is described in Chapter 12.

Following a period of healing, new casts must be made, mounted in the articulator and diagnostic waxing carried out in order to determine the form of the final restorations, to construct templates to guide tooth preparation and to allow the all-important temporary restorations to be made. Diagnostic waxing will also show how much the vertical dimension must be increased. The wax-up is presented to the patient for discussion and agreement on the treatment plan, including the type of restorations that are to be provided.

Sequence of preparation

A decision has to be made about which teeth must be prepared first, and at what stage the new occlusion should be established on the temporary coverage. There are a number of ways in which this can be done. However, when dealing with the elderly patient it is important to consider whether they will be able to tolerate the clinical procedures that may be involved in what might be considered in theory to be the 'ideal' treatment.

It is generally sensible to deal with the anterior teeth first, because these provide the guidance on mandibular movement. However, when the temporary restorations are constructed at an increased vertical dimension, the posterior teeth will be taken out of contact. It is undesirable to allow them to remain so between appointments. There are four ways by which posterior occlusal contacts can be achieved and maintained during the treatment of the anterior sections:

- **By means of the occlusal splint** When the anterior temporary crowns that have been made from the diagnostic wax-up have been placed, the front part of the maxillary splint is cut away and the posterior part adjusted to give contacts against the lower teeth.
- **By using composite resin** With the anterior temporaries in place, enamel and dentine bonding agents may be used to allow com-

posite resin to be placed on the posterior teeth in one arch, so as to provide occlusal contacts.

- **By placing temporaries on the posteriors first** The posterior teeth in one arch are prepared first and temporaries fitted to provide the increase in vertical dimension. At the same visit, composite resin can be placed on the anterior teeth to maintain occlusal stability. The anterior teeth are prepared at the next visit. This approach is, in some ways, more difficult to control, and is, therefore, considered only when there is a clear need to improve short-term stability of the posterior occlusion.
- **The preparation of one arch at one visit** This technique speeds treatment and allows the vertical dimension to be increased easily. However, it is a major undertaking, and demands expertise of the dentist and resilience from the patient.

The preparation and construction of crowns in stages is perfectly acceptable and in general makes treatment easier. The anteriors crowns may be fitted and temporarily cemented before restoring the posteriors, provided that occlusal stability is maintained as described above.

When treatment is provided in stages, it is preferable to restore opposing quadrants of posterior teeth as a group, rather than to restore one arch and then the other. The former approach enables the preparations to be controlled more easily and is likely to lead to a better occlusal form on the finished crowns. Once again the need for well-made temporary restorations, conforming to the diagnostic wax-up, cannot be over-stated.

Impression procedures

It can be difficult to record impressions of multiple preparations simultaneously. It is our standard practice to make several impressions, each of a limited number of teeth. From these, electro-plated dies and acrylic resin transfer copings are made (Figs 10.14–10.17). The copings are returned to the preparations in the mouth, checked for fit, and a locating impression taken to produce the working cast.

An alternative approach may be possible if reversible hydrocolloid is used. This material allows the accurate transfer of wax patterns between dies of the same teeth made from different impressions. In this method, quadrant impressions are taken of the preparations so that individual dies can be produced. A full arch impression is made next, which does not necessarily have to record the margins of the preparations. The full-arch cast made from this impression is not sectioned and is used for most of the waxing procedure. The almost completed wax patterns are then transferred to the individual dies for finishing of the margins.

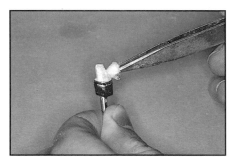

Figure 10.14 Electro-formed die of preparation

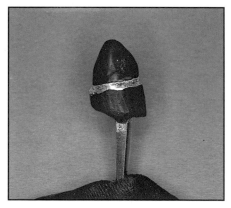

Figure 10.15 Acrylic resin transfer coping

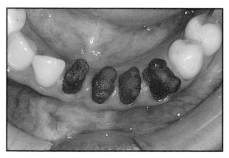

Figure 10.16 Copings seated on preparations

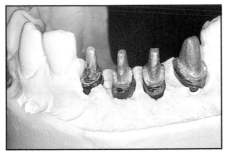

Figure 10.17 Completed cast with individual dies

Jaw relations for working casts

The method of recording the mandibulo-maxillary relationship is critical, because inaccuracies at this stage will be reflected in the amount of adjustment required when the crowns are fitted. Cast restorations should require little if any adjustment when they are fitted. This demands accurate working casts and accurate occlusal records.

A face-bow transfer is used to mount the maxillary cast in the articulator. Additionally, the bite fork can be used to check the accuracy of the working cast. If the cast does not fit the shallow indentations in the bite fork exactly, either the record is distorted or the cast inaccurate. It is worth while to use a second bite fork to check the accuracy of the lower cast.

The record must be taken at the final working vertical dimension. This means having some restored teeth in contact with antagonists. If all the teeth have been prepared, some of the temporaries will have to be in place. The registration cannot accurately be made using a full arch wax squash-bite, because the opposing teeth will not be in contact. Such an approach will result in an error when the casts are mounted. A better method is to use a recording medium placed between the prepared teeth, whilst using contacts between teeth elsewhere to control the vertical dimension at which the record is made. Extra hard wax can be used to make the registration. When metal dies are being used, acrylic resin transfer copings can be employed. When the record is made there will be a reduced number of occlusal contacts. Thus, the mandible must be guided into position by the dentist. The casts should be mounted as soon as possible so as to minimize distortion of the recording materials.

Laboratory fabrication of the restorations

A skilled crown and bridge technician is a prerequisite of rehabilitation work. The breaking down of the procedure into a number of stages will usually benefit the technician as well as the clinician.

Trial cementation

Following the try-in and any necessary adjustments of the aesthetic or functional form of the restorations, á period of temporary cementation is highly advisable to check the response of the patient to the final crowns. Final cementation should not be undertaken until both the dentist and patient are satisfied.

Maintenance

It is often said that treatment does not really begin until the crowns are finally cemented. Vigilance and care is required from both parties. The patient's responsibilities are to maintain an appropriate standard of home-care. The dentist must regularly monitor both the integrity of the restorations and the maintenance of hygiene. It is important to realize that patients who had previously damaged their teeth as a consequence of parafunctional activity may continue these habits. Such patients should be advised before treatment begins that once the crowns are placed, if signs of continued wear become evident, they may be expected to wear a splint in order to protect the restorations (Figs 10.18, 10.19).

Specific problems of the short clinical crown

Many of the difficulties that are encountered when attempting to provide cast restorations for a patient with a worn dentition derive from the shortness of the clinical crowns.

The shortening results in broad flat functional occlusal surfaces. In addition, there will be some loss of contour interproximally, with an increase in size of the contact area and a reduction in the embrasure space between adjacent teeth.

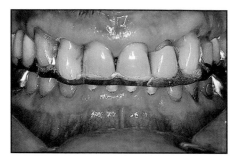

Figure 10.18 Maxillary occlusal splint provided following posterior reconstruction

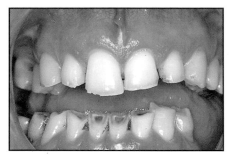

Figure 10.20 Worn anterior teeth

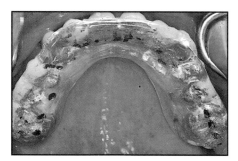

Figure 10.19 Occlusal view of splint

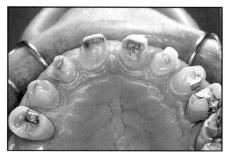

Figure 10.21 Teeth prepared for ceramo-metal restorations

Reduction of the clinical crown length results in a decrease in the potential height of the axial walls of the preparation, so that adequate levels of retention and resistance may not be achieved. In addition, there is likely to be little scope for improving the contour, or appearance, of the finished restoration due to the limitation in vertical space.

The approximation of adjacent teeth as a result of interproximal tooth tissue loss makes the preparation of the axial surfaces difficult. Inadequate axial reduction will result in over-contoured restorations which may exacerbate problems of plaque control.

If the clinical crown length is reduced, then considerable care and skill must be exercised to achieve sufficient retention and resistance form. The influence of taper on retention is well known and the preparation of short teeth gence between opposing axial surfaces. A tapered diamond bur, such as a Hi-Di 501 or 556[a] will produce axial walls with a 5–6° total convergence angle when maintained parallel to the desired long axis of the preparation (Figs 10.20, 10.21). A taper greater than this

[a]Hi-Di, Ash Instruments, Gloucester

will result in a significant loss in retention which cannot be accepted where the axial walls of the preparation are short.

In those cases where the vertical dimension is not to be increased as part of the rehabilitation, the choice of material from which the occlusal surface of the restoration is to be constructed will determine the length of the axial walls, because of the need for vertical reduction of the preparation. It will thus also influence the retention and resistance form of the preparation.

A porcelain occlusal surface requires greater inter-occlusal clearance than cast metal alone. Thus, for a given tooth, a crown with a porcelain occlusal surface will exhibit less retention and resistance form than one made entirely of metal.

Accessory retention features

The preparation of parallel axial surfaces is important. However, these may be insufficient to retain a crown on a short tooth. Even if the taper is 'ideal', such teeth will possess short axial walls and broad occlusal surfaces. This will give the crown a relatively large radius of rotation and consequently poor resistance form. Features to improve the resistance form should be incorporated into all such preparations as a standard procedure. Strategically placed supplementary features, such as axial grooves or boxes, will enhance resistance form considerably. These should be placed in areas of the preparation where there is an adequate bulk of dentine. They should be cut so that the radius of rotation of the casting about the preparation is reduced (Fig. 10.22).

Increasing vertical space

If improvements in the appearance and function of worn anterior teeth are to be achieved using full coverage restorations, the existing crown height will often be unacceptable. This is also often true for posterior teeth if any improvement in the occlusal relationship is intended, or if the tooth is so short that a retentive preparation cannot be cut. In all such cases, greater vertical space for the

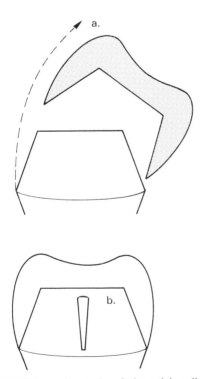

Figure 10.22 Where the angle of the axial wall of the preparation lies inside the arc of rotation (a), displacement of the restoration is likely. The risk can be reduced by the provision of axial retention grooves which lie within the arc of rotation (b)

restoration must be found. The following methods may be used:

Crown lengthening

Indications

A surgical crown lengthening procedure will provide a greater height of axial wall and allow improved retention and resistance form to be achieved in the finished preparation. The technique may also provide an opportunity to improve the appearance of the tooth. However, there are limitations to what can be achieved due to the presenting form of a worn tooth. In posterior teeth, the increased width of the occlusal surface will be unaffected, whilst the appearance of anterior teeth will remain compromised unless there is scope to increase the incisal edge length to some degree.

Increasing the overall length of an anterior tooth without a full assessment of the factors which caused it to become worn in the first place is a procedure that is fraught with problems and should be avoided. Nevertheless, crown lengthening can be an invaluable way of providing increased axial wall height to improve retention and resistance form, or to place the margins of crowns in a position which is accessible for finishing and maintenance.

Crown lengthening should be performed for groups of teeth. If an isolated tooth is treated, there will result some elongation of the teeth adjacent to the one for which treatment was undertaken. This approach will result in unfavourable gingival architecture.

Caution is required when considering the crown lengthening of multi-rooted teeth, because the surgical procedure may expose furcations. This may be undesirable on periodontal grounds and because it results in a cervical architecture that may complicate margin placement. It is also possible that following tooth lengthening, lateral root canals may be exposed, leading to pulpal involvement. The patient should be warned of this, of the possible aesthetic disadvantages, and of the likelihood of sensitivity from the newly-exposed root surfaces.

This list of problems may seem sufficient to deter even the keenest operator from ever considering crown lengthening. However, in

practice the procedure can be highly advant-
ageous in changing a situation in which provision of a crown with adequate retention would
be impracticable, into one where a successful
result can be achieved.

The surgical procedure is described in detail
in the Chapter 12. The problems associated
with the procedure, especially when done for
an old person, should be borne in mind.

Preparation margins

Where the root surfaces of the teeth are
exposed following a crown lengthening
procedure, the character of the axial profile
following reduction will be altered. The finishing line, as it is moved apically, will lie on a
narrower part of the tooth. If its width is to be
maintained at the 'classically' described proportions, fairly destructive axial reduction will
be necessary. This carries with it the risk of
pulpal exposure. The problem is of particular
relevance when making porcelain fused to
metal crowns. One answer to the problem is
to use a metal bevelled or knife-edged margin,
rather than attempting to make insufficient
space for an all-porcelain margin (Figs. 10.23
and 10.24). The effect of a high or low lipline
should be assessed and the patient warned
that a small collar of gold will be visible upon
close inspection.

Modification of the vertical relationship

Another approach to the provision of adequate axial wall length is to increase inter-
occlusal space between opposing teeth, so that
the need for occlusal reduction of the shortened tooth during crown preparation is
avoided. If this is done, the excessive width of

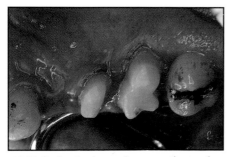

Figure 10.23 Occlusal view of preparations where the
finishing line lies well apical to the cement–enamel junction

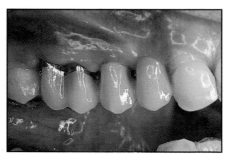

Figure 10.24 Buccal view of completed ceramo-metal
restorations showing the use of a metal collar

the occlusal surface of the worn tooth, as
described above, will be less of a problem
because it will be possible to place the occlusal
surface of the new restoration more coronally
than the worn surface. The reduction in the
width of the occlusal table will facilitate the
production of smaller, more precise points of
contact with the opposing dentition.

Local modification

Modification of the vertical relationship can
be achieved either in a local area, or for the
whole arch. It is possible to modify the vertical relationship of teeth utilizing a local appliance when only a few teeth are involved in
the pathological toothwear, as may be seen
when acid erodes the upper anterior teeth.
The increased vertical space may be achieved
by fitting an onlay onto the palatal surfaces of
the teeth involved (Figs 10.25–10.30). In this
way inter-occlusal contact will occur at an
increased vertical dimension on the onlay
alone, leaving the patient with the remainder
of their teeth out of contact. Over a period of
a few months, the opposing teeth gradually
come into contact as a result of a combination
of eruption of those teeth that do not occlude
against the appliance and intrusion of those
that do. It is important to note that the intruded teeth do not disappear into the alveolus, reducing their crown length, but
rather that the tooth/alveolar complex is intruded, crown length being maintained.

When sufficient clearance has been obtained, the onlay is discarded and the teeth
are restored. The clinical procedures involved
in making a Dahl appliance are considered in
more detail in Chapter 11.

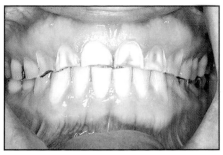

Figure 10.25 Anterior teeth showing erosive wear (posterior teeth relatively unaffected)

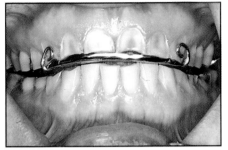

Figure 10.26 Anterior removable chrome–cobalt appliance resulting in separation of posterior teeth

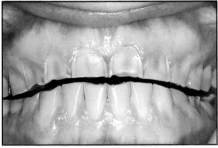

Figure 10.27 Following 10 weeks, full-time wear, posterior teeth in contact, anterior teeth no longer in contact

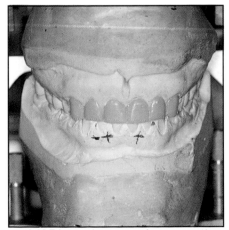

Figure 10.28 Diagnostic wax-up of upper anterior teeth

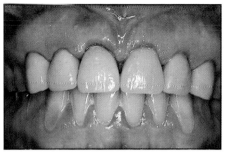

Figure 10.29 Anterior view of completed crowns

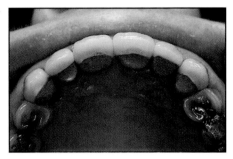

Figure 10.30 Palatal view of completed crowns

General modification

A generalized increase in vertical dimension may be required in cases where there is uniform severe wear when reconstruction is going to involve restoration of a large number if not all the standing teeth.

It may be necessary to use a combination of crown lengthening and an increase in the vertical dimension to achieve the desired result of a stable and efficient occlusion with restorations exhibiting adequate retention and resistance form. The use of crown lengthening affords two further advantages: first, that the crown margins may be placed in areas which are more accessible for maintenance by the patient and second, that sufficient vertical space is provided to allow strong connectors, aesthetic pontics and acceptable embrasure spaces.

New materials

The provision of restorations where space is limited has been made easier by the development of new dental materials. Although at a relatively early stage of assessment, some success has been achieved by the cementation, using enamel etching and dentine bonding agents, of oxidized or tin-plated gold onlays, directly onto the worn surface of back teeth.

Elective endodontics

Another way of increasing retention when the clinical crown is short is elective devitalization of pulps in order to utilize the root canal for retention. This procedure has nothing to commend it. Elective devitalization is likely to worsen the prognosis for the tooth when compared with the methods of restoration described above, where vitality is maintained.

References

1 Kayser A.F., Minimum number of teeth needed to satisfy functional and social demands, in: *Public health aspects of periodontal disease*, ed.: A. Fransen, Quintessence Publishing Co., Chicago 1984; 135–47
2 Wise M., *Occlusion and restorative dentistry for general practitioners*: second edition, British Dental Association; 1982
3 Dahl B.L., Krogstad O., Karlesen K., An alternative treatment in cases with advanced localised attrition, *J. Oral. Rehab. 1975*; 2: 209–14

11

Toothwear: space creation with the Dahl appliance

Robert Wassell

Treatment of the worn dentition can often be made easier if space can be created between opposing groups of teeth. The Dahl appliance and its modifications provide an effective means of doing this, through selective intrusion and extrusion of the dento-alveolus. Dentists need to be aware of the potential problems, but generally speaking the technique is straightforward and should be undertaken in appropriate cases.

The problems of localized and generalized toothwear, and their treatment have been discussed in the previous chapter. Some patients will present with localized wear, often of the lingual surfaces of their upper anterior teeth (Fig. 11.1). Usually, the lower teeth remain in contact because of a continued growth of the alveolus. When this occurs, the dentist is faced with the difficulty of providing sufficient space for restorative material, be this a crown, onlay or overdenture. Further reduction of

the worn palatal surfaces would often result in pulpal exposure and/or an unretentive crown preparation because of the inadequate height of the axial wall. In such circumstances it can be very helpful if space is created by depressing the less worn teeth, usually the lowers. The technique can also play a part in the treatment of generalized tooth loss.

A number of methods of creating space are available (see Table 11.1), of which one of the most effective is Dahl appliance.[1] This is a partial coverage splint designed to depress the opposing teeth against which it contacts, and to allow the unopposed teeth to overerupt (Fig. 11.2). Alveolar remodelling ensures that the teeth are not intruded into the bone, with a resulting loss of crown height.

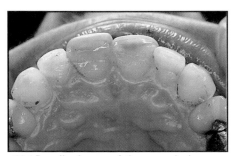

Figure 11.1 Localized wear of the upper incisors can produce a difficult restorative problem due to the lack of space for restorative material

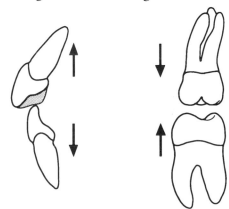

Figure 11.2 A partial coverage splint 2–4 mm thick attached to the upper anterior teeth will induce intrusion of the anterior dento-alveolar segments and extrusion posteriorly

Dahl described the use of cobalt–chrome appliances, but acrylic and bonded composite have also been used successfully. These options are discussed below. Whatever material is chosen to construct the device, it is essential that the opposing teeth are not loaded at an angle to the long axes of the roots. If they are, the oblique forces will cause them to be tilted rather than depressed. Thus, the occluding surface of the splint must be shaped to contact the opposing teeth at a right angle to their long axes (Fig. 11.2).

Patients must be advised that the appliance may have to be worn continuously for several months. However, sufficient space is often created in 10–14 weeks (Fig. 11.3).

Dentists were aware of the capability of partial coverage splints to induce dento-alveolar remodelling before Dahl devised his appliance. The anterior bite plane has been used for many years to produce an overbite reduction in the treatment of Class II division I malocclusions. Moreover, partial coverage splints used for the treatment of temporo-mandibular dysfunction have sometimes been observed to cause massive unwanted disruptions to the occlusion, especially when worn over an extended period (Fig. 11.4). Nevertheless, Dahl's idea of using a partial coverage splint to create space for restorative material was a significant development and has allowed otherwise difficult or near-impossible cases to be treated in a relatively straightforward manner.

Many questions which might otherwise deter from the use of such appliances have been answered by Dahl's meticulous measure-

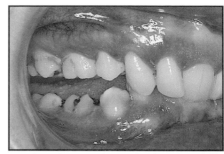

Figure 11.4 Unplanned dento-alveolar remodelling can produce devastating effects. This TM dysfunction patient wore an inappropriate posterior partial coverage splint for several years

ments. A series of four cephalometric analyses were made on 20 patients suffering from wear of the anterior teeth. These patients were aged from 18 to 50 years and wore cobalt–chrome splints ranging in thickness between 2 mm and 4 mm. Tantalum implants were inserted into the midline basal portions of the upper and lower jaws to act as reference points. The studies reported the following main findings:

- Only transient discomfort and speech impediment occurred after the splint was fitted.
- After the appliance had been worn for six months the mean intrusion was 1.05 mm (range 0.2 to 2.1), and the mean overeruption was 1.47 mm (range 0.4 to 2.4). Younger patients showed slightly more posterior eruption than the old patients. However, age was not correlated with the amount of anterior space that was created.[2]
- The thickness of the splint was correlated with the amount of anterior tooth intrusion.[3]
- Most of the space had been created within two and four months.[2]
- The appliance produced insignificant protrusion of the upper incisors or retroclination of the lower incisors.[4]
- After 5 years, the increase in vertical dimension obtained by eruption of the posterior teeth and restoration of the anterior teeth, had been maintained in most patients.[5]
- None of the patients reported problems with temporo-mandibular dysfunction.

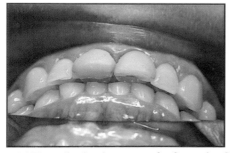

Figure 11.3 The splint has been worn for 3 months. Sufficient space has been created between the anterior teeth to allow the upper incisors to be crowned without palatal reduction

Construction of the Dahl appliance

The original Dahl appliance consisted of a 2–4 mm thick cobalt–chromium onlay for the upper incisors, retained bilaterally with clasps on the canines and premolars (Fig. 11.5).

The appliance is best made on a semi-adjustable articulator with the casts mounted in the retruded axis position (RAP), because the patient will usually function on this relationship when the posterior teeth are lifted out of occlusion. After mounting the casts, the jaw record is removed and the incisal guide pin adjusted to obtain a suitable amount of space between the occluding surfaces of the upper and lower incisors. The anterior space should be judged in relation to the space created between the molars. A greater amount of opening has been found to be beneficial if there is minimal clearance between the molar teeth, for example in patients with a steep occlusal plane or a marked curve of Spey.

The appliance should be waxed-up so as to direct occlusal forces axially through the lower incisors in RAP. A shallow anterior guidance ramp should also be incorporated in order to guide the patient into RAP.

Design modifications

The appliance may be retained satisfactorily with canine clasps, provided these teeth have sufficient buccal undercut. Buccal recontouring with composite can be used to supplement retention if necessary (Fig. 11.6).

The appliance may also be cemented to the teeth with a glass ionomer cement (Fig. 11.7). This approach does away with the clasps and ensures patient compliance but is not without

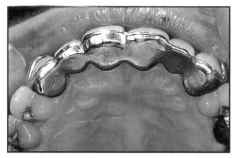

Figure 11.6 Premolar clasps may be omitted if the canine clasps are sufficiently retentive

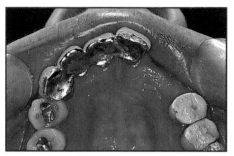

Figure 11.7 An appliance retained by glass ionomer cement

problems. First, oral hygiene can be compromised, so it is important to contour the appliance so that it does not encroach unnecessarily on the gingival tissues. Second, it is impossible to gauge the amount of space that has been created between the anterior teeth. Usually, 10–14 weeks' wear will be sufficient. The splint can be removed with a sharp tap applied to a strategically positioned chisel.

The original chrome–cobalt Dahl appliance may be less than ideal in two situations:

- Where the appliance is unduly visible and unaesthetic
- Where the appliance is bulky in cross-section (it will also be unduly heavy).

It also is highly dependent on high-quality technical support and can be time consuming, if not impossible to fit if poorly made.

Aesthetic problems occur when the incisors are in Class III relationship, with a minimal overbite. One solution to the problem is to veneer the occluso-labial aspect of the metal appliance with acrylic or composite (Fig. 11.8). An even simpler solution is to make the appliance out of acrylic. Clasps may not be necessary if the appliance is made to

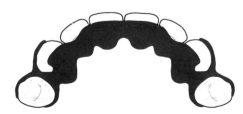

Figure 11.5 Diagrammatic representation of the original Dahl appliance. The occluding surfaces are designed to load the lower teeth along their long axes

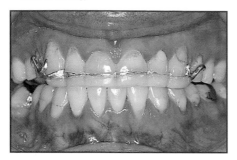

Figure 11.8 Composite resin or acrylic may be incorporated into the design to reduce aesthetic problems

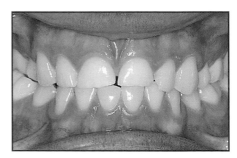

Figure 11.11 A 21-year-old woman with severe localized wear of the upper central incisors

partially overlap the labial aspects of the teeth (Fig. 11.9). A bulky appliance is best made in acrylic as this will avoid the excessive weight and porosity problems associated with a metal casting (Fig. 11.10).

A logical extension of the acrylic appliance is to build up the affected teeth with acid-etch/dentine bonded composite (Figs 11.11, 11.12, 11.13). The teeth are not splinted together and so it is particularly important that the palatal aspects are contoured so as to direct forces down the long axes of the lower incisors. If this is not done the upper anterior teeth may be loosened, drift anteriorly or

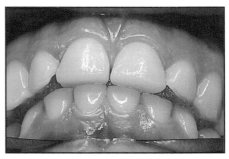

Figure 11.12 The central incisors have been built to the required length with composite. The composite cinguli have been shaped so as to provide a localized 'Dahl appliance' against the four lower incisors

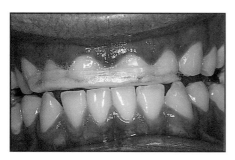

Figure 11.9 An all-acrylic design used in an Angles Class III incisor relationship. The incisors have been overlapped buccally and palatally to provide retention

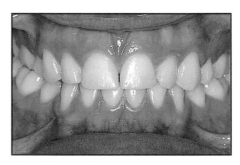

Figure 11.13 The completed case. After three months the cinguli were reduced and the occlusion adjusted to give anterior guidance and posterior stability

become uncomfortable. After a suitable period of time the large composite cinguli are reduced in size to allow the posterior teeth to occlude and to create a harmonious anterior guidance. The composites may be either used as semi-permanent restorations or replaced by crowns.

Posterior cast metal appliances have been used experimentally in a small number of cases to correct the overeruption of unopposed posterior teeth. The appliance is

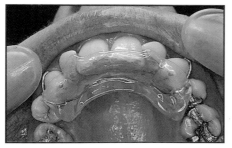

Figure 11.10 An appliance constructed in acrylic; note the bulk

cemented to the occlusal surfaces of the teeth either side of the space into which the opposing tooth has overerupted. A flat occlusal surface is used so as to avoid the creation of deflective contacts. Currently, this type of treatment cannot be recommended for general use because its long-term effects are unknown.

Problems

The possibility of creating an unstable occlusion must be borne in mind before the appliance is prescribed. Caution should be exercised where teeth are tilted or crowded because differential dento-alveolar movements could result in future occlusal problems.

Although Dahl reported no instances of temporo-mandibular dysfunction before, during or after appliance wear, it has been the author's experience that at least one patient has had problems. Pain and clicking of the left temporo-mandibular joint started after two months of splint wear when the right molars erupted into partial occlusion. The patient was treated by the removal of the resulting non-working side interferences. This patient had a history of mild temporo-mandibular joint dysfunction before treatment. Similar patients should be warned that their dysfunction might be exacerbated.

The patient should be warned that speech is usually affected for a few days after placement of the device, and that there may be some transient minor discomfort in the teeth and muscles of mastication.

The clasps should be adjusted carefully because most patients will not tolerate a loose appliance. It should be possible to clean the embrasures of a cemented appliance with Super Floss and the palate must remain uncovered. An appliance should not be cemented if it is evident that oral hygiene is likely to compromised.

In those cases where tooth movement does not occur, the reason is usually non-compliance. The patient should be instructed that the appliance must be worn at all times, though dispensation may be made for meal times. Dahl's studies were made in patients with low Frankfurt mandibular plane angles. The possibility that other skeletal patterns may respond differently has to be borne in mind.

After appliance therapy, the posterior occlusion needs time to 'settle' before stable contacts are re-established. Usually, the most posterior teeth are the first to come into contact, followed by the others. Anterior restorations can be made before all the teeth have come into contact, but care should be taken to create a definite cingulum stop to direct forces axially. If occlusal adjustment of the posterior teeth is deemed appropriate, it should be remembered that this procedure could decrease the amount of inter-incisal space. The dentist should be familiar with the principles of occlusal adjustment,[6] and any adjustments should be planned on casts mounted on a semi-adjustable articulator in the retruded axis position.

References

1 Dahl B.L., Krogstad O., Karlsen K., An alternative treatment in cases with advanced localised attrition,

Table 11.1 Methods of obtaining space to restore worn anterior teeth

Method	Comment
Dahl appliance	Method of choice if wear localized
Grind opposing teeth	Possible aesthetic and pulpal problems
Increase vertical dimension	Indicated only if majority of posterior teeth need full occlusal coverage restorations
'Distalize mandible'	Extensive occlusal adjustment needed to eliminate slide from RCP – ICP; only appropriate if large horizontal component of slide present
Crown lengthening	May be required to increase axial wall height to aid crown retention
Post and core	Occasionally suitable for change of angulation of worn anterior teeth. Risk of root fracture if occlusion incorrect
Extraction or surgical repositioning	Rarely indicated but may be required where gross over-eruption has occurred

J. Oral Rehab. 1975; 2: 209–14

2 Dahl B.L., Krogstad O., The effect of a partial bite raising splint on the occlusal face height. An X-ray cephalometric study in human adults, *Acta Odontol. Scand. 1982*; 40: 17–24

3 Krogstad O., Dahl B.L., Tooth intrusion and facial morphology. A cephalometric study in adults, using the implant method, *Eur. J. Orth. 1987*; 9: 200–203

4 Dahl B.L., Krogstad O., The effect of a partial bite-raising splint on the inclination of upper and lower front teeth, *Acta Odontol. Scand. 1983*; 41: 311–14

5 Dahl B.L., Krogstad O., Long-term observations of an increased occlusal face height obtained by a combined orthodontic/prosthetic approach, *J. Oral Rehab. 1985*; 12: 173–6

6 Setchell D.J., Periodontal diagnosis and occlusal analysis. in, *Companion to dental studies*, eds: A.H.R. Rowe, R.B. Johns, Blackwell, Oxford 1986; 417–519

12

Toothwear: Crown lengthening procedures

David Smith

Crown lengthening procedures may be neces-sary prior to repairing worn teeth or denti-tions, where the loss of coronal tooth tissue is such that retention of a restoration, usually a crown, would otherwise be compromised.

Background

Several writers have described what is known as a 'biologic width' which represents the soft tissue (epithelial and dentogingival fibre) attachment to the tooth.[1,2] As can be seen from Figure 12.1, a 'normal' gingival crevice may be 0.5–1 mm in depth, the junctional epithelium 1–2 mm or more and the dento-gingival fibre attachment 1–2 mm or more. Thus, there exists from the base of the 'normal' clinical gingival crevice to the alveo-lar bone crest, a 'biologic width' of 3–4 mm or more. In health, this overall length usually remains constant for a given tooth, although it may vary from tooth to tooth in the same individual. If the configuration of the marginal tissues are altered surgically then this 'biologic width' of tissues tends to re-establish.

In patients who have periodontal pocketing, whether supra- or infra-bony, crown lengthen-ing is achieved relatively easily by reducing or eliminating the soft tissue pocket wall, and, if necessary, the hard tissue pocket wall. In such circumstances there will be little trespass onto the 'biologic width' (Fig. 12.2). However,

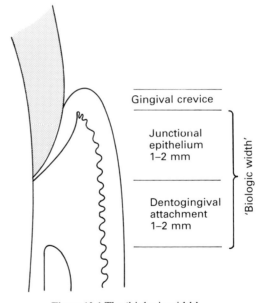

Figure 12.1 The 'biologic width'

where there has been little or no destruction of the periodontal tissues and no pocketing, as is often the case in patients with a worn denti-tion, adequate hard tissue removal must be performed in order to preserve the 'biologic width' for a given tooth (Fig. 12.2). Any attempt to site a restoration margin within the 'biologic width' will tend to result in persistent gingival inflammation, discomfort, and oc-casionally marked bunching or overgrowth of the marginal gingival tissues (Fig. 12.3).

(a)   (b)

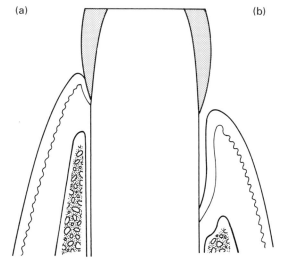

Figure 12.2 Toothwear (a) without attachment loss, (b) with attachment loss and pocketing. Crown lengthening is easier and less destructive in (b)

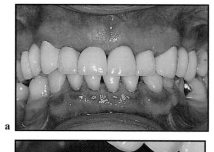

a

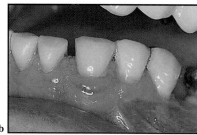

b

Figure 12.3 Gingival bunching following crown lengthening with inadequate preparation of the 'biologic width': (a) 3 months, (b) 6 months post-surgical

Preoperative assessment

Preoperative assessments should include some or all of the following:

- Periodontal probing depths around all the teeth involved
- Transgingival probing to assess the height and thickness of the alveolar crest and marginal gingival tissue
- Exposure of long cone radiographs to assess the alveolar bone contour and presence of angular bony defects as well as radicular and apical integrity
- Determination of pulp vitality
- Determination of the width of keratinized and attached gingivae
- Determination of the smile line, and thus the likely exposure of marginal tissue especially in the upper labial segment
- The preparation of study models to assess the extent of any direct dental trauma to the gingival margins, to aid in planning the extent of surgery, and to act as a permanent record.

In addition to the above it is essential to warn and demonstrate to the patient the extent of gingival recession that is to be expected and the likely consequences. These can include a marked change in appearance as a consequence of the wide interdental spacing, and the different colour of some parts of the newly exposed dental tissue. In addition, an increase in dental sensitivity may be anticipated. If the procedure is prolonged or if there has been extensive flap retraction or bone removal, then post-operative pain and swelling can be troublesome.

Surgical techniques

The surgical techniques used in crown lengthening procedures can be one of the following:

- Gingivectomy, where largely soft tissue pocketing or gingival overgrowth has occurred
- Mucoperiosteal flap procedure, with thinning by resection of the marginal tissues (filleting)
- Apically repositioned flap.

Gingivectomy

Indications

A standard gingivectomy procedure is indicated in the following circumstances:

- Where pocketing exists which is largely supra-alveolar in nature (Fig. 12.4a)

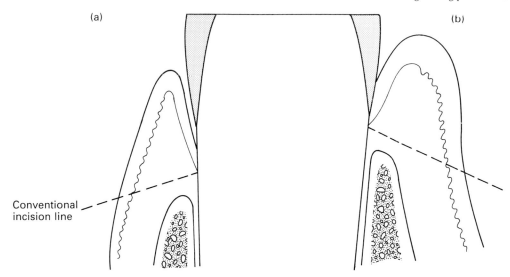

Figure 12.4 Gingivectomy for crown lengthening (a) with suprabony pocketing, (b) with gingival overgrowth

- Where some reduction of clinical crown height has occurred because of marked gingival overgrowth (Fig. 12.4b)
- Where the post-surgical presence of keratinized gingiva is not an important aesthetic or restorative consideration.

Gingivectomy cannot be recommended where controlled apical relocation of the alveolar crest is required.

Surgical technique (Fig. 12.5)

Under local anaesthesia the soft tissue pocket depths are marked on the external mucosal surface in the usual way and, where possible, a classical gingivectomy incision performed. Root planing and debridement is carried out. Final adjustments to the incision contour can be made using either a scalpel blade or slowly rotating burs. The maintenance of an even

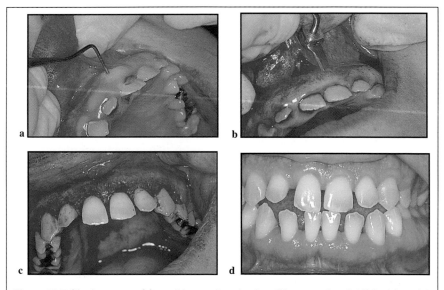

Figure 12.5 Gingivectomy: (a) marking pocket depths, (b) conventional 45° incision, (c) finished gingival contour, (d) 6 months post-surgical

gingival contour is desirable, especially if performed in the front of the mouth.

Mucoperiosteal replaced flap

Indications

A full thickness mucoperiosteal flap may be raised when the marginal tissues are particularly bulky, and/or on all palatal surfaces (where an apically repositioned flap cannot be done). Submucous thinning of the marginal tissue (filleting) is then performed, together with any necessary osseous recontouring.

Surgical technique

If a satisfactory assessment of the thickness of the marginal tissue and underlying bone can be made, the experienced operator may be able to make an inverse bevel incision in the tissues at a distance from the tooth which is taken down to alveolar bone so as to allow the removal of a substantial collar of soft tissue and removal of marginal bone if necessary. The remaining tissue margin is then sited more apically (A, Figs 12.6a, 12.6b).

Alternatively, a full thickness mucoperiosteal flap can first be raised by using a crevicular incision so as to allow direct visual assessment of the thickness of the marginal tissue and the underlying bone, before reducing their bulk (B, Figs 12.6a, 12.6b). A second inverse bevel, colleted incision is then made at an appropriate distance from the free margin of the flap, being extended to resect enough submucosa to achieve the desired amount of thinning and apical positioning (Fig. 12.6c). Finger support on the outside of the flap is a useful means of control while this filleting process is carried out.

Both envelope and two- and three-sided flaps may be used with the technique. When using the envelope design, a sufficient length of flap must be created to allow manipulation of the marginal tissues. The surgical technique is illustrated in Figures 12.7a–j.

Apically repositioned flap

Indications

This technique is particularly suitable when there is existing pocketing, a shallow adjacent buccal or lingual sulcus, or a need to reduce the overall height of the alveolar margin when the dentition is worn with little or no periodontal disease. The procedure can be very expensive in terms of supporting crestal bone and should be undertaken only in selected cases.

Surgical technique

The flap may be developed by either a crevicular or inverse bevel incision, depending upon the requirement for thinning of the marginal soft tissues. Sufficient teeth must be included to ensure the creation of an even and aesthetic gingival contour. A two-, or more usually, a three-sided full thickness mucoperiosteal flap is fully retracted and mobilized to allow apical displacement without tension at the vertical relieving incisions (Fig. 12.8a). When necessary, root planing and debridement is performed, as is osseous recontouring of the alveolar crest (Fig. 12.8b). It is also recommended that residual dento-gingival fibres be curetted from the cemental surface in order to prevent reattachment and coronal creep of the gingival margin.

In the case of the worn dentition, alveolar crestal bone is removed by a combination of burs and hand instruments. The final adjustment of bone immediately adjacent to the periodontal ligament is done with chisels, margin trimmers, curettes or sharp excavators, in order to avoid unnecessary damage to the root surface by burs.

In order to accommodate the 'biologic width', sufficient bone should be removed to allow a minimum of 3 mm of root surface to be exposed between the alveolar crest and the envisaged final position of the healed gingival margin. Enough tooth structure should be exposed to allow placement of restorative margins without encroaching on the 'biologic width'. A recent study concluded that this approach led to stable periodontal tissue levels over a six-month period.[3]

Figure 12.6a Mucoperiosteal replaced flaps – (A) is a conventional inverse bevel incision, (B) is a crevicular incision

Figure 12.6b Bony reduction follows removal of a collar of tissue (A) or a second thinning (filleting) incision (B)

Figure 12.6c Flap replacement to cover reduced bony margins

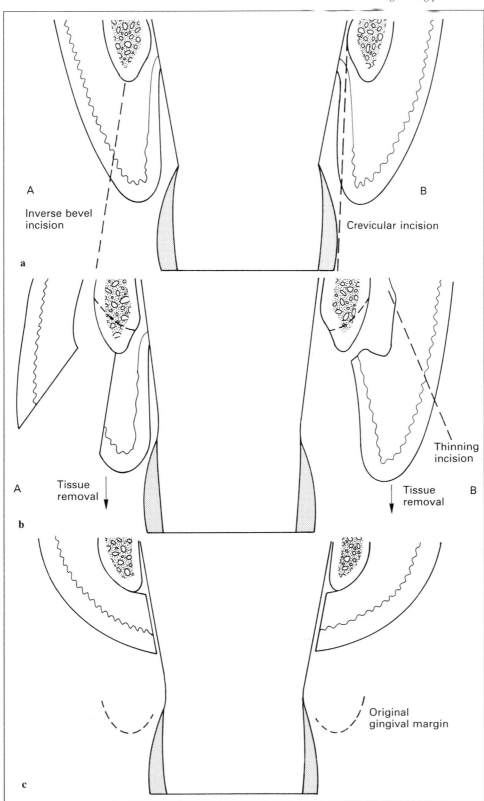

A Inverse bevel
incision

B Crevicular incision

a

A Tissue
removal

Thinning
incision

Tissue
removal B

b

Original
gingival margin

c

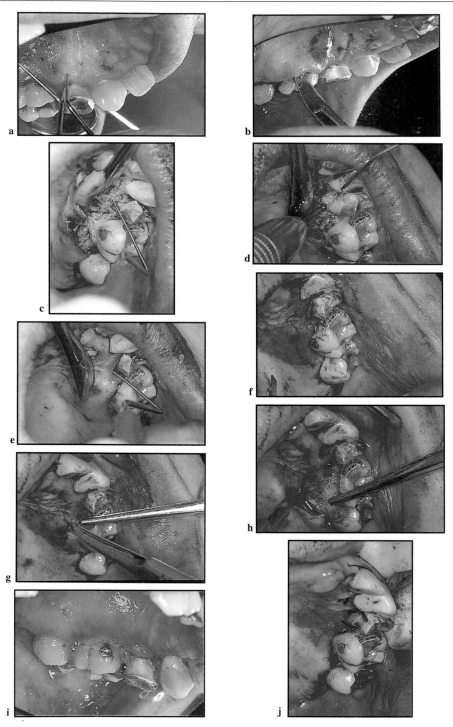

Figure 12.7 Mucoperiosteal replaced flap |3–6. (a) |4 for palatal crown lengthening, transgingival probing. (b) Crevicular incision. (c) Flap elevation and probing to assess 'biologic width' (temporary crown removed). (d) Bone margin reduction. (e) Assessing depth and height of tissue removal prior to second incision. (f) Location of thinning incision marked. (g, h) Thinning (filleting) incision. (i) Flap replaced with interrupted sutures. (j) 2 weeks post-surgical

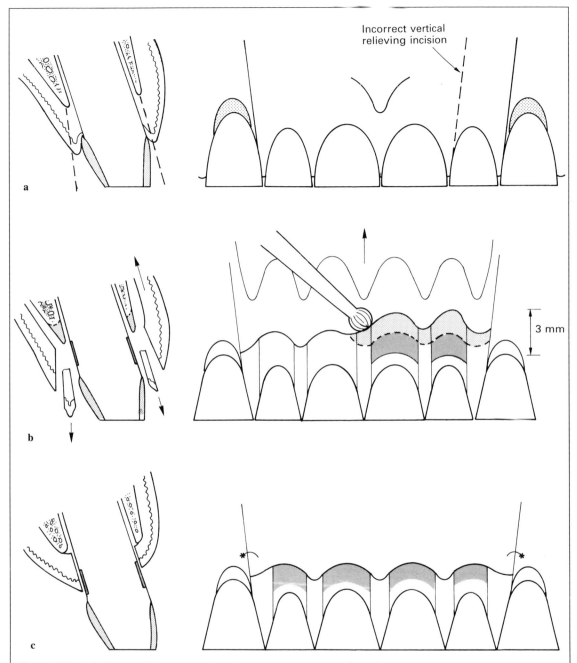

Figure 12.8a Apically repositioned flap (ARF) made labially from 21|12. 3|3 are not included because of existing recession. Note the need to include |2 to ensure an even gingival contour around all incisors

Figure 12.8b Labial ARF fully mobilized. Bone is removed to a level 3 mm apical to the final healed gingival contour. The shaded zone indicates the area of root planing necessary to remove dentogingival fibre attachment. Note that the palatal flap is replaced after a thicker collar of tissue has been removed to allow 'apical' replacement

Figure 12.8c The labial ARF is secured with anchoring sutures – then interrupted or continuous sutures are placed so that the alveolar crest is fully covered

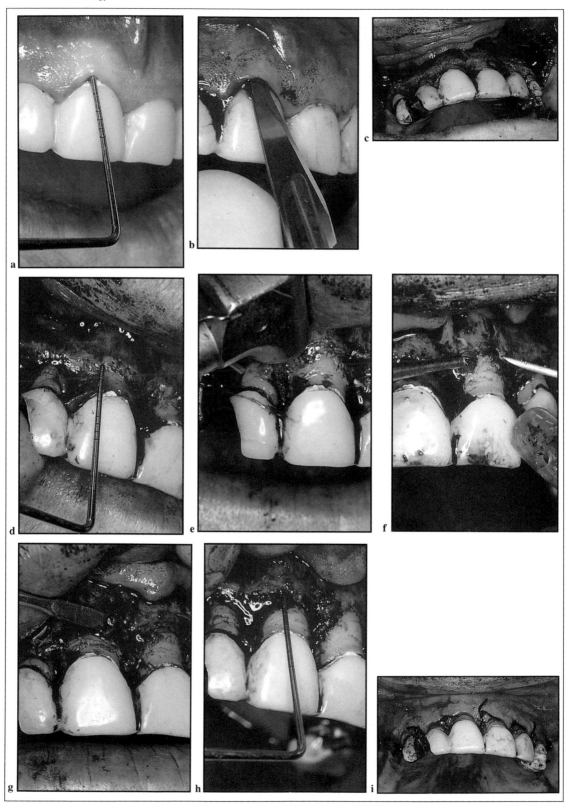

It is also necessary to remove bone from adjacent teeth so as to produce a flowing bony contour and avoid the creation of a step between the lengthened teeth and their neighbours. Otherwise, the results may be unaesthetic, create difficult access for cleaning, and even encourage periodontal pocket formation.

The flap is repositioned apically to the desired level and is secured by one or two retaining sutures in the vertical relieving incisions. The marginal tissue can be held by interrupted interdental sutures or a continuous suture (Fig. 12.8c). A periodontal pack is usually necessary in these cases.

Once initial healing has taken place, a gentle revision of the gingival contour by means of electrosurgery may be helpful. The clinical technique is illustrated in Figures 12.9a–i.

Complications

- Exposure of furcations may occur as a direct result of lengthening molar teeth and occasionally premolars. In the case of worn teeth where there has been little existing periodontal disease, this can complicate tooth cleaning. In the writer's experience, such an exposure is rarely a prelude to the development of periodontal disease at the site, provided that the restorative superstructure does not contribute further to the retention of plaque. However, in the presence of existing periodontal disease at that site, a grade II or III furcation involvement may require the resection of a root in order to improve access for cleaning. Endodontics will be necessary prior to tooth restoration.
- Tooth mobility after surgery is usually transient. Provided that the remaining periodontal support and gingival margin can be maintained in health, the tooth may be crowned or used as a bridge retainer.
- Aesthetics can be impaired. The operator must be careful not to create steps in the gingival contour as a consequence of lengthening only one or two teeth. If this is likely, other alternatives to crown lengthening should be considered, such as orthodontic tooth extrusion, or extraction and replacement of the worn tooth or teeth.
- Damage to the root surface during surgery can provoke hypersensitivity and the deficiency may impinge on the area where the crown margins require to be placed.
- In a recent study, 12% of sites which had undergone crown lengthening surgery demonstrated further gingival recession in the period between 6 weeks and 6 months after.[3] Therefore, in aesthetically-sensitive locations it would be wise to delay final crown margin preparation until monitoring indicates that the gingival margin is stable.

References

1 Ingber F.J.S., Rose L.F., Coslet J.G., The 'biologic width' – a concept in periodontic and restorative dentistry, *Alpha Omega* 1977; 10: 62–5
2 Palomo F., Kopczyk R.A., Rationale and method for crown lengthening, *J. Am. Dent. Assoc. 1978*; 96: 257–60
3 Bragger U., Lauchenauer D., Lang N.P., Surgical lengthening of the clinical crown, *J. Clin. Periodontol. 1992*; 19: 58–63

Further reading

Kieser J.B., *Periodontics – A practical approach*, Wright Publishers; London: 1990
Rateitschak K.H., Rateitschak E.M., Wolf H.F., Hassell T.M., *Colour atlas of dental medicine – Periodontology*, second edition, Thieme Medical Publishers Inc.; New York: 1989

Figure 12.9 Apically repositioned flap 3|3. (a) Assessment of pocket and tissue depth. (b) Crevicular or inverse bevel incision. (c) Flap elevated and fully mobilized by vertical relieving incisions distal to 3|3. (d) 3 mm 'biologic width'. (e, f) Initial interdental and bone removal. (g) Fine bone removal done with chisels adjacent to the root surface will reduce the risk of damage. (h) 2 mm apical reduction of alveolar crest. (i) Flap closure with interrupted sutures

13

Endodontic treatment of the old tooth

Chris Stock

Endodontic treatment is increasingly being undertaken for old patients, for a variety of reasons. These are chiefly, to retain teeth as part of a reasoned treatment plan, because of the patient's wishes, and as a less traumatic alternative to extraction for the debilitated patient. The techniques are similar to those for younger teeth, though the problems encountered may be greater.

The number of endodontic treatments undertaken for patients of all ages has increased dramatically during the last ten years. What may not be appreciated is the change in the age distribution of these treatments. Figure 13.1 shows the large numbers of endodontic treatments being carried out in the older age-groups. It is often more difficult to do endodontic treatment for an old person than for a younger person. Notwithstanding, the same problems may be encountered when treating younger teeth whose pulps have received repeated insults due to caries, restorations or trauma. It is for this reason that the term 'old tooth' has been used in the title. The difficulties that may be encountered when treating the 'old tooth' should not deter the dentist from attempting treatment, provided that he or she is aware of the problems that may be encountered, and has sufficient knowledge and patience to deal with them.

The problems that may occur in the endodontic treatment of the old person can be divided into general and local.

General problems

Many old people cannot tolerate long appointments, and find it onerous to keep their mouths wide open, even for short periods. Some cannot open their mouths wide at all, which obviously impedes access to the posterior part of the mouth. Jaw tremor may make the taking of radiographs difficult. Finally, some patients will not tolerate the supine position.

Local problems

In heavily restored teeth the original anatomy may be disguised so that it is difficult to locate the root canals. Large patched restorations may disintegrate when access is made, making it difficult to place a rubber dam clamp.

Attempts to gain access into the root canals may be made particularly difficult because of the virtual absence of a pulp chamber and the presence of pulp stones (Fig. 13.2). Even when the entrances to the root canals have been identified, the narrow canals may be difficult to negotiate and can easily be blocked with dentine chips during instrumentation.

Spontaneous vertical root fractures, particularly of premolars and molars, are a common occurrence, and can be difficult to diagnose and treat. The incidence of perio-endo lesions increases with age, and this too can present

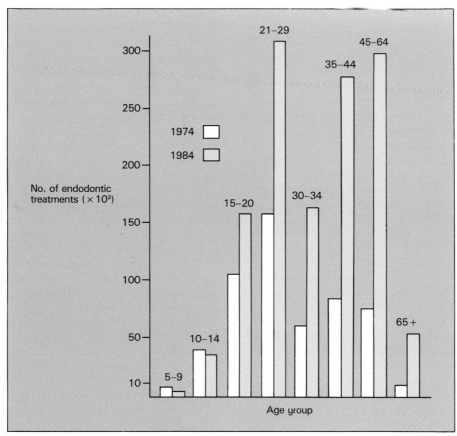

Figure 13.1 Change in age distribution of canal treatment in the UK (courtesy Dr J. Lilley, Department of Conservative Dentistry, Manchester Dental School)

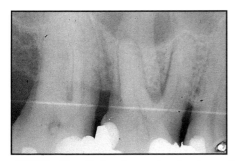

Figure 13.2 Maxillary first and second molars in an elderly patient. The pulp chambers are small and contain pulp stones

the operator with difficult treatment decisions.[1]

Indications for treatment

There are many medical conditions where root canal treatment, rather than extraction,

would benefit the patient. For example, root canal treatment is less likely to produce a bacteraemia than a tooth extraction,[2,3] consequently, patients with a history of rheumatic fever or congenital valvular heart disease will be less compromised. Patients with high blood pressure or those on anti-coagulant therapy may bleed excessively following extraction; the healing process may be impaired following extraction in diabetics, those on long-term steroid therapy or following radiotherapy to the jaws. These problems may be avoided if the tooth can be root filled rather than extracted. Pulp extirpation and root filling may be less traumatic than extraction, both physically and emotionally, particularly for the old person who is debilitated.

The principal indication for root treatment in the elderly patient is the pain of a pulpitis or an apical periodontitis. On the other hand, symptomless non-vital pulps may, in many cases, not require to be treated, unless there is evidence of active pathology, or where the crown of the tooth requires to be restored.

In the absence of pain the benefits of endodontics must be weighed against the distress that may be caused. Thus, treatment would be justified in the case of a single standing posterior tooth or a critical bridge abutment, whereas it might be reasonable to extract a tooth whose loss would not appreciably disrupt function or aesthetics.

Some elderly patients have a psychological dread of losing teeth and will go to any lengths to retain them. These people must be handled sympathetically and their teeth treated if practicable.

There may be situations where elective devitalization is the treatment of choice. For example, the canal space may be required to accommodate a post in a case of toothwear in which there is insufficient coronal tissue to accommodate a conventional crown, or a molar tooth may have to be resected if it is fractured or periodontally compromised. Similarly, when planning an overdenture the retained supporting teeth will in most cases require to be root filled.

Treatment planning

The importance of the medical history cannot be overemphasized. It is not sufficient simply to ask the patient if they have any medical problems. It is best to ask specific questions from a checklist (Fig. 13.3). The patient's general medical practitioner should be contacted if there is any doubt about a systemic condition or if the patient is on long-term medication. It may be necessary to alter the dosage of drugs (after consultation with the medical adviser). For example, a patient who has been taking systemic corticosteroids for some time may require an increase in dosage for a period of 24 hours during treatment. Antibiotics may require to be prescribed. On occasion it may be in the patient's best interest to recommend extraction.

Local anaesthetic is the preferred method of pain control, but an elderly patient may also wish for sedation. This can be administered by means of Diazepam preoperatively in tablet form. Alternatively, intravenous Midazolam can be administered by an anaesthetist. Patients thus treated are particularly relaxed and co-operative, and the apparent recovery time is short. However, the residual effects of any of the benzodiazepines may last for up to 24 hours, and should not be ignored.[4] Hospitalization with a general anaesthetic may be required for extremely nervous patients or when long and difficult surgical procedures are to be undertaken. However, the risk must be balanced against advantage.

Appointments must be carefully planned. For example, long appointments should be

PREVIOUS MEDICAL HISTORY

RHEUMATIC F (Suspect, confirmed)	YES	NO
In bed for ..... weeks, months		
HYPERTENSION OR CARDIAC DISEASE	YES	NO
HEPATITIS	YES	NO
PREGNANT	YES	NO
UPPER RESP. TRACT INFECTIONS	YES	NO
ALLERGIES TO	YES	NO
ANTIBIOTICS	YES	NO
LOCAL ANAESTHETICS	YES	NO
OTHER DRUGS..................................	YES	NO
TAKING ANY DRUGS NOW?	YES	NO
ANTICOAGULANTS	YES	NO
STEROIDS	YES	NO
INSULIN	YES	NO
TRANQUILIZERS	YES	NO
OTHER	YES	NO
UNDER TREATMENT BY GP OR HOSP.	YES	NO
SERIOUS ILLNESS PAST 3 YEARS	YES	NO

Figure 13.3 Medical case history suggested checklist

made when antibiotic cover is to be given, so as to complete as much treatment as possible. If further treatment is required, a minimum period of one week should be left between appointments.[5] Amoxycillin is the cover of choice.

Generally, appointments should be no longer than forty-five minutes, preferably at a convenient time of day for the patient.

Treatment

Root canal treatment on the 'aged tooth', in which little pulp chamber remains and canals are very fine, can be described in five sections.

Preparation of the tooth

A good preoperative radiograph must be available. The size of the pulp chamber is assessed and the position and direction of curvature of the roots are noted, as is evidence of periradicular pathosis. Caries or leaking restorations must be removed. Whenever possible the tooth must be built up sufficiently to allow the placement of a rubber dam. Glass ionomer cement is a useful material for this purpose. The crown need not be restored to its original contour. Dentine pins should be used with caution because they may weaken the remaining tooth substance, and may have to be removed and new pins inserted before the final restoration is placed.

Cast restorations and crowns must be examined carefully to see if they are decemented or leaking before access is made into the pulp chamber. This precaution is particularly relevant in the case of bridge retainers. A particular problem may be the tooth in which the crown has fractured off at the gingival margin, or worse, subgingivally. Modified clamps may hold the dam and it can help to groove the root surface. If this cannot be done, then careful isolation with cotton wool rolls, good aspiration, and speedy treatment using retained instruments, may be necessary.

The access cavity

The shape of the access cavity in an 'old tooth' is similar to that described classically for the 'normal tooth', though it will be smaller as a result of the reduction in size of the pulp chamber and diameter of the root canals. The pulp chamber may be very small, and on occasion absent, because of the formation of reparative dentine or pulp stones. This can make the location of canal entrances very difficult.

Access is made with a tungsten carbide cross-cut fissure bur which is used to remove the roof of the pulp chamber. In posterior teeth when the preoperative radiograph shows the pulp to be small, it is useful to hold the bur in the handpiece against the radiograph to offer some guidance as to the required depth of penetration (Fig. 13.4). This will reduce the risk of perforating the floor of the pulp chamber. When the initial penetration is being made in single rooted teeth, care must be taken to direct the bur in a straight line towards the canal. In posterior teeth, access is

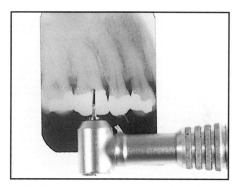

Figure 13.4 Judging depth of penetration with a bur held against the preoperative radiograph

made towards the largest part of the pulp chamber, which usually lies above the largest canal, which is the distal in lower molars and the palatal in the upper molars. When access is being made through a bonded crown, it is better to use a round diamond bur to cut through the porcelain, prior to using a purpose-designed, tungsten carbide metal-cutting bur for the gold subframe. Once the pulp chamber has been located, a high speed, tapered non-end-cutting diamond bur[a] is used to remove the remainder of the roof and

---

[a]FG 332/018, Hopf, Ringleb and Co. GMBH., Kronprinzenstrasse 5–11, D-4000, Dusseldorf 1, Germany

complete the access cavity shape. The floor of the pulp chamber is darker than the surrounding dentine and is usually easy to recognize. On occasion the pulp chamber may have receded to the extent that the roof is in contact with the floor. In these cases, it may be helpful to use a slow speed round bur to aid access. The use of surface silvered mirrors in which a double image is not produced, is also an invaluable adjunct.

Location and negotiation of root canals

It is often difficult to locate the fine canals, and care and patience must be exercised. More important perhaps is the subsequent negotiation of the canals, and a successful initial penetration is critical.

In posterior teeth the root canal entrances are located at the corners of the pulp chamber. The operator must be aware of their likely position and number. This information can be found in the standard texts.[6,7,8]

The entrances to fine root canals are often masked by overlying pulp stones or debris and they can often be successfully detected by probing or scratching the likely area of chamber floor with a fine canal probe. Good eyesight is essential for the search and as the age of the operator advances so does the need for binocular loupes. If the coronal length of the root canal is sclerosed, the only way to locate it will be by using a bur. Great care has to be exercised and radiographs taken frequently with the bur in position so as to ensure the correct angle of attack (Fig. 13.5). Fibre optic lighting may also be used in the search for these small entrances. The dental operating light is switched off and the fibre optic light-tip placed at the gingival margin so

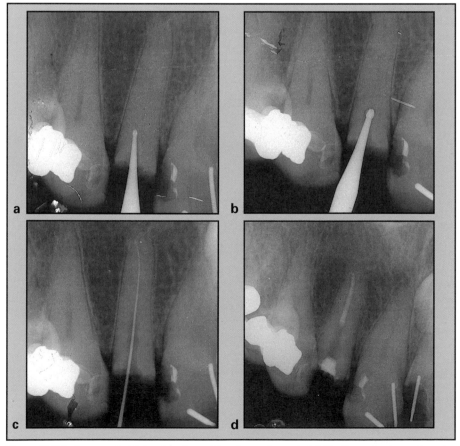

Figure 13.5 A decoronated lateral incisor with sclerosed canal. (a) Radiograph shows that the direction of cut with the small round bur is incorrect. (b) The direction was altered, (c) the canal located and finally (d) the root filled

that the beam is transmitted through tooth substance across the floor of the pulp chamber. The canals should appear as small brown spots.

The initial penetration must be made slowly with fine instruments, lubricated with an agent such as Hibiscrub. Instrument sizes 06, 08 and 10 are appropriate for this initial penetration and are readily available. Size 08 will show on radiographs. A small curve is placed at the end of the instrument (Fig. 13.6), which is dipped in lubricant and placed into the canal. It is then advanced with very gentle apical pressure, at the same time being rotated backwards and forwards through 90° to allow the tip to negotiate any fine obstructions within the canal. It is often recommended that ethylene diamine tetra-acetic acid (EDTA) is used as a chelating agent to soften the dentine walls of fine canals. It is available either as a liquid or as a paste (R C Prep[b]). When used as a paste, the material may be more controllable, without the risk of penetrating the periapical tissues associated with the liquid version. The main danger with EDTA is that its function is to soften dentine and it may allow

the operator to make his own canal, rather than follow the natural one. The main use for EDTA is to help to widen a narrow canal, once it has been fully negotiated. If the material is used in a paste form, it will act as a lubricant during canal preparation in addition to its chelating activity. The instrument must be maintained within the canal during the initial penetration, the depth of which must, therefore, be determined by the estimate of root length made from the preoperative radiograph.

An efficient way of measuring the working length of a root canal is to attach an electronic apex locator to the fine exploratory instrument. When the locator shows the instrument tip to be at the apex, a confirmatory radiograph is taken, and the depth of insertion is recorded. The working length should be 1 mm less than the recorded length so that an apical stop may be placed at the constriction.

Preparation

The objective when preparing the root canal is the removal of all canal debris by way of the access cavity, and the shaping of the canal so that it can be obturated. Secondary dentine will have been laid down in the older tooth so that the root canals have become relatively small in diameter. It may not be possible to negotiate and prepare some of these fine canals to their full length and in these cases preparation and obturation should be made as far as is possible. This will often be sufficient to secure a successful outcome.[9]

The method of preparing these fine canals is the same as those used in the larger root canal. Current thinking is that a step-down approach should be made. The technique consists first of widening the coronal two-thirds of the canal by means of Hedstrom files and then by Gates Glidden burs; and finally of using a step-back technique to prepare the apical third of the canal.[10] By using this technique, a deeper penetration of irrigant is facilitated; the amount of debris extruded through the apex is reduced; and preparation of the apical one-third is made easier. The final shape of the root canal should be a smooth taper with an apical stop 1 mm short of the radiographic apex. The master apical file should be a minimum size of no less than no. 25 or 30. The

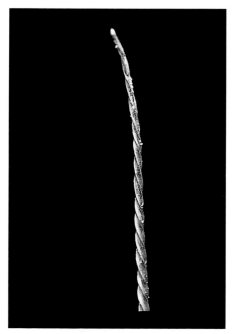

Figure 13.6 A small curve placed at the end of the instrument to help in the negotiation of fine canals

[b]R C Prep, Premier Dental Products, Philadelphia, USA

technique is more fully described in the standard endodontic texts.

Copious irrigation during preparation is essential, using a syringe with a fine irrigation needle (guage 27) loosely inserted into the root canal. Irrigation is facilitated by the initial coronal widening which is a feature of the step-down technique. The irrigant of choice is sodium hypochlorite in 2–3% concentration. Preparation of the canal may be carried out either by hand, or using sonically/ultrasonically powered instrumentation. Current practice favours the use of sharp yet flexible filing instruments which have a non-cutting tip. Reamers are no longer recommended because they cut only when rotated within the canal, held in contact against the dentine wall. K-type files cut when they are either rotated or used in a push-pull action. The cross-sectional shape of root canals is irregular, no canal is round, and few may be prepared to a round shape. It is logical, therefore, that a canal should be prepared predominantly using a filing action to plane all parts of the canal wall. This is particularly applicable to fine, curved, canals where a reaming action is likely to produce an 'hour glass' shape (zip) in the apical parts of the prepared canal. Several effective designs of file have become available, including K-flex files, safety Hedström files, and in particular, for narrow curved canals, Flexofiles. These instruments are used with a filing action only, being moved gradually clockwise around the circumference of the canal wall.

Obturation

The aim of obturation is to fill the prepared root canal system with a biocompatible insoluble material. Currently, the only material which is universally accepted is gutta percha. A sealer is also used to fill the minute spaces that inevitably remain between the filling material and the walls of the root canal. When the root canal has been prepared there is no difference between the old and the young tooth in the choice of filling technique. The initial step, whatever the technique chosen, is to fit a master gutta percha point which is one size larger than the master apical file. It is a common complaint that gutta percha points tend to buckle and do not reach the correct length in fine canals. There are two ways of over-

coming this problem. The first is that the canal should be prepared with sufficient taper to permit easy passage of the trial point to the apical region. Second, the point can be fitted in a wet canal. Copious irrigation is used during preparation of the canal, and the master cone can be fitted into the canal before it is finally dried prior to filling. The lubricating effect of the irrigant allows the point to pass up to the apical portion of the canal without buckling. The point should fit the full working length, and to have a slight resistance to withdrawal or 'tug-back'.

Following the trial fit, the master point is removed and the root canal dried with paper points. The gutta percha point is then coated lightly with the sealer of choice and reinserted into the canal. Only the apical half of the point need be coated. Obturation of the canal is next achieved by means of a laterally condensed multiple cone technique. Optimum results can be achieved by modifications of this basic technique, for example, by the use of the Endo-Tec.[c]

The battery operated Endo-Tec spreader has two heatable plugger tips, sizes 45 and 60. The control over heating of the tip is an On/Off button. The appropriate sized plugger is chosen and checked in the canal; it should reach to within 2–3 mm of the working length. A rubber stop is placed on the shank of the plugger tip to mark the point of maximum depth of penetration. The master gutta percha point is then inserted into the canal, coated with sealer, as described previously. Several accessory cones are then inserted into the canal. The plugger is placed in the canal opening and the plugger tip is heated by pressing the On/Off switch. The plugger will gradually sink into the gutta percha, under gentle pressure, until the desired depth of penetration is achieved. The instrument is then moved with a rotational action to spread the softened gutta percha. The On/Off switch is released and the plugger is withdrawn from the root canal. An accessory point, coated with sealant, can then be inserted into the channel produced by the heated instrument. A conventional finger spreader is then used to provide space for the insertion of several more accessory points. The heated plugger may be reapplied, followed by the insertion of more accessory points until the canal is fully obturated. The Endo-Tec technique is simple, convenient and the instrument is easy to control. Other techniques introduced more recently comprise a central rigid core of plastic or titanium that is coated with gutta percha. The points are warmed in an electrical heater before use. There are two main types. The first is more expensive, being custom made, with the gutta percha already applied around the core, and available in a range of sizes[d]. The second presents with blank cores and a syringe filled with gutta percha[e]. The syringe is placed in an electrical heater, and the warmed gutta percha is syringed around the blank core. Root canal sealer is wiped around the canal walls and the point is inserted to the working length. The core can either remain in the canal, or in some systems will be rotated out, leaving the gutta percha in place[f]. The advantage of this system is that the rigid core is more simply and quickly placed into the root canal than are laterally condensed multiple gutta percha cones. There may, additionally, be some advantage to be gained from the use of the technique in the narrow curved canals found in molar teeth. The main problem with the technique is that when a failure does occur the core can be difficult to remove from the canal.

The vertical root fracture

An increasing problem facing the general dentist treating old dentitions is the diagnosis and treatment of vertical root fractures. This problem most commonly affects the first and second mandibular molars. Early symptoms are those of a pulpitis with a non-localized sensitivity to thermal changes. Another early symptom, which is diagnostic, is occasional sharp pain on eating, particularly when the teeth part at the end of the chewing cycle. There are usually no radiographic changes, even when the fracture has been present for some time. The diagnosis may be confirmed by removing any restoration (Fig. 13.7) that may be present, and examining the tooth with a fibre optic light, which is placed at the gingival margin and directed through the tooth. If a fracture is present it will either be revealed as a dark line, or the light will brighten the tooth up to but not beyond the

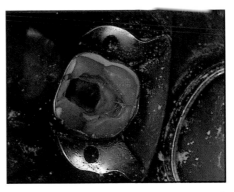

Figure 13.7 Vertical root fracture in distal part of mandibular molar

fracture because of the interruption of the passage of light. If the pulpitis is reversible, the condition may be treated by crowning the tooth; first placing a temporary crown as a diagnostic and prognostic measure. Provided that the periodontal tissues have not been compromised, an irreversible pulpitits may be treated by means of root filling and the provision of a cuspal-coverage onlay or a crown. Where the fracture is complete, and the periodontal attachment is affected, treatment, other than extraction, is seldom possible; though in 'favourable' cases hemisection or root resection might be considered.

The success rate of root canal treatment in the elderly patient is generally considered, to be the same as in a younger person.[11,12] However, in a recent study Smith *et al.* found there to be a greater success rate in the older patient.[13]

References

1 Lindhe J., *Textbook of clinical periodontology*, Munksgaard, Copenhagen 1983; 235–53
2 Bender I.B., Naidorf I.I., Garvey G.J., Bacterial endocarditis. A consideration for physician and dentist, *J. Am. Dent. Assoc. 1984*; 109: 412–20
3 Baumgartner J.C., Hegger J.P., Harrison J.W., The

[c]Endo-Tec, Dentsply, Weybridge, Surrey KT15 2SE, UK
[d]Thermafil, Tulsa Dental Products, 6804 S. Canton, Suite 600 Tulsa, OK 74136, USA
[e]SuccessFil, The Hygienic Corporation, 1245 Home Avenue Akron, Ohio 44310, USA
[f]JS Quick-Fill, JS Dental Manufacturing Company, P.O. Box 904, Ridgefield, CT 06877, USA

incidence of bacteraemias related to endodontic procedures. 1 Non-surgical endodontics, *J. Endod. 1976*; 2: 135–40

4 Ryder W., Wright P.A., Dental sedation; A review, *Br. Dent. J. 1988*; 165: 207–16

5 Scully C., Cawson R.A., *Medical problems in dentistry*: second edition, Wright, Bristol 1987; p. 65

6 Harty F.J., *Endodontics in clinical practice*: second edition, Wright, Bristol 1982: 23–49

7 Stock C.J.R., Nehammer C.F., Endodontics in practice, *BDJ 1985*: 53–69

8 Cohen S., Burns R.C., *Pathways of the pulp*: fourth edition, C.V. Mosby, St Louis 1987: 100–155

9 Grossman L.I., Oliets, S., del Rio, C.E., *Endodontic practice*: eleventh edition, Lea and Febiger, Philadelphia 1988: 219

10 Goerig A.C., Michelich R.J., Schulz M.M., Instrumentation of root canals in molars using the step-down technique, *J. Endodont. 1982*; 8: 550–4

11 Strindberg L.Z., The dependence of the results of pulp therapy on certain factors, *Acta Odont. Scand. 1956*; vol. 14, suppl. 21

12 Ingle J.I., Taintor J.F., *Endodontics*: third edition, Lea and Febiger, Philadelphia 1985: 32–3

13 Smith L.S., Setchell D. J., Harty F.J., Factors influencing the success of conventional root canal therapy– a five year retrospective study. *Int. Endod. J. 1993*; 26: 321–333

14

The partially edentulous patient

Jim Ralph and Robin Basker

Because old people are retaining their teeth, it is likely that the provision of partial dentures will increasingly be part of a considered treatment plan. However, problems, often associated with ageing, such as gingival recession, dry mouth, poor oral hygiene and root surface caries, make it important that case assessment and treatment planning are carefully considered.

Introduction

For many years the prevailing high level of edentulousness amongst elderly people gave rise to the view that gerodontics was firmly linked with the provision of complete dentures. Times, though, are changing and the information in other chapters illustrates the wide range of treatment possibilities. Recent evidence[1] confirms the continuing improvement in dental health in all age groups. This has been discussed in Chapter 1. With teeth being retained for so much longer it is likely that the provision of removable partial dentures will, increasingly, become a common form of restorative treatment for elderly patients.

Let us look more closely at the recent evidence under the following headings:

- Retention of teeth
- Current provision of partial dentures
- Attitudes and expectations.

Retention of teeth

Whether or not partial dentures need to be provided for an old person depends to a large extent on the number and location of the teeth which they have retained. One way of looking at the matter is to make the broad assumption that if 21 or more teeth are retained, there is a reasonable basis for an adequate functional dentition, particularly if the anterior teeth are retained as an intact group. Such an assumption receives forceful backing if one examines the current pattern of partial denture wearing. Only 5% of those people with 21 or more standing teeth have some of the missing ones replaced by partial dentures. This figure compares with 78% of those who have fewer than 21 teeth remaining. Looking specifically at the potential needs of the elderly, it is interesting to note that 1 in 4 of those dentate patients aged 65–74 and nearly 1 in 7 of those aged 75 had 21 or more standing teeth; as many as 90% of patients with this complement of teeth did not have spaces restored by dentures or bridges.

Taking the argument a stage further, it is interesting to refer to the work carried out by the research group in Nijmegen who have studied extensively the effectiveness of the shortened dental arch.[2] They have shown that the functional and aesthetic requirements of patients can be well satisfied if teeth anterior up to and including the second premolars are retained. This of course assumes that there is a satisfactory occlusal relationship and that steps are taken to maintain good periodontal

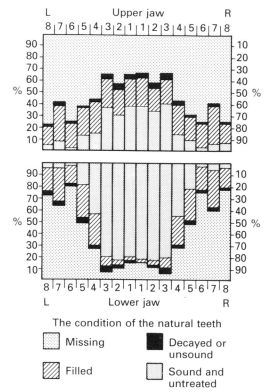

Figure 14.1 The condition of natural teeth for adults aged 55 or more. (*Adult Dental Health 1988*. UK)

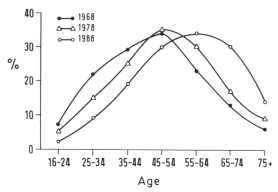

Figure 14.2 Proportion of all adults with natural teeth and dentures

health. If this viewpoint is borne in mind when looking at the state of teeth in adults over 55 (Fig. 14.1), it is interesting to see that an intact shortened lower dental arch is likely to be found in just under half the population, and an upper arch in nearly a third.

Current provision of partial dentures

The wearing of partial dentures is clearly age-related. Figure 14.2 shows the proportion of all adults with natural teeth and dentures recorded in 1968, 1978 and 1988. The shape of each curve clearly indicates a steady increase in partial denture provision towards middle age. The subsequent decline is because many patients progress to complete dentures. What is of particular interest is the shift in peak demand. The results from the 1988 Adult Dental Health Survey show the peak to have advanced ten years. Looking more closely at this curve it is apparent that fewer partial dentures are being worn by younger people and more by elderly patients.

Attitudes and expectations

Whether or not a partial denture will be worn depends on the patient's positive attitude towards the proposed treatment. Of course, if a partial denture is to be provided for a patient who has previously grappled successfully with the challenge, it is more than likely that the replacement denture will be accepted. Convincing the new wearer may not be so easy.

Evidence has been produced which gives some insight into people's attitude towards dentures. In the Adult Dental Health Survey, those people who only had natural teeth were asked whether they found the thought of having a partial denture to replace some teeth very upsetting, a little upsetting or not at all upsetting. It is interesting to note that 27% of those aged 65 and over found the idea very upsetting and that the level of concern increased with age. One possible reason for this is that young people believed that such a form of treatment was so far away that they could not identify with the prospect. Another possible explanation is that if the older people had reached the age of 65 without the need for dentures, the prospect of having to rely on an artificial appliance was a sign of failure. Whatever the reason, it is quite clear that if the dentist is faced with having to provide a first-time partial denture for an older patient, he or she must remember that 1 in 4 people view the prospect with a degree of apprehension. Of some comfort is the finding that the level of concern regarding partial dentures is markedly different to that expressed about complete dentures, where 69% of elderly people were very upset about the thought of such treatment.

Returning to the theme of the shortened dental arch introduced earlier, it is enlightening to learn of the reactions of people to the question, 'If you had several missing teeth at the back would you prefer to have a partial denture or manage without?' Whilst just over half of the younger age-groups would prefer to manage without, the proportion rose to 79% of those in the 65 and over age-group. Again, this is striking evidence of the negative attitude that older people feel towards partial dentures and suggests that the dentist is wise to gauge very carefully the motivation of the patient before embarking on treatment.

Remembering that the above evidence on attitudes and concerns has been obtained from people who rely only on natural teeth, it is useful to identify their changing expectations in respect of retaining some of their natural teeth for all their lives. The figures obtained in the 1988 survey showed that 87% of people with natural teeth and no dentures expected always to retain some teeth; the comparable figure in 1978 was 67%.

From all the evidence presented in this section, it seems reasonable to conclude that if a dentate elderly patient has to lose teeth and be provided with a partial denture, there is a very good chance that the dentist will have to work particularly hard to encourage the patient to accept the proposed form of treatment. Of course, the task is likely to be easier if the denture is needed to replace anterior teeth – the restoration of appearance is a powerful motivating factor. Nevertheless, it is very important to remember that ultimate success will depend not simply on the provision of a well-designed and constructed denture, but also on the patient's willingness to come to terms with the 'feel' of the denture and to be prepared to put a good deal of effort into learning how to control it.

The remainder of this chapter will be devoted to some of the specific problems of providing partial dentures for the elderly patient, and to a description of a realistic approach to such treatment. In a book of this nature it is not appropriate to provide details of clinical technique and details of the design of partial dentures. The bibliography at the end of the chapter offers guidance on further reading.

Specific problems of the elderly in relation to the provision of partial dentures

A number of specific problems relating to the ageing dentition have been covered in detail in previous chapters. Wear of the teeth, root surface caries, xerostomia and the general health status of the patient are all important factors which will have an influence on treatment planning decisions.

Tooth wear

Loss of tooth substance may take place because of attrition, abrasion or erosion and, in fact, frequently seems to be due to a combination of these factors. Toothwear may accelerate if tooth numbers become depleted and no replacement is provided for the missing teeth. If tooth loss is judged to have left a deficiency in occlusal support, the provision of partial dentures should be considered as a preventive measure.

The effect of wear will often be a shortening in length of the teeth, which in the anterior region is likely to provoke a request for treatment to improve their appearance. If there is adequate substance remaining to allow the teeth to be maintained as they are, or to be restored by means of crowns, partial dentures may form part of the reconstruction of the dentition, replacing the missing units and providing some of the occlusal support necessary to prevent a recurrence of the problem (Fig. 14.3). If wear is further advanced, it may be inappropriate to think in terms of crowns and it may be helpful to provide dentures which overlay the remaining tooth structure in order to achieve the desired improvement in function and aesthetics (Fig. 14.4). The most

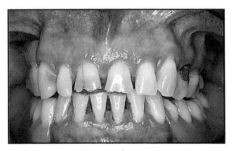

Figure 14.3 Stress on the anterior teeth may be controlled by the provision of partial dentures

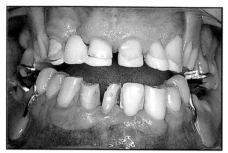

Figure 14.4 Restoration of the upper arch with a removable overlay denture

severe cases of toothwear are likely to require the use of overdentures, as described in Chapter 15.

Root surface caries

The recession of gingival tissue in older patients leads to the risk of root surface caries and there is some evidence that the incidence and severity of this problem is likely to increase in association with the wearing of partial dentures[3] (Fig. 14.5). This is in some measure a reflection of the standard of oral hygiene, but it also reflects on denture design. Those teeth which are covered by, or closely related to, components of the denture base, have an increased tendency to plaque accumulation and studies of elderly patients wearing partial dentures have shown that such teeth tend to have more extensive carious lesions.

Xerostomia

Diminution in salivary flow may be found in some elderly patients (see Chapter 4). The problem may be particularly severe when patients have had radiotherapy or are taking

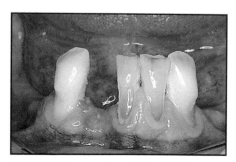

Figure 14.5 Marked recession of gingival tissues around abutment teeth

drugs such as antidepressants. Tolerance of dentures is likely to be poor in such circumstances and this may influence the decision as to whether or not a denture should be provided. There may also be a higher risk of carious damage to the abutment teeth.

General health

The general health status of patients will also influence treatment planning decisions in relation to the provision of partial dentures. If patients are severely debilitated or are unable to cope with maintenance procedures because of physical or mental infirmity, it may be best to avoid the fitting of partial dentures unless a very high quality of care and supervision can be provided by family or ancillary personnel.

It can be seen therefore, that pre-operative assessment is of importance and the following factors should be considered:

- The ability of the patient to adapt to wearing partial dentures, especially if none have previously been worn
- The ability to achieve good plaque control, given the likely increase in plaque accumulation which will accompany the wearing of even the best designed partial denture
- The general state of health and the prognosis for improvement.

An approach to the prosthetic assessment of existing partial denture wearers

There are a number of reasons why a patient may seek a replacement partial denture. The more common ones are:

- A design error in the existing denture leading to difficulty in adaptation
- The existing denture has ceased to fit because teeth have been extracted, or their shape has been altered drastically by large restorations or there has been resorption of the alveolar bone in the saddle areas
- The denture has ceased to function effectively because of 'wear and tear'; for example, components have fractured, artificial teeth have worn down or have come off the denture base.

When examining the problem it is important to assess:

- The design and construction of the denture
- The tissue reaction to the wearing of the denture
- The level of plaque control of the mouth and denture.

The questions that should be asked are:

- Is there an error in design which, when corrected on the replacement, will overcome the patient's complaint?
- Is the design of the troublesome denture so different from a previous well-tolerated one that the elderly patient has been unable to adapt to the change?
- Does the design satisfy the well-established principles which promote good tissue reaction; namely effective support, clearance of gingival margins where possible, simplicity, and a rigid connector?

An estimation of the tissue reaction to the existing denture will be necessary. This will involve an examination of the health of the teeth, the periodontal tissues and denture-bearing mucosa.

A favourable reaction to a relatively poor design (Fig. 14.6) indicates either scrupulous plaque control, a good tissue resistance, or a combination of both. Conversely, a poor tissue reaction to a good design suggests poor plaque control or perhaps a poor tissue resistance to a normal level of function.

There are a number of well-documented methods of measuring plaque control of oral tissues so that the effect of advice and treatment might be assessed. The O'Leary plaque index (Fig. 14.7) is easy to use and allows a simple percentage value to be calculated.

A recently introduced denture plaque index,[4] illustrated and described in Figure 14.8, has been found to be a convenient way of monitoring denture hygiene. A disclosing tablet is chewed in the normal way and the two plaque scores calculated in the manner described.

Many more factors, in addition to the three mentioned above, need to be taken into account before a treatment plan can be finalized. They are listed below:

- The patient's wishes and motivation
- The age and general health of the patient
- Domestic circumstances affecting the patient's ability to attend for treatment
- Health of the oral tissues.

For wearers of partial dentures the options for treatment are likely to be:

- Do nothing other than maintain the mouth and existing dentures
- Provide replacement dentures whose design will play an effective part in maintaining the health of the mouth. This can be achieved by constructing tooth-supported, clasp-retained partial dentures following the principles established by Bergman,[5] which are:
  - Effective support
  - Clearance of gingival margins
  - Simplicity of design
  - Rigid connector

- Provide dentures which are capable of being added to as and when further teeth have to be extracted, with the objective of effecting a gradual transition from a natural to an artificial dentition
- Extract the remaining teeth and provide complete dentures.

The considerations to be made when treatment planning for a new partial denture, which have been discussed above, are summarized in Table 14.1.

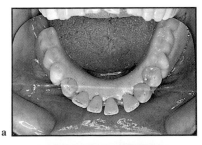
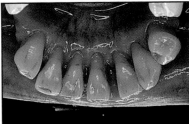

Figure 14.6a, b Favourable tissue reponse to a tissue-borne acrylic partial denture

The O'Leary plaque control record

At the initial appointment, a suitable plaque disclosing agent is used. The operator then charts any tooth surface (mesial, distal, lingual, buccal/labial) where plaque is present in contact with the gingival margin.

The operator also indicates on the chart any missing teeth.

The total number of surfaces is obtained by multiplying the number of teeth present in the mouth by four.

The total number of surfaces where plaque is present ×100 divided by the total number of available surfaces gives the percentage of affected surfaces. The patient is given oral hygiene instruction and plaque and calculus are eliminated from the mouth.

At each subsequent visit, the procedure is repeated, the charts being utilized to educate the patient.

In general, a reduction in plaque score to around 10–15% is desirable. There will be patients whose tissue responses, in terms of inflammation, will require a reduction beyond this level.

At future visits, the charting can be repeated to ensure that adequate control is maintained.

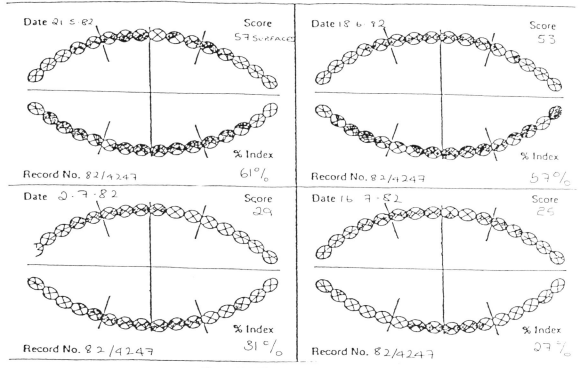

Figure 14.7 The O'Leary plaque index

Partial denture plaque score

The partial denture plaque score is the number of fitting surfaces of components on which plaque is present, expressed as a percentage of the total number of fitting surfaces for any particular denture.

Method

To calculate the total number of fitting surfaces score each component in contact with tooth/tissue surfaces as follows:

Saddle	1	Minor connector	1
Proximal surface of saddle	1	Major connector	2
Rest/overlay	1		
Clasp arm – retentive	1		
Clasp arm – bracing/reciprocal	1		

Figure 14.8 A denture plaque index

Note: Ring clasp (excluding rest) score 3.

Major connector score of 2 can be considered as right and left or as anterior and posterior components, e.g. anterior and posterior palatal bars – score 2 only.

Plate design – score 1 for each tooth covered.

Lingual plate – score 2 as major connector and 1 for each tooth covered.

Dental bar – best scored as 1 for each tooth contacted

Inevitably uncertainty may arise in scoring some designs. The important point is that the established total surface score is used consistently.

Disclose the partial denture in the mouth using a disclosing tablet. This enables both teeth and denture to be monitored at the same time.

Wash the denture under running water.

Count the number of fitting surfaces on which plaque is disclosed. Express this as a percentage of the total number of surfaces counted.

Carry out the plaque score on the natural teeth.

An example of the scoring system is shown below.

	Total score
Saddles	1
Proximal surfaces	1
Rests	5
Clasp arms retentive	3
Bracing	3
Minor connector	3
Major connector	2
	18

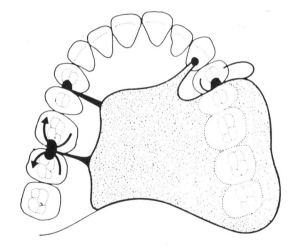

	Total score
Saddles	3
Proximal surfaces	5
Rests	5
Clasp arms retentive	4 (ring clasp 3)
Bracing	
Minor connector	1
Major connector	2
	20

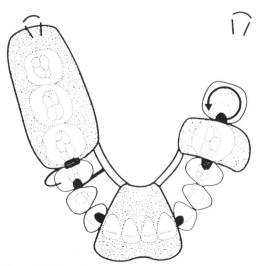

Figure 14.8 Contd

Table 14.1 Treatment planning for a new partial denture

Existing design	Tissue response	Treatment outcome
Satisfactory	Satisfactory	Maintain existing situation or make new denture of similar design
Satisfactory	Unsatisfactory	Endeavour to improve plaque control. In event of failure, design transitional denture
Unsatisfactory	Unsatisfactory	Endeavour to improve plaque control. If improvement hampered by existing design, make new denture. If no improvement, design transitional denture
Unsatisfactory	Satisfactory	Maintain present denture design. Do not try to 'improve on well tolerated shape'

In conclusion, it should be restated that the provision of removable partial dentures for old people is likely to figure more prominently in the future. It cannot be over-emphasized that there is a danger in providing such dentures for high-risk mouths. In these circumstances, discretion is often the better part of valour and a decision not to provide partial dentures, but to concentrate the effort on preserving the remaining teeth, may be the best one for the future welfare of the patient.

References

1 Todd J.E., Lader D., *Adult dental health 1988. United Kingdom*, HMSO, London
2 Käyser A.F., Witter D.J., Oral functional needs and its consequence for dentulous older people, *Community Dental Health 1985*; 2: 285–91
3 Wright P.S., Hellyer P.H., Beighton D., Heath N.R., Lynch E., Relationship of removable partial denture use to root caries in an older population., *Int. J. Prosthodont. 1992*; 5: 39–46
4 Powell K., Witt S., Personal communication 1991
5 Bergman B., Hugoson A., Olsson C.O., Caries, periodontal and prosthetic findings in patients with removable partial dentures; a ten-year longitudinal study, *J. Prosthet. Dent. 1982*; 48: 506–14

Further reading

Davenport J.C., Basker R.M., Heath J.R., Ralph J.P., *A colour atlas of removable partial dentures*, Wolfe Medical Publications Ltd; London 1988
Walter J.D., *Removable partial denture design*, second edition, British Dental Association; London 1990
Bates J.F., Adams D., Stafford G.D., *Dental treatment of the elderly*, Wright; Bristol 1986
Eds: P. Holm-Pederson, H. Loe, *Geriatric dentistry; A textbook of oral gerontology*, Munksgaard; Copenhagen 1986

Further viewing (video)

The Alliance: removable partial denture design, *Dental Progress no. 13*, British Postgraduate Medical Federation and Department of Health

15

The role of overdentures

Jim Ralph and Robin Basker

It seems inevitable that many elderly people will be partially dentate at an age when, in previous times, the edentulous state was the norm. The overdenture has a part to play in the treatment of such patients, particularly to ease the transition to complete dentures. It is a relatively simple, inexpensive prosthesis, but will provide long-term success only if the patient and the mouth have been assessed with care and a rigorous after-care programme is instituted.

An overdenture may be described as a prosthesis which derives some of its support from complete coverage of one or more natural 'abutment' teeth. In some instances it may be appropriate to cover the entire clinical crown of such abutments but more usually the crown height is reduced and the overdenture is supported by the root face.

The extraction of teeth is followed, initially, by resorption of the alveolar bone. The extent of bone loss will vary from patient to patient and is likely to be greater in the mandible than in the maxilla, leading to the higher incidence of complaints of pain, and instability in relation to lower complete dentures. Changes in ridge height were followed over a large number of years by Tallgren,[1] who demonstrated that the extent of resorption in the mandible was almost four times that in the maxilla. A radiographic study by Crum and Rooney[2] (Fig. 15.1) has demonstrated the value of root abutments in reducing the rate and degree of resorption in the mandible. The

maintenance of bone improves the functional efficiency of dentures, and more evenly distributes the load to the denture-bearing tissues. The role of overdentures is particularly important when a patient is faced with wearing a complete denture in one jaw opposed by a substantial number of natural teeth in the opposing jaw.

The role of overdentures in the treatment of the old edentulous patient

Overdentures often have a valuable role to play in the dental treatment of elderly patients, and there are a number of indications for this approach.

- Transition to the edentulous state
- Compensation for severe toothwear
- Additional support for partial dentures
- Positive retention.

Transition to the edentulous state

Increasing numbers of old people are retaining part of their natural dentitions, although in the UK many of the most elderly are edentulous. One possible consequence of retaining the natural teeth for a greater number of years may be that a significant number of older patients will be faced with the transition to

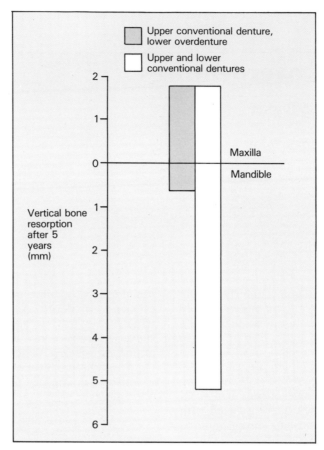

Figure 15.1 Bone resorption rates with conventional dentures and overdentures. The lower overdentures were supported on canine root abutments; their value is well demonstrated

wearing complete dentures when they may be physiologically less well able to adapt to change. They may also have been conditioned by their previous dental experience and by their attempts to retain their natural teeth, to view the prescription of dentures as a sign of failure and something to be resented. The level of anxiety with which people view complete dentures is well illustrated in Figure 15.2, which comes from the Adult Dental Health Survey of 1988.[3] Even a large proportion of people who expect to lose their teeth and be provided with complete dentures view the prospect with considerable alarm.

At the outset it is important to evaluate the dentition of elderly patients and to judge whether it has such a good prognosis that the patient is unlikely ever to face wearing complete dentures (Fig. 15.3). Sometimes the remaining teeth will be showing such signs of deterioration that the loss of some of them will be inevitable well within the likely life-span of the patient (Fig. 15.4). In the latter case the timing of any necessary extractions and the design of the most appropriate form of replacement should be considered very carefully. It is better to embark on such treatment as a planned procedure than to wait until intervention may be less favourable, perhaps when the general health of the patient makes extractions hazardous. The use of overdentures will allow the patient to gain confidence in the wearing of dentures, because the retained root abutments contribute significantly to support the stability of the prosthesis. In this way the eventual transition to complete dentures may be made gradually and more easily. The practical application of this philosophy is illustrated by the treatment of the patient shown in Figure 15.5.

Percentage of people questioned

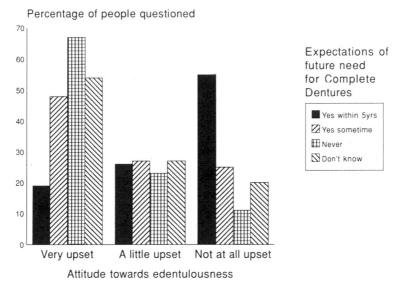

Expectations of
future need
for Complete
Dentures

- ■ Yes within 5yrs
- ▨ Yes sometime
- ▦ Never
- ▧ Don't know

Attitude towards edentulousness

Figure 15.2 Attitude towards edentulousness

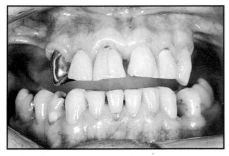

Figure 15.3 The periodontal health of these upper teeth is excellent in spite of the considerable loading. The patient has been without posterior teeth in the upper jaw for over 20 years

Compensation for severe toothwear

It is not uncommon to find that considerable toothwear has taken place on the dentition in older patients. This is often associated with, though it is not necessarily caused by, widespread tooth loss (Fig. 15.6). A low incidence of symptoms from the remaining teeth, an absence of functional problems, a lack of concern about appearance, and possibly economic factors, often contribute to a neglect of regular dental care and treatment. When the request for treatment is eventually made there is often little realistic prospect of restoring the

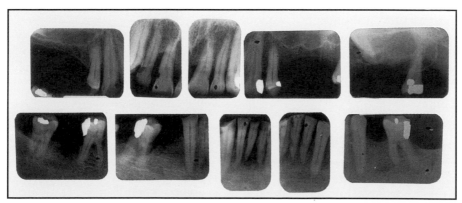

Figure 15.4 The periapical radiographs of this dentition show how poor is the prognosis

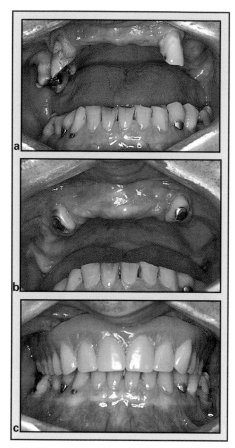

Figure 15.5 Planned treatment with an overdenture: (a) a residual upper dentition opposed by many lower teeth, (b) canine teeth prepared as overdenture abutments, (c) overdenture fitted

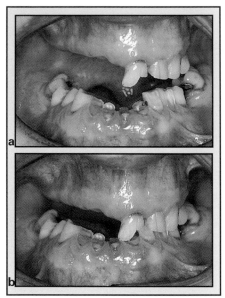

Figure 15.6a, b A severely worn dentition resulting from widespread tooth loss and a habit of chewing lumps of coal

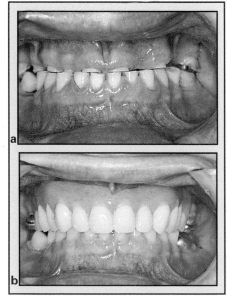

Figure 15.7 Worn teeth used as abutments without the need for root canal treatment: (a) gross wear of upper teeth due to parafunction, (b) very little tooth preparation was needed before the overdenture was fitted

worn teeth, and it may prove difficult to provide a conventional partial denture which the patient can tolerate.

It is often possible to prepare the remaining tooth structure of some of the badly worn teeth as overdenture abutments, without the need for root canal treatment. The resulting overdenture can restore aesthetics and re-establish an acceptable facial vertical dimension (Fig. 15.7). It will usually be well tolerated because of the support and stability provided by the root abutments.

Additional support for partial dentures

The motivation to wear partial dentures is strongest where one or more anterior teeth have to be replaced. Partial dentures are also more likely to be worn successfully when they involve the provision of small bounded saddles whether in the anterior or posterior region. Problems of support and retention become greater as more teeth are lost and the edentulous area becomes more extensive.

Damage to coronal structure, or deterioration in periodontal support, can make it impractical to retain individual teeth as abutments for conventional partial dentures. However, the teeth often provide valuable support for a lengthy saddle if they are reduced to serve as root abutments (Fig. 15.8).

Positive retention

The concept of using root abutments to contribute to the retention as well as the support of overdentures is attractive, and a large number of devices have been developed for this purpose. Stud attachments are probably the most familiar and the most popular. It must be recognized that the use of these attachments will transmit considerable additional loading to the root, and that not all such potential abutments, particularly in older patients, will be able to withstand these forces. Many attachments take up considerable space within the denture base and so increase the possibility of fracture or make it difficult to place the artificial teeth in their correct positions (Fig. 15.9).

The development of the Zest[a] anchor is an attempt to overcome these problems by gaining retention from a nylon peg which fits into a machined housing located within the root canal (Fig. 15.10). Unfortunately, many patients find it difficult to prevent plaque from accumulating around the margins of the housing and, as a result, there is often a high incidence of recurrent caries. The nylon pegs also tend to become brittle with use, although they are relatively easy to replace.

The use of rare earth magnets as a means of providing additional retention has become popular in recent years. The early magnets were rather large and could not always be accommodated in the available space but miniaturization of components, as in the Dyna magnet system[b], has largely overcome these difficulties. The system involves the provision of a palladium–cobalt alloy coping on the root face (Fig. 15.11a). The magnet is housed

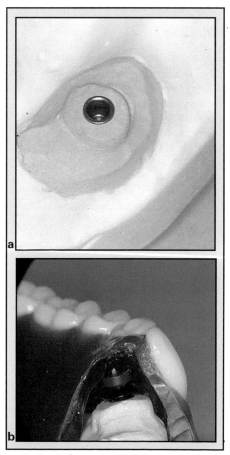

Figure 15.10a, b Components of the Zest anchor system

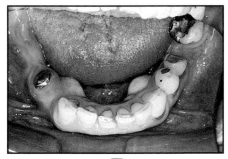

Figure 15.8 Preservation of 5| improves the support for an extensive free-end saddle

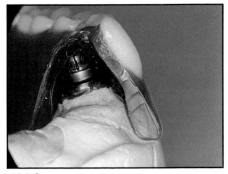

Figure 15.9 Cross-sectional view of a denture to show the space occupied by a Ceka attachment

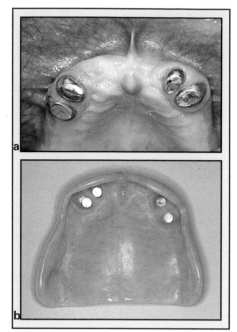

Figure 15.11 The Dyna magnet system: (a) copings constructed in a palladium–cobalt alloy, (b) magnets housed in the upper denture

within the denture base (Fig. 15.11b). Magnets offer positive retention without the transmission of potentially damaging lateral forces to the abutment teeth. Oral hygiene and denture cleansing are simple and straightforward. This is appreciated by the older patient who may have suffered deterioration in visual acuity and manual dexterity.

Additional retention is not always required, because the contribution of the root abutment in providing positive support and maintaining ridge shape is often sufficient to enhance the retention and stability of the prosthesis.

Patient selection

When deciding upon whether or not an overdenture would be an appropriate form of treatment, it is important to make a careful assessment of the patient. The attitudes and expectations that people have in relation to dental treatment is influenced by their experience of previous treatment procedures, and possibly by those of friends and relations who may have undergone treatment of a similar nature. In this respect, it is important to evaluate the quality of earlier dental care.

Previous lack of success in wearing partial dentures will often leave patients reluctant to face up to the prospect of embarking upon more complex treatment.

If there are features in the design of old dentures which have contributed to their failure, they should be pointed out to the patient in order to reassure them. Patients must receive the fullest possible explanation of the proposed treatment. The use of study models and visual aids may be helpful.

The retention of roots to serve as abutments will impose additional demands on the patient to maintain a high standard of oral and denture hygiene. Age in itself is no barrier to the selection of this technique, but the general state of physical and mental well-being is a critical factor. Unless an adequate level of patient co-operation can be predicted, it may be wiser to select a simpler form of treatment.

Selection of abutment teeth

Frequently, the abutment teeth will tend to select themselves, particularly if the dentition is already reduced in numbers.

The periodontal status is probably the single most important factor in the selection procedure. In older patients there will often be considerable recession of the gingival tissues, leaving the teeth relatively elongated and possibly mobile (Fig. 15.12). This need not rule them out as potential root abutments because the preparation will eliminate the clinical crown and reduce the unfavourable leverage on the root, often resulting in the reduction of mobility. It is important, however, to eliminate active periodontal disease and to establish

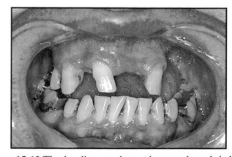

Figure 15.12 The loading on these elongated teeth is likely to be reduced if they are prepared as overdenture abutments

an adequate standard of oral hygiene, otherwise deterioration in the periodontal condition is likely to continue, leading eventually to loss of the root abutment.

When the teeth have suffered extensive wear, slowly over many years, there will often have been deposition of a substantial thickness of secondary dentine. In these circumstances it may be possible to complete any required preparation without the need for root canal treatment (Fig. 15.13). When root canal treatment is necessary, there can be some difficulty in achieving a successful result in older patients . Deposition of secondary dentine may virtually eliminate the pulp chamber and root canal, making endodontics problematical (see Chapter 13).

Some clinical and technical procedures

In the context of overdentures for elderly patients it is commonly the case that there are relatively few natural teeth remaining, that there has been significant loss of periodontal attachment, and that those teeth already lost have been replaced by removable partial dentures. We shall, therefore, concentrate on the following:

- The provision of immediate overdentures
- The conversion of existing dentures
- The inclusion of magnetic retentive devices.

The provision of immediate overdentures

The amount of periodontal destruction that has occurred in the remaining upper anterior teeth shown in Figure 15.14, led to a decision

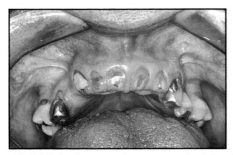

Figure 15.13 Minimal preparation was required for these severely worn anterior teeth. An overdenture has been worn for 5 years

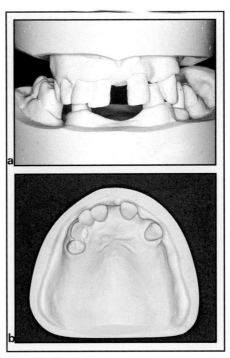

Figure 15.14 Periodontal destruction: (a) study casts demonstrate occlusal collapse and periodontal deterioration, (b) occlusal view of upper arch illustrates labial drift of incisors

that the incisors and the upper right first premolar should be extracted, but that the canines should be retained as overdenture abutments. After the canines have been root-treated successfully, prosthetic treatment can be commenced. It is important to ensure that the impression covers the maximum denture-bearing area and that the shape of the functional sulcus in the labial area is accurately recorded. Because the guiding influence of posterior teeth has long been lost, the jaw relationship is recorded with the mandible in the retruded contact position. After the try-in, the cast is prepared for the immediate overdenture. The teeth to be extracted are moved from the cast and the ridge is prepared. Each canine tooth is then shaped so that the apex of the dome is approximately 3 mm above the level of the gingival margin (Fig. 15.15). A measurement of this height may be recorded with dividers. The artificial teeth are then added in the conventional manner.

At the appointment when the denture is to be fitted, the canine teeth are prepared so that the apex of the dome is approximately 2 mm

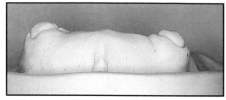

Figure 15.15 Domed preparation of canines as root abutments

above the level of the gingival margin. Use of dividers and reference to the previous measurement will help guide the preparation. The tooth surface is smoothed and an amalgam or glass-ionomer cement restoration placed in the root canal. The remaining teeth are then extracted and the denture fitted. One day later the denture is checked and an accurate fit located on the abutment teeth. This is done by cutting a vent-hole in the denture (Fig. 15.16), placing a mix of cold-curing acrylic resin in the appropriate area of the denture before seating it in the mouth and re-establishing correct occlusal contact. The vent-hole allows most of the excess resin to escape. Relief for the gingival tissues around the newly-prepared abutment must be provided by removing the cold-curing acrylic resin that forms a negative replica of the gingival crevice around the abutment. Subsequent recall visits follow routinely.

The conversion of existing dentures

An existing partial denture can be converted into an overdenture by adding teeth, using conventional laboratory techniques. The abutment teeth may be prepared before an impression is taken with the denture in situ, or

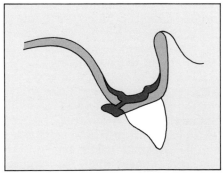

Figure 15.16 Use of cold-curing acrylic resin to refine fitting surface of immediate overdenture

the immediate procedures described above can be adopted.

An alternative approach is a chairside conversion. In the example shown in Figure 15.17, the remaining lower canine teeth have been root-treated. An impression is taken of the arch with the partial denture in situ using silicone putty; the denture is left in the impression. The teeth are then prepared as overdenture abutments. Tooth-coloured cold-curing acrylic resin is poured into the impressions of the canines (Fig. 15.18) and the impression and denture are then reseated in the mouth. Once the resin has cured, the denture is removed from the silicone putty and the new artificial crowns are polished. A labial flange may be added by adapting a cold-curing butyl methacrylate resin directly in the mouth.

The inclusion of magnetic retentive devices

Retentive devices are usually provided only when a conventional overdenture has been found to lack adequate retention. An example is shown in Figure 15.19, where the preservation of abutment teeth has created a ridge

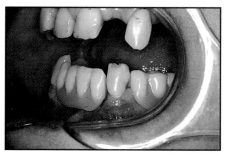

Figure 15.17 In this case the partial denture already replaces all the teeth in the lower jaw with the exception of the canines which have been root-treated and will be prepared as root abutments

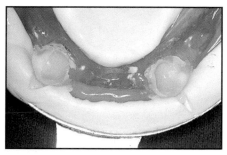

Figure 15.18 Partial denture converted to complete overdenture. Cold-curing resin adapted to root faces of the abutment teeth

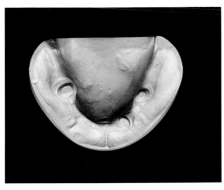

Figure 15.19 The preservation of abutments has retained undercuts especially on the lingual aspect

which is markedly undercut in certain regions. Because the flanges of the denture could not engage this depth of undercut, the patient experienced some loss of retention. The root faces of the abutment teeth were covered by gold copings in which were placed stainless steel keepers (Fig. 15.20). When fitting the denture, the magnets were placed on the keepers, cold-curing resin was placed in previously created cavities in the denture and the denture was localized in the mouth. An alternative approach is to construct the coping in an alloy which itself is attracted to the magnet (see Fig. 15.11).

Problems

Overdenture abutment teeth are at risk of:

- Carious attack of the root face
- Periodontal disease
- Infection of the pulp or pulpal remnants.

Caries and periodontal disease are the most

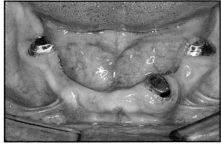

Figure 15.20 Root abutments restored with gold copings and stainless steel keepers

significant risks, because the abutment teeth spend much of their time covered by a denture. There have been a number of studies of the prevalence of caries and although it is difficult to make close comparison because of differing experimental protocols, a summary of the results (Table 15.1) clearly indicates the level of risk.

A comparison of the various studies into the prevalence of periodontal disease is also difficult to make. However, reports, from different studies, of obvious inflammation occurring around 12% of abutment teeth after three years, around 21.2% of abutment teeth after 5 years, and of gingival bleeding around all teeth after four years, emphasise the problem.

Prevention and maintenance

The chief precaution to be taken is the selection of suitable patients, with motivation and the ability to respond to advice on prevention. Subsequent measures are as follows:

- Plaque control of teeth
- Plaque control of the overdenture
- Dietary advice
- Fluoride treatment
- Maintenance of abutment teeth
- Maintenance of overdentures.

Plaque control

Teeth

Although the smooth, simple shape of the abutment teeth should be easy to clean, it

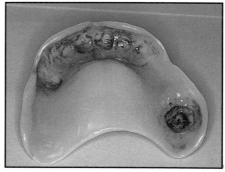

Figure 15.21 Application of disclosing solution to overdenture reveals inadequate plaque removal, especially around the molar abutment (illustration reproduced from *The Dental Annual, 1988*, courtesy Butterworths)

Table 15.1 Prevalence of caries in overdenture adutment teeth

Survey	Duration (years)	No. of patients	Caries prevalence (%)
Fenton and Hahn[4]	1.3	17	15.2
Toolson and Smith[5]	2	74	19
Davis et al.[6]	2	11	20
Ettinger et al.[7]	5	44	13.6
Renner et al.[8]	4	7	35.7
Hussey and Linden[9]	3	40	22

must be remembered that the state of the remaining dentition is the result of previous neglect and that the elderly patient may have difficulty in seeing the tooth surface. Careful instruction in plaque control must be given and frequent checks should be made on the patient's performance.

Overdentures

The shape of the impression surface of an overdenture may present obstacles to efficient plaque control. It is sensible to monitor the level of care by using a disclosing solution on the denture surface (Fig. 15.21). Normal brushing techniques should be backed up with the regular use of a proprietary hypochlorite denture cleanser.

Dietary advice

Bearing in mind that elderly patients may be inclined to eat more of the cheaper carbohydrates, it is important to warn them of the inevitable danger of frequent ingestion of cariogenic foods when the tooth surface is living in a sheltered environment under an overdenture.

Fluoride treatment

Previous studies have shown the beneficial effect of fluoride treatment in reducing the level of caries in overdenture abutment teeth. The daily use of fluoride toothpaste goes without saying, but this measure should be backed up with the regular application of a fluoride varnish at the maintenance visits and with the use of a proprietary fluoride rinse. A weekly rinse with a product containing 0.2% sodium fluoride is a regimen which will be acceptable to most elderly patients.

Maintenance of abutment teeth

Carious attack of the root face may be treated either with a carefully contoured amalgam or glass-ionomer cement restoration or with a gold coping. It is our view that a coping should be provided only when a concave surface, arising from a previous restoration, from cervical erosion or from parafunction has to be corrected, when the abutment teeth are opposed by natural teeth in a patient who indulges in occlusal parafunction, or when it has been decided to enhance retention by the use of an attachment or magnet. In any event we prefer to wait for several months after the overdenture has been fitted to allow the position of the gingival tissue to stabilize before contemplating such a restoration.

Maintenance of overdentures

One of the more common types of complete overdentures is the lower which covers canine abutment teeth. Such a denture is not dissimilar in concept to a bilateral free-end partial denture. Although the abutment teeth reduce the rate and amount of bone resorption, particularly anteriorly, there is the possibility of resorption occurring in the molar region, with the result that an antero-posterior rock is created. Unless this movement is corrected by rebasing the denture, undue stress will be applied to the denture-bearing tissues, further resorption will be encouraged and the abutment teeth may become mobile.

References

1 Tallgren A., The continuing reduction of the residual alveolar ridges in complete denture wearers: a mixed-longitudinal study covering 25 years, *J. Prosthet. Dent. 1972*: 27; 120–32

2 Crum R.J., Rooney G.E., Alveolar bone loss in overdentures: a five-year study, *J. Prosthet. Dent. 1978*; 40: 610–13

3 Todd J.E., Loder D., *Adult Dental Health: United Kingdom*, London, HMSO 1988

4 Fenton A.H., Hahn N., Tissue response to overdenture therapy, *J. Prosthet. Dent. 1978*; 40: 492–8

[a]Zest anchor: APM Sterngold, Attleboro, MA 02703, USA
[b]Dyna magnet: Dyna Dental Engineering, Bergen-op-zoom, Netherlands

5 Toolson L.B., Smith D.E., A two-year longitudinal study of overdenture patients. Part I: Incidence and control of caries on overdenture abutments, *J. Prosthet. Dent. 1978*; 40· 491

6 Davis R.K., Renner R.P., Antos E.W., Schlissel E.R , Baer P.N., A two-year longitudinal study of the periodontal health status of overdenture patients, *J. Prosthet. Dent. 1982*; 45: 358–63

7 Ettinger R.L., Taylor T.D., Scandrett F.R., Treatment needs of overdenture patients in a longtudinal study: five-year results, *J. Prosthet. Dent. 1984*; 52: 532–7

8 Renner R.P., Gomes B.C., Shakun M.L., Braer P.N., Davis R.K. Camp P., Four-year longitudinal study of the periodontal health status of overdenture patients, *J. Prosthet. Dent. 1984*; 51: 593–8

9 Hussey D.L., Linden G.J., The efficacy of overdentures in clinical practice, *Br. Dent. J. 1986*; 161: 104–7

Further reading

Basker R.M., Harrison A., Ralph J.P., Watson C.J., *Overdentures in general dental practice*, 3rd edn, British Dental Association, 1993

Preiskel H.W., *Precision attachments in prosthodontics: overdentures and telescopic prostheses*, vol. 2. Quintessence, Chicago, 1985

16

Full dentures for the ageing patient

David Murray

The aim of the dentist will be that his or her patient should retain a functional natural dentition throughout life. Nevertheless, at least in the near and mid-future, some of our older patients will require the provision or the replacement of full dentures.

Introduction

The provision of complete dentures requires a team effort on the part of the dentist, the technician and the patient. The dentist must make a diagnosis, formulate a treatment plan, undertake the clinical work, and monitor the result. The technician must interpret the prescription. The success of the patient in adapting to a new prosthesis will relate to their ability to learn, to their muscular skills and to their motivation. These qualities may well be reduced in the old person.

The edentulous ageing patient

There is a continuing trend for an increase in the number of people who retain some teeth.[1] Notwithstanding, it is anticipated that by the end of the century, approximately 10% of the population will be edentulous.

It is important to be aware of the profound changes which occur in both the oro-facial tissues and the central nervous system as a result of ageing and pathology.[2] These changes are discussed more fully in earlier chapters. It is the biological age, rather than the chronological age[3] that is important in the context of complete dentures, and which may influence both the treatment planning and the prognosis for the satisfactory management of a prosthesis.

Ageing in the oro-facial region

Facial tissues

Age changes in the facial tissues produce wrinkling of the skin (Fig. 16.1) which can make difficult the estimation of the correct lip support of a new prosthesis. It is impossible to eliminate all these wrinkles. Consequently, the naso-labial angle is a more useful guide to correct lip support.

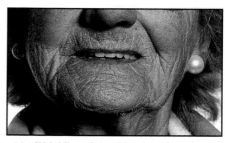

Figure 16.1 Wrinkling of the skin of the face due to ageing

The denture-bearing tissues

The denture-bearing tissues consist of bone covered with mucosa of varying thickness and compressibility. In most areas of the mouth there is no underlying fatty tissue to undergo degeneration. The submucosa will be affected by the coarsening of collagen fibres and the reduced elasticity that is seen throughout the bodily connective tissues. These alterations in the submucosa are probably responsible for some of the clinically recognizable changes in mucosal elasticity, and its apparent thinning.

Alveolar bone is lost in the period following extraction of the teeth at a rate which varies with individuals. The height of the anterior mandible is reduced by four times that recorded in the maxilla.[4] One result of mandibular alveolar resorption is that patients may be left with a flat or even a concave alveolar ridge so that the muscle attachments that are sited on basal bone become superficially placed and obtrusive. Surgical correction may be necessary in order to extend the usable denture-bearing area (see Chapter 18).

Muscles and temporo-mandibular joint

The oral musculature undergoes a reduction in bulk as well as in the number of functional motor units.[5] Arthritic changes and deterioration of the meniscus of the temporo-mandibular joint have been described.[6] It is unclear whether these are age changes or a consequence of local trauma or systemic disease.

Saliva

In order to achieve the best conditions for denture retention it is necessary to have an adequate volume of saliva, of medium viscosity, which can be reduced to a very thin film by normal intra-oral forces. Diminution of salivary secretion will make denture wearing more difficult.

Current evidence suggests that ageing by itself is not responsible for a reduction in salivary flow. However, many elderly people take medication or have a concurrent systemic disease which impairs salivary function[3,7] and which may lead to dry mouth. A reduction in the function of the taste buds will also tend to increase the problem of satisfactory denture wearing.

The mechanisms of denture wearing

If a first complete denture is to be accepted, the patient must learn to accommodate the bulk of a prosthesis in place of their natural dentition. Most people are able to surmount this hurdle and learn to master the altered muscular activity that is required for the use of dentures. They will also come to terms with the reduced masticatory efficiency that ensues. However, the adaptation is more difficult for old people, as a result of a reduction in the skills of remembering, the speed of reasoning, and short-term learning abilities.

It is impossible to predict whether a person will be capable of adapting to complete dentures. The greatest caution must, therefore, be exercised before taking the irrevocable decision to extract all the remaining natural teeth. Consideration should be given to the alternatives of rendering the patient edentulous. The advantages and disadvantages of transitional dentures, overdentures and immediate dentures must be fully explored with the patient.

Transitional (trainer) dentures

In an ageing individual, especially one who has had little or no experience of the use of partial dentures, there are advantages in making temporary use of mobile teeth as abutments for partial acrylic dentures retained by wrought wire clasps. Such prostheses serve two functions. First, they allow the few remaining teeth to stabilize the denture, and so aid chewing. They give the patient time to acquire the skills necessary to control the appliance, as well as adapting to the new patterns of speech. Second, they can be converted gradually into complete dentures as the abutment teeth fail, by the immediate addition of individual teeth. Such dentures are referred to as transitional or trainer dentures (Fig. 16.2). Most patients adapt readily to transitional dentures, and having done so can usually convert to complete dentures without major problems.

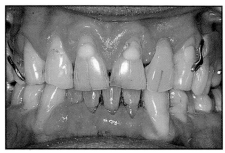

Figure 16.2 A transitional or trainer partial denture with simple stainless steel clasps

Overdentures

The use of overdentures may also help the older patient to adapt to the prosthesis.[8] The retention of some roots offers the advantages of increased support and proprioception, as well as the maintenance of some alveolar bone around the abutment teeth.

The first denture

Circumstances will arise when extractions are inevitable and where partial dentures arc not possible. Alternatively, the patient, either for medical reasons or simply as a result of personal preference, may opt for what is thought by them to be the simple solution of a clearance, followed by a waiting period to allow resorption to take place. This course of action incurs several major disadvantages. These include tongue enlargement, the development of imprecise mandibular movements, and the loss of all natural landmarks to aid with denture design (Fig. 16.3). It is important, therefore, that the patient should be counselled carefully before embarking on this line of treatment.

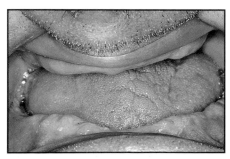

Figure 16.3 The edentulous mouth, demonstrating tongue spread and a loss of natural anatomical landmarks

Treatment planning and denture design

Having taken a history, and carried out a clinical examination, it is necessary to draw up a definitive treatment plan.

Extension of the denture

The upper denture-bearing area is approximately twice the size of the lower, consequently, loading forces are likely to cause more discomfort in the lower jaw. The upper denture should be designed to provide maximum coverage, particularly over the tuberosities and by distal extension on the palate to the compressible tissue just anterior to the vibrating line.

It is even more important that the lower denture be extended to its maximum usable limit. The distal extension should extend on to the so-called 'pear-shaped pad' at the distal ends of the residual ridge (Fig. 16.4). The flanges of the lower denture should extend disto-lingually to the full depth and width of the lingual pouch, with proper allowance being given for elevation of the mylohyoid muscle during swallowing. Where there is little or no alveolar ridge remaining, these vertically directed flanges offer stability to the denture base.

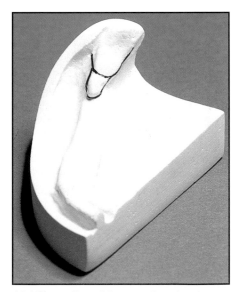

Figure 16.4 The outline of the pear-shaped and retromolar pads on a lower working cast. The pear-shaped pad is anterior to the retromolar pad

Ridge shape and form

Lower jaw

Mandibular atrophy may result in a small residual alveolar ridge in which the remaining tissue is composed almost entirely of fibrous tissue (Fig. 16.5). Resorption is an ongoing process, and it is advisable periodically to examine the fitting surface of full dentures. It will often be observed that there is a disparity in the reverse morphologies of the fit surface of the denture and of the alveolar ridge against which it should adapt. Much of the load that was once transmitted by the fit surface of the denture to the alveolar ridge is now transmitted by the flanges of the denture. The 'redundant or unemployed' ridge no longer supports the prosthesis (Fig. 16.6). In these circumstances it is sensible, when remaking the denture, to consider the use of one of the several impression techniques which compress the tissues at the periphery of the denture but which do not load the crest of the ridge.[9,10] Failure to do this often results in complaints of pain which suggests that the crest of the ridge is no longer capable of being loaded.

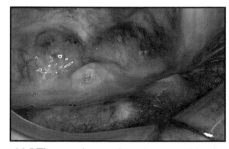

Figure 16.5 The anterior portion of an atrophic mandible. Note the prominent genial tubercles, rising above the residual alveolus in the mid-line

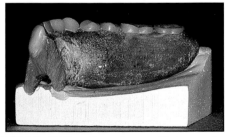

Figure 16.6 A section through an old lower denture, placed on a plaster cast of the patient's alveolus. Note the discrepancy between the fitting surface of the denture and the plaster cast

Upper jaw

The most common support problem seen in the upper jaw is the so-called 'flabby ridge', which may extend over the whole arch to include the maxillary tuberosities. It is, however, most commonly seen in the anterior region, classically under a complete denture opposed by natural teeth.

Surgical removal of the flabby fibrous tissue is relatively easy, but the procedure may result in an unacceptably reduced ridge, and scarring can make the post-surgical condition more difficult to treat than was the original one. Some authorities recommend a simultaneous sulcoplasty to deepen the labial sulcus to overcome this problem but this option should be used only if it is felt that the need for stability of the denture is overwhelming.[11] Recent work in which flabby ridges are treated surgically by augmentation with hydroxyapatite has reported encouraging results.

The condition is dealt with prosthetically by recording an impression of the ridge in such a way as not to displace or distort the flabby area. This may be achieved by using a loose-fitting tray spaced by about 3 mm, and by recording the impression using a fluid material such as a low viscosity alginate or impression plaster. Alternatively, a two-stage technique can be used. Here, a preliminary impression is recorded in a stock tray using alginate, and on the resulting cast a special close-fitting self-cure acrylic tray (0.6 mm space) is constructed. A window is cut in the tray in the area of flabby tissue, so that when the tray is placed this area is left uncovered (Fig. 16.7). The borders of the tray are corrected, and an impression is recorded of the firm areas of the ridge using a mucocompressive material such

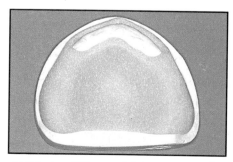

Figure 16.7 A close-fitting special tray, cut away from the flabby area of the ridge to permit a two-stage impression technique

as zinc oxide/eugenol. Any material that flows into the window area is excised with a scalpel, and the impression is reinserted (with the patient placed in the supine position). A mucostatic impression is then made of the area of flabby tissue left uncovered through the window in the tray, by applying a thin mix of impression plaster with a spatula.[12]

The mental nerve and mental foramen

Mandibular resorption can result in the mental foramen and nerve lying on the surface of the alveolus, causing pain when the patient closes his/her teeth together. Several techniques are available to overcome this problem. The simplest is to tin foil the lower cast in the areas of the foramina, or to use a localized box-shaped relief in the denture.

Recourse is often made in this clinical situation to one of the permanent acrylic or silicone soft lining materials. The rationale for their use is simply to avoid direct pressure over the mental nerve by the hard denture base. A more common indication for the use of such linings is, however, where there are ridge irregularities or other bony prominences, covered by thin mucosa. The lack of sufficiently thick and resilient tissue is compensated for by the resiliency of the lining material. If this line of treatment is to be successful it is imperative that the dentures should be correctly balanced with respect to both muscular and occlusal forces. Sufficient saliva should be present to provide lubrication and so allow for any slight movements of the lower denture which may occur.

The best solution to the problem is probably the tin foiling of the cast prior to processing, and the provision of a high polish to the fitting surface of the denture.

Design of a prosthesis

Free way space

Whether the approximation of the mandible to the maxilla seen in the elderly edentulous patient is due solely to age changes in the tissues, or is in part an adaptive response, is unclear. Whatever, any attempt to restore the vertical dimension to so-called classical proportions is unlikely to succeed and it is advisable to allow an old person rather more free way space (4–5 mm) than would be used in the treatment of someone younger.

Occlusion

The occlusion of the artificial teeth should be arranged so as to give a wide range of balance during functional movements of the jaws, including protrusion.

The use of shallow-cusped teeth is recommended because they are said to facilitate movement between centric and eccentric occlusal contacts and thus reduce the risk of creating forces which would produce displacement of the denture bases. Narrow posterior teeth are also indicated because this allows greater tongue space and the easier production of favourable polished surface shapes.

Stable bases to the wax rims must be used when registering the occlusion. In this context permanent bases are ideal, offering the prospect of accurate registration and assessment of the trial tooth arrangement. They are however sometimes contra-indicated, not only on the grounds of cost, but also because it is necessary either to complete the dentures using self-cure acrylic, or to risk a second cure which may produce warpage of the base. Warpage of the upper dentures is likely to adversely affect the post-dam seal. Well-fitting shellac bases will suffice if properly used.

Muscle function

Fish conclusively demonstrated that a patient is given the best possible opportunity to adapt successfully to a new prosthesis if the polished surface of the denture is properly shaped.[13] These surfaces should be modelled into a series of inclined planes, each of which presents itself to the muscle with which it comes into contact, at such an angle that when the muscle moves it pushes the denture into place. It is also necessary to position the teeth so as to provide maximum space for the tongue.

The immediate replacement denture

The transition from the dentate to the edentulous state can be made easier by the provision of immediate replacement dentures. In many instances these dentures should be designed so that the denture teeth occupy the same spatial relationship as their natural predecessors. However, when chronic periodontal disease has resulted in drifting and splaying of the natural anterior teeth it is often more appropriate to correct the position of these teeth on the immediate denture. A patient is more likely to accept an explanation that correction of markedly proclined teeth is necessary to achieve denture stability, at this stage, rather than later, when the definitive dentures are being made.

The replacement denture

The statement has been made that 'complete denture wearing in the context of time exerts a biological price from the tissues that support the prosthesis'.[14] More concisely, dentures can cause damage.

A time will come in the life of a denture when its deficiencies cannot continue to be remedied by modification. It will need to be replaced. If it is not, damage will be done, including the development of denture-induced stomatitis, denture-induced hyperplasia and alveolar resorption.

If a patient can manage complete dentures satisfactorily, then they should be able to adapt to replacement dentures. Regular review of complete dentures is a relatively uncommon practice. Many denture wearers attend their dentist only when they become aware of faults in their dentures that are becoming unacceptable. Looseness, repeated bouts of soreness, or the inability to chew satisfactorily are the most usual reasons for seeking professional advice. It is common to see gross wear of the occlusal surfaces of dentures, which combined with resorption of the alveolar ridges has produced an unacceptable reduction in occlusal face height and a gross change in facial appearance (Fig. 16.8). Surprisingly, such dentures are often well tolerated. This is probably because the occlusal wear and alveolar resorption has occurred so gradually that the patient's reflex patterns have been able to adapt to the changes produced.

In such cases most of the retention and stability of the denture comes from the control exerted by the oral musculature on the polished surfaces.[13] Significantly, these patients

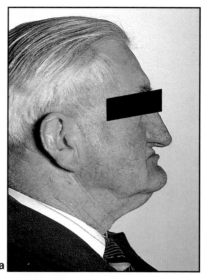
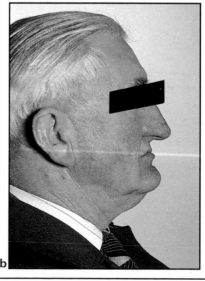

Figure 16.8 Gross change in facial appearance: (a) occlusal wear on the complete dentures has led to a gross reduction in occlusal face height, with relative apparent protrusion of the mandible, (b) the facial profile subsequent to correction of the occlusal wear, using a copy technique, with an inter-occlusal wax wafer to restore the vertical dimension

manage to function with such dentures, albeit at a reduced level of efficiency. They have been able, subconsciously, to adapt to the position of the teeth, the shape of the polished surfaces and the nature and timing of tooth contacts. Wearing the dentures has become a reflex rather than a conscious effort. If an attempt is made to make new dentures using 'conventional' techniques, disregarding the basic design of the old dentures, then failure is likely, because the patient is faced with a task that is too demanding for their declining abilities to cope with.

A successful outcome will usually follow when replacement dentures are constructed utilizing those features of the dentures which have proved to be acceptable to the patient, modifying only those areas of the prostheses that have caused the patient to seek advice (Fig. 16.9). This is the philosophy behind the 'Copy Technique'. If modifications must be made, they should be within the old person's reduced limit of tolerance.

Copy techniques

Many methods for copying or duplicating dentures have been described.[15-19] Most rely on the production of replica dentures from impressions of the existing dentures, the form of which are used as a basis for the new appliances. The replicas are constructed from a wide variety of materials including self-cure acrylic resin, modelling wax, and various combinations of these two materials.

The production of replicas usually involves the use of flexible moulding materials so that any undercuts that may be present in the old dentures are recorded. Silicon polymers, reversible (agar) and irreversible hydrocolloids (alginate) can be used as the mould impression material. To contain and adequately support the flexible moulding materials numerous types of vessels have been used, both improvised and custom-built.

Experience shows that the most satisfactory type of replica denture is one which has a rigid base, and wax teeth which make the technician's job easier when setting up.

Alginate is commonly used as the investing material, supported in a rigid container such as a modified soap box (Fig. 16.10), or a specially designed aluminium flask (Fig. 16.11). Alternatively, stock impression trays can be used with silicone putty as the investment material of choice (Fig. 16.12). This method has the advantage that it allows a shellac base to be adapted and secured to the

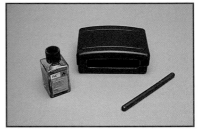

Figure 16.10a A modified soap box used to invest the patient's dentures in alginate

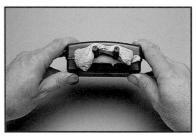

Figure 16.10b A window is cut in the side to provide an exit for the sprues

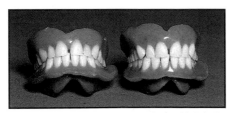

Figure 16.9 Original (left) and duplicate (right) dentures. Modifications were performed to the fitting surface and the teeth. The polished surfaces and the occlusal relationship were left unchanged

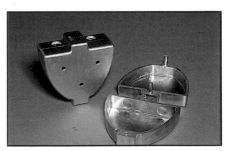

Figure 16.11 Aluminium flask specifically designed for the copy technique. Stainless steel

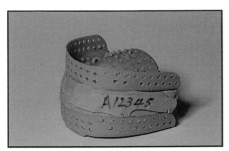

Figure 16.12 Stock impression trays are used with silicone putty to invest the dentures. Sprue holes are cut into the heels of the impression

putty impression material prior to pouring the molten wax to form the polished surfaces and teeth.

The chief indication for the use of a copy technique is that the dentures have in the past been satisfactory, and that the problems that have caused the patient to attend are of recent onset. All the denture surfaces must be carefully examined to enable the operator to decide which features of the prostheses should be modified and which features retained. At this stage it should be possible to decide if a copy technique is feasible.

Careful modifications to the existing denture morphology, during the process of duplication, can greatly improve the retention and stability of the new denture, and will reduce the effort required by the patient to relearn the skills of denture wearing. The fitting, occlusal or polished surfaces can all be so modified, but alterations should be confined to those areas of the dentures that have caused problems.

Fitting surface

The fitting surface is probably the most common site requiring modification to compensate for resorption of the alveolar ridge.

Occlusal surface

Modifications to the occlusal surface are determined by the amount of wear of the existing dentures. Varying amounts of increase in occlusal height may be indicated. Three ways by which such increase can be achieved are as follows:

Minimal wear

When only a small amount of wear has occurred, it may be sufficient to make use of new denture teeth with a similar morphology to that of the originals. This, together with the modest increase in vertical dimension that results from the impression technique, may well restore the occlusal face height to its previously satisfactory level.

Moderate wear

Moderate amounts of wear are best dealt with by incorporating a wax wafer of appropriate thickness between the replica dentures when recording the vertical relationship (Fig. 16.13). The replicas are then articulated using this wax registration. Once this has been done the clinician can then determine how the increase in occlusal face height (OFH) should be distributed between the dentures. If a registration stage is required, the use of the replica dentures as record blocks has been found to have many advantages over conventional blocks with wax rims which are traditionally designed to be oversized to permit trimming.[20] The size and shape of the replicas will be familiar to the patient who will be more likely to give a correct registration than with a bulky block.

Severe wear

When a considerable amount of wear has occurred the increase in occlusal face height necessary to restore the vertical dimension should be established by adding cold-cure acrylic resin to the occlusal surfaces of the existing prostheses (Fig. 16.14). The additions are made in small increments over the space of a few days or weeks, ensuring that the patient's adaptive capacity is never exceeded. Once the patient has adapted to the modified prostheses the dentures can be duplicated at the increased vertical dimension.

It is important when constructing complete dentures for an elderly patient to look carefully for any wear patterns which may be present in the old dentures. Wear not uncommonly produces free sliding movements in articulation: such patterns must be copied. If they are not the patient may experience problems in eating.

Figure 16.13 (a) An interocclusal wax wafer between acrylic replicas, prior to try-in. (b) The increase in vertical dimension is being divided evenly between the replicas as the denture teeth are set up on the replicas. The casts have been removed from their articulator to improve the clarity of the illustration

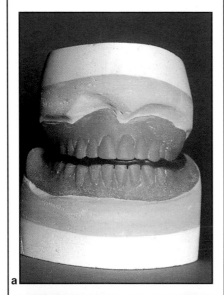

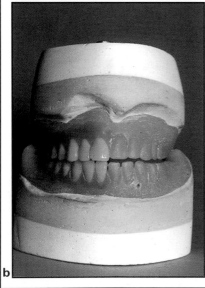

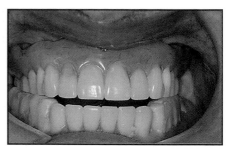

Figure 16.14 Temporary increase in the vertical dimension using self-cure acrylic resin on the occlusal surface of the posterior teeth of the patient's existing dentures. This technique is used to establish a satisfactory vertical dimension prior to duplication

extended originally, and resorption has occurred, then the borders of the denture will have become overextended. In this situation, it is necessary to trim away any overextension on the replica denture. It is inadvisable to carry out this procedure on the existing dentures, lest the practitioner is blamed for spoiling their fit! It is a good general rule not to extend a denture that is theoretically underextended, provided that the long-standing underextension has not been detrimental.[21] This rule is particularly appropriate to the distolingual area of a lower denture. An elderly patient will often be unable to tolerate in this area a flange which has been newly extended to a theoretically correct position.

Areas of underextension that require correction can be dealt with by modifying the patient's existing denture with low-fusing tracing compound (green-stick) prior to duplication. This can then easily and quickly be removed from the dentures after duplication, without causing any damage.

Old people will often request that the denture be 'built up' so as to support the upper lip and remove facial wrinkles. This can be achieved either by alteration of the tooth position, or by an increase in bulk of the labial polished surface (Fig. 16.15). The latter approach has the advantage that a temporary addition of wax or of green-stick can be placed as a 'trial'. The result can then be assessed by the patient, in respect of the appearance; and by the operator, in terms of retention and stability.

The use of copy techniques has long been recognized as ideally suited to the hospital environment where in-house laboratory facilities are readily available. There is evidence to

Polished surfaces

Modifications to the polished surfaces will include alterations to the periphery of the denture. If the existing dentures were correctly

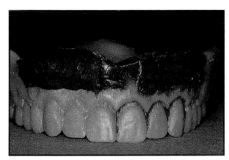

Figure 16.15 An upper replica denture with additions of green-stick and wax to illustrate one method of improving lip support

suggest that the value of this type of treatment is becoming recognized in general practice, particularly for domiciliary treatment.

There are many reputable methods for copying dentures, all employing the same basic principles. The copy technique must not be regarded by either the dentist or the technician as a short cut to denture construction, where little care is needed. Unless the decision to use the method is based on a sound diagnosis, and the clinical and technical procedures are undertaken with the greatest care, the treatment is likely to fail.[21] The method described below has been in regular use at Newcastle Dental Hospital for the last eight years, and is extensively undertaken in NHS practice.

First clinical stage

After carrying out a thorough clinical examination of the patient, and an analysis of their dentures, a treatment plan is formulated. Those features of the existing dentures which are to be retained are identified, and areas in which modifications are to be made are noted. If a clinical decision has been made to compensate for any moderate occlusal wear of the existing artificial teeth, then an interocclusal wax record of appropriate thickness should be taken at this stage and stored for use later.

The upper and lower dentures are duplicated separately. The shapes of the polished, occlusal and fitting surfaces of the dentures to be copied are recorded using alginate impression material inside two-part duplicating boxes.

The duplicating box (Fig. 16.11) is of aluminium construction, and the two halves fit accurately together by means of stainless steel locating pins both front and rear. The base of the box has two holes at the rear, one to act as a pouring hole, the other as an escape hole. The top of the box is provided with holes to allow escape of excess impression material.

Sufficient alginate is used to fill the lower half of the box and the denture is inserted into the mould teeth first. Care must be taken to prevent the formation of air blows. The alginate is allowed to set and is then trimmed with a wax knife so that 2–3 mm of the border and all the fitting surface of the denture are exposed. Once set, Vaseline is applied to the surfaces of the alginate to prevent mechanical locking and water loss (Fig. 16.16). A second mix of alginate is prepared and the majority is used to fill the upper half of the box, whilst the remainder is applied to the fitting surface of the denture in order to avoid trapping air when the flask is closed. The top of the flask is guided down into position on the lower using the locating pins, the surplus alginate escaping through the holes placed for that purpose. When set, the surplus alginate is trimmed, the boxes opened, the dentures removed and the moulds checked for accuracy. After consulting with the patient as to the mould and shade of tooth to be used, the dentures are returned to the patient and a further appointment made. The moulds are closed and if there is to be any delay in pouring the replicas the duplicating boxes should be kept moist and stored in self-seal polythene bags.

The production of the impressions is easily undertaken by a dental nurse or technician. The patient needs only be without their dentures for about 20 minutes whilst this process is carried out.

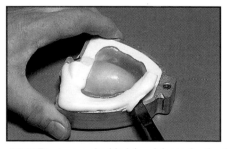

Figure 16.16 Denture embedded in alginate in the lower half of the flask. A wax knife is used to trim the excess alginate so that 2–3 mm of the border and all the fitting surface is exposed

First laboratory stage

The moulds are opened and examined. A tubular stainless steel sprue cutter is used to cut a pouring hole and an escape hole through the holes provided in the box into the polished surface side of the mould (Fig. 16.17). Before closing the moulds the surface of the alginate should be thoroughly dried with either compressed air or paper towelling because retained moisture can be the cause of inaccuracies in the resulting replicas. Self-cure acrylic resin is mixed in the proportion of 30/35 g resin to 15 ml monomer and is vibrated into the mould. Pouring should cease when acrylic can be seen near the surface of the escape hole. The moulds are left until the acrylic polymerizes. The moulds are then opened and the self-cure replicas with their attached sprues are removed without damaging the alginate. The two halves of the mould are then re-sealed and dental stone or plaster poured to produce plaster replicas. These will be used by the clinician and the technician (Fig. 16.18).

The sprues attached to the acrylic replicas are removed and the occlusal and fitting sur-faces of the replicas are checked for any roughness or pimples, which are removed. Any undercuts in the fit surfaces are blocked out using wet paper and base casts poured. The replica dentures are then mounted on an articulator. Various type of articulators can be used for this technique ranging from the simple hinge to the fully adjustable articulator. The plasterless articulator and the average value articulator (Rational) are suitable.

If an inter-occlusal record has been used, it is incorporated when mounting the replicas (see Fig. 16.13). The clinician must decide how the increase in OFH should be distributed between the dentures.

It is important at this stage to search for wear patterns in the old dentures. These should be replicated. When only a small amount of wear has occurred, it may be sufficient to make use of new denture teeth with a similar morphology to that of the originals. This, together with the modest increase in vertical dimension that results from the impression technique, may well restore the occlusal face height to its previously satisfactory level.

The replica teeth are carefully removed from their base either singly, which is the safest, or in sections if the technician is skilled. The replacement teeth are waxed to the base using the replicated plaster models as a reference when necessary.

Before final waxing up is completed, the upper denture is removed from the cast and two slots are cut through the palate as shown in Figure 16.19. These slots should extend to within 2 mm of the posterior border and leave 2 mm of intact resin anteriorly. These slots are

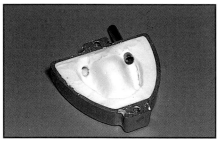

Figure 16.17 A tubular sprue cutter is used to cut pouring and escape holes in the polished surface of the mould

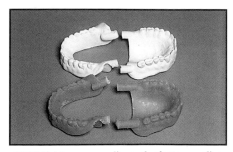

Figure 16.18 Cold-cure acrylic and plaster replicas with sprues attached

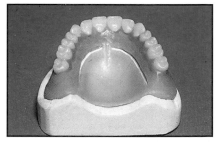

Figure 16.19 Slots are cut through the palate as shown to enable a single thickness palate to be adapted after the impressions are recorded in the replicas. The slots are filled with wax

filled with wax prior to the try-in stage. Their function is to allow the acrylic palate and underlying impression material to be cut and prised away from the plaster base that will be cast at the next laboratory stage. If this is not done, the new palate will be unduly thick.

Second clinical stage

The replica dentures are tried in the patient's mouth. Any errors in occlusion or tooth position must be corrected and modifications made to the borders if necessary. If the existing borders were originally correctly extended and resorption has occurred, then the borders of the dentures will have become over-extended and it will be necessary to trim away any overextension on the replica denture.

When the trial dentures are judged satisfactory, all undercuts present in the fit surfaces of the replicas must be removed by the clinician in order to prevent damage or fracture of the major casts at the flasking stage. Removal of undercuts not infrequently leads to the production of a knife edge along the border of the denture. In order to compensate for this and to produce a rolled border on the finished denture, carding wax can be placed as shown in Figure 16.15. The wax acts as a matrix over which the impression material can be adapted when muscle trimming is carried out. Care must be taken when recording the impressions not to allow the borders to become over-extended.

The fitting surface is probably the most common site requiring modification to compensate for resorption of the alveolar ridge. This may be done by using a low-viscosity wash impression taken within the replica dentures. It is best performed using a closed mouth technique, so as to ensure that no unwanted alteration to the vertical dimension or the horizontal relationship occurs.

The use of a closed mouth technique allows minor occlusal errors to be adjusted.[22] The impression materials of choice are zinc oxide/eugenol paste, or low-viscosity addition or condensation-cured silicone rubbers (Fig. 16.20). The latter are clean, well tolerated by the patient and can be removed easily from the fit surface of the replica in the laboratory. They are particularly useful for domiciliary work.

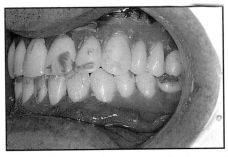

Figure 16.20 A closed mouth impression for the copy technique. Note the low-viscosity condensation-cured silicone rubber impression

When the impression material has set, the replicas are removed from the mouth and the impressions checked for deficiencies. The flange thicknesses should also be compared with those of the existing dentures or the plaster replicas. This comparison will help to detect any movement of the replicas relative to the basal tissues which may have taken place. The width and depth of the post-dam is indicated to the technician and the replicas are returned to the laboratory.

Second laboratory stage

Casts are poured, care being taken whilst trimming to preserve the functional width of the border. Surplus impression material is removed from the teeth and polished surfaces. The dentures are retained on the new casts and the palate and underlying impression material is detached and discarded by cutting through the three 2 mm retaining strips of acrylic (Fig. 16.21). The remaining edges are chamfered and a single thickness wax palate laid down.

The dentures are checked to ensure that no teeth have become loosened during the try-in stage, and the wax of the gingival margins and polished surface are given a final finish.

The replicas are flasked in the standard fashion. If severe tissue undercuts are present, damage to the casts can be prevented by careful tilting when flasking. After flasking, the wax is boiled out and the replica bases are discarded. The flasks are packed and processed by conventional methods, and the resultant dentures trimmed and polished ready for insertion.

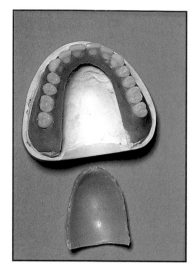

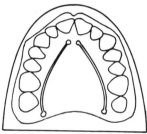

Figure 16.21 Cold-cure palate and impression material removed prior to laying down a single thickness palate

Third clinical stage

The dentures are inserted using the same criteria and techniques as for a denture produced by a conventional replacement technique.

Some reservations have from time to time been expressed about the dimensional accuracy of the replicas produced.[15] A number of workers have shown that it is possible to produce clinically acceptable replicas,[23] using alginate as the investing material, provided it is supported in a rigid container.

Unless major modifications are to be made, only three relatively short clinical visits, well tolerated by the frail patient, are required. It has been found that the use of a copy technique produces fewer requests for denture eases and adjustments than would be anticipated had conventional replacement techniques been used.[24]

The clinical use of a copy technique in the situation of replacing complete dentures for elderly patients has proved its value. It gives an exact method for copying the old dentures, or an exact point of departure for a planned and controlled alteration.[22] However, it must be stressed that the successful use of any denture technique depends on an accurate assessment of the patient and their old dentures. A careful history and examination is required to determine which aspects of the prosthesis should be modified and which should be retained.

Summary

The treatment of the elderly edentulous patient offers a challenge to the practitioner. The provision of complete dentures for this group of people may be difficult and time consuming, and success is not always attainable. It is important to recognize that any changes made to existing prostheses should be made gradually, in order to allow the patient to adapt.

References

1 Todd J.E., Lader D. *Adult dental health 1988 United Kingdom*, HMSO, London: 1991

2 Flint S., Scully C., Orofacial age changes and related disease, *Dental Update 1988*; 15: 337–42

3 Storer R., The effect of the climacteric and of ageing on prosthetic diagnosis and treatment planning, *Br. Dent. J. 1965*; 19: 349–54

4 Tallgren A., The continuing reduction of the alveolar ridge in complete denture wearers: a mixed-longitudinal study covering 25 years, *J. Prosthet. Dent. 1972*; 27: 120–25

5 Drummond J.R., Newton J.P., Yemm R., Dentistry for the elderly: a review and an assessment for the future, *J. Dent. 1988*; 16: 47–54

6 Carlsson G.E., Kopp S., Oberg T., Arthritis and allied diseases of the temporomandibular joint, in: *Temporomandibular joint: function and dysfunction*, eds: G.A. Zarb, G.E. Carlsson, Munksgaard, Copenhagen; 1979

7 Sreebny L.M., Schartz S.S., A reference guide to drugs and dry mouth, *Gerodontology 1986*; 5: 75–99

8 Basker R., Harrison A., Ralph J.P., *Overdentures in general dental practice*, British Dental Association, London 1988

9 Appleby R.C., Technique for difficult lower impressions, *Practical dental monographs 1957*; January, Year Book Publishers Inc., Chicago

10 Watt D.M., McGregor A.R., *Designing complete dentures*; first edition, Saunders, London 1976: 116–18

11 Howe G.L., *Minor oral surgery*; third edition, Wright, Bristol 1985: 287

12 Watson R.M., Impression technique for maxillary fibrous ridge, *Br. Dent. J. 1970*; 128: 552

13 Fish E.W., *Principles of full denture prosthesis*; fourth edition, Staples, London 1948: 30–75

14 Boucher C.O., Hickey J.C., Zarb G.A., *Prosthodontic treatment for edentulous patients*; seventh edition, Mosby, St. Louis 1975: 35–8

15 Cooper J.S., Watkinson A.C., Duplication of full dentures, *Br. Dent. J. 1976*; 141: 344–8

16 Duthie N., Lyon F., Sturrock K.C. *et al.*, A copying technique for replacement dentures, *Br. Dent. J. 1978*; 144: 248–52

17 Davenport J.C., Heath J.R., The copy denture technique, *Br. Dent. J. 1983*; 155: 162–3

18 Duthie N., Yemm R., An alternative method for recording the occlusion of edentulous patients during the construction of replacement dentures, *J. Oral Rehabil. 1985*; 12: 161–71

19 Murray I.D., Wolland A.W., New dentures for old, *Dental Practice 1986*; 24: 1–6

20 Duthie N., Yemm R., New occlusion from old dentures, *Dental Practice 1982*; 20: 1–4

21 Basker R.M., Davenport J.C., Tomlin H.R., *Prosthetic treatment of the edentulous patient*; third edition, McMillan, London 1992: 107–10

22 Farrell J.H., *Full dentures, a personal view*; first edition, Henry Kimpton, London 1976: 25–37 and 53

23 Basker R.M., Heath J.R., The dimensional variability of duplicate dentures produced in an alginate investment, *Brit. Dent. J. 1978*; 144: 111–14

24 Murray I.D., *Proceedings of BSSPD*, British Society for the Study of Prosthetic Dentistry, Leeds 1989

17

The role of osseointegrated dental implants in the treatment of elderly people

Richard Johns

The use of intraosseous implants can be a great help in the treatment of elderly patients who cannot retain their dentures, or who have undergone ablative surgery.

The association of toothlessness with old age is often regarded as an inevitable fact of life and all too frequently it is true. The high incidence of failure of complete dentures for many old people is apparent when visiting homes for the elderly, particularly at meal times.

Many words have been written, books published and reputations made on the design and making of complete dentures. However, one of the fundamental causes of failure is sometimes almost forgotten, namely the abuse to which the mucosal lining of the mouth is subjected. Because of the nature of this tissue and the reduced area of the fitting surface of the lower denture, compared with that of the upper, the inadequacies of the lower denture are usually pre-eminent. It is not difficult to appreciate that the mucous membrane and underlying connective tissue is poorly equipped to resist the trauma of being squeezed between hard plastic on the exterior surface and the bone below. The ability that these tissues have to withstand trauma is known to deteriorate with age, so that with less and less bony support, due to resorption, the unfortunate patient is frequently driven to discarding the lower denture when attempting to eat. To add to the elderly patient's problems there is often a decrease in the amount

of saliva present. This dryness of the mouth not only increases the susceptibility to ulceration but also interferes with the retention of the upper denture. Difficulties such as these are further compounded by the deterioration in muscle control and the associated tremors of old age.

It is a sad observation on the dental profession that the psychological damage which edentulism and inadequate dentures inflict on some patients, particularly but not exclusively the elderly, is often ignored. It is all too easy for dentists to give patients the idea that the problems of complete dentures are a fact of life which has to be accepted as part of being old. It is equally sad to observe that those dentures which are made, often bear no resemblance to the type of dentition which should be consistent with the patient's age. For example, the arrangement of the teeth is frequently standardized on some hypothetical dentition perceived in the mind of the technician. Poor appearance, inadequate retention of and discomfort from their dentures can be extra burdens on an elderly patient who may be trying to cope with the numerous other problems of old age.

Osseointegration

The work of Brånemark and his co-workers on the microcirculation of blood, in the late

1950s,[1] was meticulous and thorough, and led naturally to a study of bone and the reaction of bone to thermal trauma. This work culminated in a paper by Brånemark *et al.*[2] and Lundskog[3] which demonstrated that if a temperature of more than 47 °C is maintained for more than one minute, delayed healing results. The device that they designed to identify this and other *in-vivo* reactions in bone, was made of titanium, a metal noted by Bothe *et al.*[4] in 1940 and Leventhal,[5] in 1951, as being inert in the tissue environment and likely to be suitable as an implant material. It was noticed by Brånemark that when the device came to be removed it had become inextricably attached to the bone. The term that he devised to describe this attachment was 'osseointegration', a description which implies a permanent dynamic relationship between living bone and an inorganic material, which in this instance is the oxide layer which surrounds commercially pure titanium.

The significance of osseointegration was soon realized and developed by Brånemark and his team (1969).[2,6] They devised and designed numerous applications for surgical techniques which made use of this new-found permanent form of attachment to bone. The concept that an artificial root could be inserted into the jawbone and used as a permanent fixture to support a dental prosthesis had immediate appeal, and was the first application to be developed in detail.

Unlike all other such devices proposed since Maggiolo[9] (1809), the Gothenberg design was tested over periods ranging from 10 years to 17 years prior to the publication of their results in 1981 when Adell reported on over 4000 implants placed in 650 jaws of 600 patients. The individual fixture survival rate over a 10-year period was 81% in the maxilla and 91% in the mandible. The achievement of stable prostheses was 90% and 100% respectively. This success culminated in the American Dental Association Council on Materials and Devices making the following statement in July 1988. 'The Brånemark system is acceptable for use in selected fully edentulous patients. Responsibility for proper selection of patients, for adequate training and experience in the placement of the implant and for providing appropriate information of informed consent rests with the dentist.'

Outline of procedure

The technique which has been evolved by the Brånemark team can be discussed only briefly.

Selection and assessment

There are few absolute contra-indications to treatment. The prospective patient must be psychologically stable and not someone who has unreal expectations. Age in itself is not a barrier provided that it is felt that an operation, either under local or general anaesthesia and lasting up to two hours, is within the patient's physical and mental capability.

A careful assessment must be made of the texture and volume of bone available. This is perhaps the cornerstone of the procedure and demands skill and experience.

Preparation of the implant site

When the mucoperiosteal flap has been raised, the intrabony implant site must be delicately prepared, particular attention being made to keeping the temperature of the bone below that which would interfere with the healing process.

Placement of the implant

A commercially pure titanium implant must be used, the surface oxide layer of which is uncontaminated by any other metal or by protein. The first 'contaminant' of the oxide layer must be the patient's own blood. The implant must exert some pressure on the bone into which it is placed but, initially, must not be subjected to functional loading. The length of time allowed for osseointegration, following this first surgical phase of the procedure, will vary according to the character of the bone. As a general rule, four months is allowed for this interaction to take place in the lower jaw and six months in the upper. During this period no radiographs should be taken and no more than a minimal load should be exerted on the implant by any denture that may be resting upon the overlying mucosa.

Exposure of the implant and connection of an abutment

The second surgical phase of the procedure is the exposure of the osseointegrated implant and the attachment of an abutment. Thus, a permanent connection has been established between the mouth and the underlying jaw bone. It is on to this abutment that a prosthesis may now be attached. Provided that the implant has osseointegrated and is immobile, the downgrowth of the epithelium will not take place. The epithelium appears to form a weak attachment to the abutment, but one which can function indefinitely.

Provision of the prosthesis

Construction of the prosthesis may be started as soon as the sutures are removed following the second surgical stage (Figs 17.1–17.4). The design of the prosthesis must take account of the length of each implant and the character of the bone in which it is placed. The exact parameters of loading individual implants are not yet known but clearly they must be related to the total area of osseointegration as well as the loading pattern which

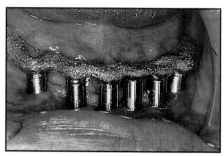

Figure 17.2 Cast gold (Stabilor G, manufactured by Degusa) bar which must fit abutments exactly. This bar provides rigid support for the bridge – note the distal cantilever design and abutment length of approximately 12 mm

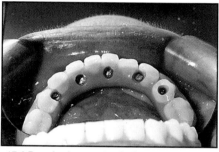

Figure 17.3 Prosthesis retained by screws embedded within the bridge. After appropriate tightening these are sealed within the structure

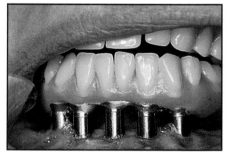

Figure 17.4 Labial view of prosthesis after 4 years in use. Note the incisal edges of the artificial teeth are placed where their natural predecessors would have been. There is wide clearance below the bridge to allow for cleaning

can be expected. It is reasonable to expect that four or five implants, ten millimetres in length, placed in the anterior region of the mandible and extending to the lower border, will be sufficient to support a prosthesis from the second premolar bilaterally. Where the support of an implant is not ideal, either because there is inadequate bone or the bone is less dense in character, there is a risk of

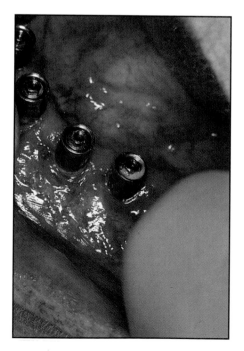

Figure 17.1 Abutment fixtures prior to impression being taken. Parallelism of implants to one another is not required

overloading. This is likely to result in either the failure of the implant to integrate, or the progressive loss of osseointegration once the implant has become integrated but is subjected to excessive functional loading. Failure is complete when all contact between the implant and the bone is lost and replaced by fibrous tissue.

As yet, the limitations of loading individual implants or those rigidly attached to one another are not known. One factor, however, which will lead to failure is the imperfect fit of a prosthesis upon its abutment. This causes a sustained force to be placed upon the various components of the implant itself as well as the bone/implant surface.

The benefits of permanent implant fixtures

With the possibility of the direct attachment of a prosthesis to the jawbone and the transmission of all functional loads directly from artificial teeth to the bone, not only is the stability of the prosthesis assured but so too is the avoidance of trauma to the soft tissue. For most patients the sensation that the artificial teeth have become an integral part of themselves is apparent as soon as the bridge is attached permanently to the implant fixtures. With this realization comes assurance and relaxation of all the muscles around the mouth. No longer are these muscles continually on guard against inadvertent displacement of the dentures when eating, speaking, coughing or sneezing. Even when the fixtures are placed in only one jaw, patients describe a sense of confidence and comfort. In purely functional terms, too, much is gained. The chewing of food is more effective,[8] and the range of foods which can be eaten is greatly increased. An improvement in taste is often reported, probably as an indication of the effectiveness of the prosthesis in crushing food which itself is associated with the restored pleasures of chewing.

Hygiene

The benefits gained bring obligations, namely, to keep the bridge and its supports clean. For older patients who have been without natural teeth for 20, 30 or 40 years this can be a problem which may be exacerbated by failing sight, impaired manual dexterity, or simply a loss of interest in attending to the demands of personal hygiene. It is of the utmost importance when the possible use of implants is being considered, that these potential difficulties are identified and discussed with the patient. The dentist clearly has a responsibility for both alerting and advising the patient about these considerations.

Partial edentulism

Further development of osseointegrated implant fixtures will provide support for fixed bridge work and will clearly benefit those patients who would otherwise have had to resort to partial dentures.

Because an implant supported bridge, or indeed a single tooth, must function alongside natural teeth, the inequality of their support mechanism must be recognized. The intrusion of a tooth into its socket is not duplicated by the implant supported tooth, and the attachment of one to the other results in stresses being introduced, with the possibility of excessive loads being imposed upon the implant. For this reason, until definitive research has been undertaken, it is prudent to have no more than simple contact between natural teeth and implant supported artificial teeth. Also, the occlusion must be adjusted so that excessive premature contact pressures are not exerted upon the implants.

With careful planning, patients who have some fixtures will be able to make the transition from partial to complete implant supported prostheses with a minimum of inconvenience should they lose more teeth. The problems of the transitional period will depend on the extent of bone loss, both prior to tooth extraction and subsequent to it. This difficulty is likely to be particularly apparent in the upper jaw where fixtures must be placed in sites where a suitable volume of bone exists. This may well necessitate fixtures being placed into those regions of the jaw which were not occupied by natural teeth. The prosthesis will then have to be designed to take such constraints into account, ensuring at the same time that the artificial teeth and the soft tissue support are both functionally and aesthetically acceptable.

Overdentures

For those patients who have worn complete dentures for many years and for whom the lack of stability of the denture is their main concern, a removable overdenture retained on fixtures is the alternative solution to a full-length fixed bridge (Figs 17.5, 17.6). Surgically, there is the advantage that fewer fixtures are required, the optimum being two in the lower jaw and four in the upper. Moreover, the complexity and cost of the prosthetic work is greatly reduced and involves techniques with which both the technician and the dentist are familiar. The patient can also clean dentures in what may be regarded as a conventional manner, requiring little training and less need for manual dexterity.

Further and significant advantages of an overdenture, particularly in the upper jaw, are those of function and appearance. There are situations where the implant abutments which support bridgework may be very apparent, particularly in patients with a high lip line. The ability of an overdenture to give support for both the oro-musculo curtain as well as providing a simple and effective anterior seal is obvious. Moreover, an overdenture affords an older patient a form of prosthesis which enhances appearance and greatly improves function.

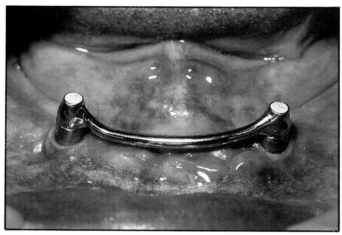

Figure 17.5 Gold alloy bar (2 mm diameter) connecting two implants to provide support and stability for overdentures

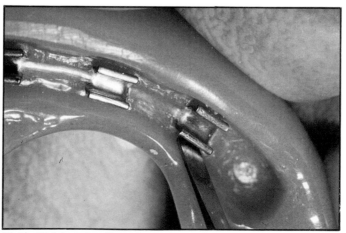

Figure 17.6 Anterior fit surface of complete lower denture showing retention clips

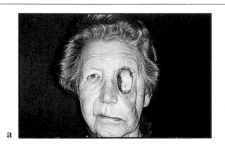

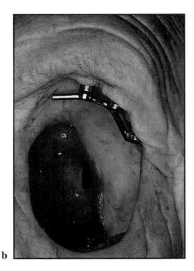

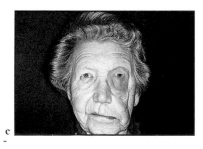

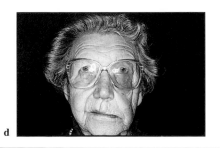

Figure 17.7a–d Implant and bar. This patient lost her eye as the result of a maxillary carcinoma (case reproduced by courtesy of Professor Anders Tjellström and Dr Kerstin Bergström; University of Göteborg)

Obturators/maxillo-facial prostheses

Traditionally, the retention of large intra- or extra-oral prostheses has relied upon the use of soft-tissue undercuts, where available, and tissue adhesives. Implant supported prostheses offer the advantage of dramatically improved retention and stability, compared to these traditional approaches.

Care must be taken during the surgical procedures involved in implant placement. It may be necessary to use specially short fixtures (a flanged 3 mm implant is available for this purpose). Osseointegration procedures should not be performed on irradiated bone until 12 months after the cessation of radiotherapy.

The forces responsible for displacement of such prostheses may be relatively low, for example, when reconstructing an ear or the orbit. The use of gold alloy or plastic clips to provide retention to a cast or wrought substructure is analogous to those employed to retain overdentures, and they therefore provide good retention for extra-oral prostheses. Cobalt–samarium magnets, however, can also be used in these circumstances as they provide adequate retention, with minimum bulk within the prosthesis.

As with all implants, the patient must take meticulous care to maintain an appropriate level of hygiene around the junction between the implant and skin/mucosa. A pulse-jet irrigation system, using 0.02% chlorhexidene, is often employed intra-orally for this purpose.

References

1 Brånemark P-I., Vital microscopy of bone marrow in rabbit, *Scand. J. Clin. Lab. Invest (suppl.) 1959*; 38

2 Brånemark P-I., Breine U., Adell R., Hansonn B-O., Lindström J., Ohlsson A., Intraosseous anchorage of dental prostheses. 1. Experimental studies, *Scand. J. Plast. Reconstr. Surg. 1969*; 3: 81–100

3 Lundskog J., Heat and bone tissue, an experimental investigation of thermal properties of bone tissue threshold levels for thermal injury, *Scand. J. Plast. Reconstr. Surg. 1972*; 9

4 Bothe R.T., Beaton L.E. Davenport H.A., Reaction of bone to multiple metallic implants, *Surg., Gynecol. Obstet 1940*; 71: 598

5 Leventhal G.S., Titanium, a metal for surgery. *J. Bone Jt. Surg. 1951*; 33-A: 473

6 Brånemark P-I., Hansonn B-O., Adell R. *et al.*, Osseointegrated implants in the treatment of the eden-

tulous jaw, *Scand. J. Plast. Reconstr. Surg. 1969*; 11 (Suppl. 16)

7 Adell R., Lekholm U., Rockler B., Brånemark P-I., A 15-year study of osseointegrated implants in the treatment of the edentulous jaw, *Int. J. Oral Surg. 1981*; 10: 387–416

8 Brånemark P-I., Adell R., Albrektsson T. *et al.*, *Osseointegreated titanium implants in the rehabilitation of the edentulous patient. Clinical applications of biomaterials*, eds: Lee, T. Albrektsson, P-I. Brånemark. John Wiley & Sons Ltd, New York 1982

9 Maggiolo, Le manuel de l'art du dentiste, Nancy 1809

18

Oral surgery for the older patient

Peter Ward-Booth

Inevitably, old people may, on occasions, have to undergo oral surgical procedures. These may be relatively minor and done by the practitioner in the surgery; for example extractions, apicectomy and small soft tissue procedures. More major surgery needing specialist care may be required as a consequence of the age-associated increase in pathological changes that occur in the oral tissues. The nature and extent of the oral surgery procedures that are done will be influenced by the systemic age changes which have affected an old person's general health, and the more localized changes that have affected the oral tissues.

Old people are often referred by a general practitioner to a hospital for specialist advice about a procedure which would be done without qualm on a younger patient. However, hospitalization may not always be the best option. The old patient may become confused and agitated by the transfer to unfamiliar surroundings, particularly if admitted overnight. If possible, treatment as an outpatient is to be preferred.

Elderly patients often tolerate treatment under local anaesthetic better than the young. Simple dento-alveolar surgery, such as root removal or difficult extractions, can safely and easily be done in this way by a suitably trained general dental practitioner. In contrast, the provision of a general anaesthetic in the outpatient environment is potentially very dangerous.

General anaesthesia for the old patient is synonymous with hospitalization.

Precautions and problems

Drugs, including local anaesthetics

The increased susceptibility of the old person to drugs has been discussed in Chapter 5. Fortunately, one group of medicaments which appears to be remarkably safe, provided that the recommended dose is not exceeded, is that of local anaesthetics. Because the effects of endogenously secreted catecholamines is likely far to exceed that done by adrenaline-containing local anaesthetics, the surgeon's attention should be directed towards reducing the anxiety of the patient, maintaining efficient pain control and keeping the surgery to short simple sessions.

Infective endocarditis

The management of infective endocarditis is becoming an increasingly difficult problem and the mortality remains depressingly high. Whilst the prevalence of rheumatic fever is falling, the incidence of valvular disease is rising, as people live longer. In many cases, as a result of a carefully taken medical history, the patient may disclose that he or she has previously been diagnosed (whether accurately or not) as having suffered from rheumatic fever. The catch-all use of prophylactic antibiotics to cover occult valvular disease is not desirable, because there is a risk of producing resistant strains of bacteria, or causing an anaphylactic reaction. However, it requires an experienced clinician to detect whether the patient has valvular disease. A number of cardiology units now offer the facility of diagnostic testing for valvular heart disease, for such patients.

Fragility of tissues

The surgeon must be aware of the increased fragility of the old person's soft tissues (Fig. 18.1). Flap elevation and retraction must be performed with care. The patient must be warned that even after minor surgery, such as extractions, there will be oozing of blood into the soft tissues which can cause dramatic and frightening bruising.[1]

The atrophic mandible and maxilla expose the surgeon to the risk either of encountering the inferior dental nerve, or entering the maxillary sinus, even when only relatively small amounts of bone are being removed. Force, which would not be considered excessive in the young person, can readily lead to the fracture of an elderly thinned mandible.

Extraction of teeth can often be surprisingly difficult as a result of bony ankylosis, and the increasing brittleness of the teeth.[2] Elevation of impacted teeth should be completed only

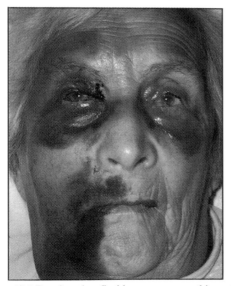

Figure 18.1 Despite the florid appearance, this patient only had a minor fall, with no facial fractures – a good example of friable tissues in the elderly

when the last few millimetres of bone have been drilled from around the tooth. If the jaws are markedly atrophic, or the teeth ankylosed or deeply buried, the patient might best be referred to hospital for advice.

Wound healing

Wound healing may be delayed as a result of an impaired blood supply caused by atherosclerosis. In addition, it has been demonstrated that the inferior alveolar artery has a limited role in the atrophic mandible. The periosteum is the chief source of nutrients for the edentulous mandible in the ageing individual. Any technique which minimizes stripping of and damage to the periosteum is beneficial.

Pre-prosthetic surgery

Pre-prosthetic surgery may be required by the elderly patient. Modern implant techniques have, however, revolutionized treatment. They are simple and effective and fewer patients now require pre-prosthetic operations. On the occasions that such treatment is required the best results will usually be obtained by the simplest procedures, many of which can be carried out under local anaesthesia.

Pre-prosthetic surgical procedures can be divided into those involving soft tissues alone, and those where some alteration to the bone architecture is involved.

'Minor' soft tissue surgery

Flabby ridge

An unacceptably flabby alveolar ridge, for example, in the maxillary tuberosity region (Fig. 18.2), can usually be treated under local anaesthesia by removing a wedge of tissue. Wound closure will produce edge-to-edge contact at the soft tissue margins.

Denture-induced granuloma

The lesion that most commonly requires to be treated is probably the 'denture-induced granuloma' (Fig. 18.3). These hyperplastic

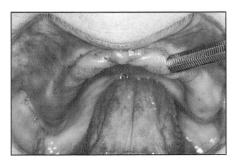

Figure 18.2 A troublesome flabby ridge for denture construction

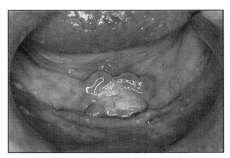

Figure 18.3 Small ridges of hyperplastic tissue which will resolve once the denture is trimmed

masses can be florid and ulcerated and sometimes mimic a squamous cell carcinoma in appearance. Initially, any over-extension of the denture flange should be eased. The lesion will usually reduce in size once the source of the trauma is removed. However, if resolution does not occur, the lesion should be excised under local anaesthetic. This often requires no more than removal of the most florid superficial part of the lesion. The excised tissue must be sent for histopathological examination. Unfortunately, in very florid lesions, removal of the mass can result in a significant loss of sulcus width and depth, and in such cases a vestibuloplasty may subsequently be required.

Sulcus deepening (vestibuloplasty)

The indication for sulcus deepening is the presence of an alveolus with minimal attached mucosa (Fig. 18.4). This is of particular detriment in the lower anterior region because movement of the surrounding musculature readily displaces the lower denture. The operation is usually performed under general anaesthetic and the patient must be warned that the postoperative period can be quite uncomfortable. Many techniques have been

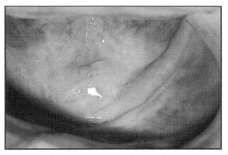

Figure 18.4 A shallow sulcus with only mobile tissues underneath most of the denture flange

described.[3] Most are designed to leave the existing attached mucosa in position, overlying the alveolar crest. A typical surgical approach is to make an incision at the level of the muco-gingival junction and then reposition the mucosa lying below this incision inferiorly (Figs 18.5, 18.6, 18.7). It is important that the mobilization takes place superficial to the periosteum. The defect thus created is covered by a split skin graft taken from the inside of the arm. The graft is stabilized using a modified lower denture or base plate, which is constructed to the anticipated depth of the sulcus. It is lined with a composition stent which is moulded at the time of the operation

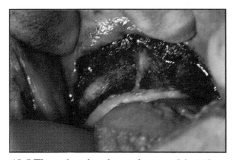

Figure 18.5 The sulcus has been deepened but the periosteum is still intact

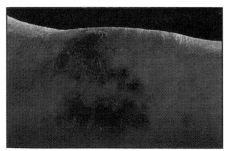

Figure 18.6 Split skin taken from the inside of the arm (at 10 days)

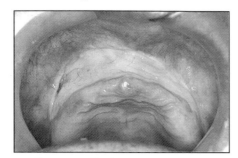

Figure 18.7 The healed split skin graft

to get a more precise impression of the re-defined sulcus. The stent is fixed with circum-mandibular wires or, more comfortably, by bone screws into the alveolus, for 7–10 days. On removal, the stent must be replaced immediately with a denture constructed to utilize the full depth of the new sulcus.

Hard tissue surgery

Surgery to the hard tissues can range from simple to extensive.

Bone spicules

The simplest procedure is, perhaps, the removal of sharp spicules of alveolar bone which prevent the comfortable wearing of a denture. Such problems should be anticipated and prevented at the time of extraction by the judicious use of bur or bone nibblers. Persistent spicules can be removed by raising a small mucoperiosteal flap and smoothing the bone with a suitable round bur thoroughly cooled and irrigated with normal saline (Fig. 18.8).

Muscle attachments

The ridges of bone produced by the attachments of muscles, particularly the mylohyoid and sometimes the geniohyoid, can become prominent as a result of resorption of the alveolus and may cause discomfort beneath dentures. In such cases surgery must be undertaken with caution. Stripping the muscle attachments in order to gain access to the bone can produce significant bleeding and oedema in the floor of the mouth. The procedure should be done by a specialist in hospital because careful postoperative observation is required.

The mental nerve

Not infrequently, patients suffer pain from the denture pressing upon the mental nerve which has become superficially placed as a result of the resorption of the alveolus (Fig. 18.9). The nerve can be repositioned under local anaesthetic. A mucoperiosteal flap is raised so that the nerve can be seen. A window of bone is created and divided horizontally. The bone is carefully dissected away to expose the path of the nerve within the bony canal. The nerve is taken out of the canal and placed more inferiorly in the soft tissues.

Implants

The use of osteointegrated implants in the elderly patient is covered in Chapter 17. The surgical technique is simple and can be performed under local anaesthetic as an outpatient procedure. The successful use of an implant technique may well eliminate the need to employ the more hazardous ridge augmentation techniques discussed below.

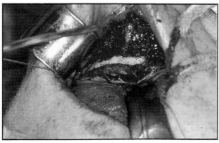

Figure 18.8 A sharp alveolar ridge prior to smoothing

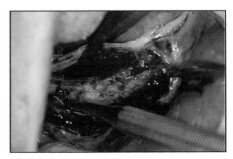

Figure 18.9 A very superficial exit of the mental nerve, prior to repositioning

Alveolar ridge augmentation

Bony augmentation of the alveolus usually requires a general anaesthetic, and involves complex surgery with high morbidity at both the donor and recipient site.

Augmentation with synthetic materials overcomes many of the problems caused by bone augmentation, because there is no donor site morbidity. One of the popular materials in current use is hydroxylapatite, which is produced in block form or as granules of differing size.[4]

The subperiosteal placement of blocks of hydroxylapatite in order to augment the alveolar ridges has not proved successful because of a tendency for ulcers to develop in the overlying mucosa. However, granular forms of the material seem to be well tolerated, and it can be demonstrated that fibrous tissue and some bone enters into the hydroxylapatite granules during healing. Unfortunately, the granules tend to become dispersed from the site of the augmentation procedure under the forces of mastication. Thus, the technique appears to be useful in well-demarcated areas of bone loss such as a localized area of ridge resorption beneath a poorly adapted denture saddle or in a broad alveolus with a

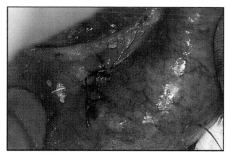

Figure 18.12 Wound closure. This simple procedure can be performed under local anaesthetic

central hollow. Under local anaesthesia a narrow subperiosteal tunnel is created into which the granules are injected (Figs 18.10–18.12). Care must be taken not to strip large areas of the periosteum lest the granules escape from the area proposed for augmentation. Recently, Vicryl tubes and collagen glues have been used to stabilize the granules, and show promise (Fig 18.13).

The other techniques for ridge augmentation involve some form of bone graft, and are usually performed under general anaesthesia. Early attempts at ridge augmentation consisted of onlaying autogenous bone over the alveolar crest. The usual donor material was a split rib (Figs 18.14, 18.15, 18.16). This technique has limited indications because of the

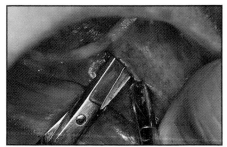

Figure 18.10 Insertion of hydroxylapatite into a posterior deficient alveolus

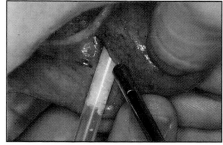

Figure 18.11 Hydroxylapatite granules are placed in a narrow subperiosteal tunnel

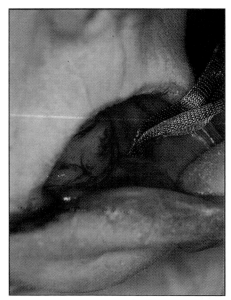

Figure 18.13 A Vicryl tube inserted prior to injecting the hydroxylapatite granules. This prevents migration of the granules from the ridge

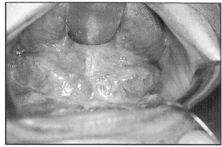

Figure 18.14 A very atrophic ridge to be augmented by rib graft

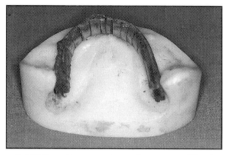

Figure 18.15 The rib is contoured to a sterilized acrylic cast

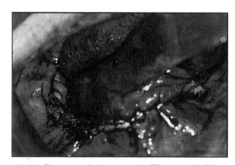

Figure 18.16 Closure of the wound. The pencil-thin mandible was too thin for sagittal osteotomy augmentation

rapid resorption of the donor bone when placed under load as the result of an overlying prosthesis.[5] Split ribs are still used to repair the fractured atrophic mandible, being strapped around the fracture site in order to stabilize it. This procedure also provides a degree of ridge augmentation.

In view of the poor results achieved with onlay grafts, a number of alternative augmentation procedures have been described in which the mandible or maxilla is divided and

the height of the jaw increased by the insertion of interpositional grafts. Thus, the occlusal forces are placed upon the residual alveolar bone which retains its blood supply virtually unaltered. The interpositional grafts act as props between the two bone fragments (Figs 18.17, 18.18).

In the original Stoelinga and Tiderman technique a vertical incision was made along the length of the mandible, dividing it into buccal and lingual sections.[6] The lingual aspect received its blood supply from its periosteum, by way of the attached musculature; the buccal side from the periosteum and buccal mucosa. The lingual section was then placed above and on top of the buccal fragment, effectively doubling the height of the mandible. Unfortunately, bone resorption of up to 30% occurred, and there were, in addition, other complications such as fracture of the mandible and damage to the inferior dental nerve. Consequently, the technique has

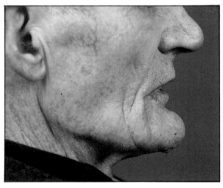

Figure 18.17 This prognathic patient had a grossly atrophic mandible

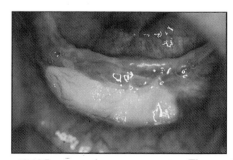

Figure 18.18 Postoperative appearance. The anterior mandible has been divided vertically and the lingual fragment wired on top of the mandible. A secondary sulcus-deepening operation demonstrates the augmentation gained

been extensively modified, primarily by shortening the splits to include just the anterior mandible so as to avoid involvement of the inferior dental nerve.[7] An interpositional bone graft is also often used to further increase the height of the anterior alveolus. Further augmentation of the untreated posterior saddle areas may be undertaken by the placement of hydroxylapatite granules.

Similar augmentations may be made in the upper jaw by means of interpositional grafts placed below a Le Fort I osteotomy. This is rather extensive surgery for an old person and fortunately is not often required because gross resorption of the maxillary alveolus is seldom a clinical problem. Bone grafts are often required to allow osteointegrated implants to be inserted.

In addition to the oral problems, the donor sites must not be forgotten. The patient is relatively immobile for 4–5 days after a bone graft has been taken from the hip, and as a consequence there is a significant risk of deep vein thrombosis, or chest infection, especially the latter if rib is used. The use of trephines into the iliac crest or tibia seems to reduce morbidity.

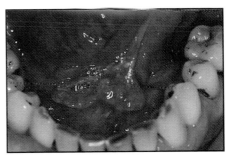

Figure 18.19 A small squamous cell carcinoma of the floor of the mouth. This may be small because it has been seen early or it may be a slow-growing tumour. For either reason the prognosis is better than for a large lesion

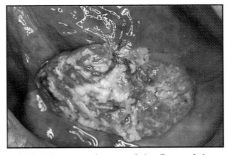

Figure 18.20 A large carcinoma of the floor of the mouth. This lesion failed to respond to radiotherapy and extensive surgery was required to excise the lesion

Oral cancer

Cancer is largely, though not solely, a disease of the elderly. Oral cancer is no exception but represents a very small percentage of the total number of malignancies reported. Sadly, the devastation and pain of the condition offsets it rarity (Figs 18.19, 18.20).

The management of a new patient is more or less standard in most cancer units. The patient is examined and a history taken, identifying possible aetiological factors such as smoking or drinking habits. An intra-oral examination is performed, and lesions are noted and photographed. A clinical evaluation is made of the extent of a suspicious area and any detectable lymphatic spread in the neck. A biopsy is performed, usually under local anaesthetic. General anaesthesia may be required if the lesions are in a difficult site in the mouth, or if they are very painful or extensive. Endoscopy may be required if another primary lesion is suspected in the oropharynx. The use of a general anaesthetic may delay

definitive surgery, or can result in significant morbidity if surgery is required for the cancer, because the patient will be subjected to two general anaesthetics within the space of a few days.

Once a diagnosis has been established, the patient is informed in a sympathetic but clear manner. It is often best if near relatives are also told, because an old person may either misunderstand or try to minimize the problem. Ideally, a trained counsellor should be involved, discussing matters on several occasions so as to give the patient and relatives a chance to understand the implications.

The prognosis for oral cancer is poor and it would be arrogant for any individual or specialty to claim a monopoly of wisdom in the treatment of such patients.[8] The patients are best seen on a combined-clinic, with surgeons and radiotherapists. Most oral cancer clinics appear to have an agreed policy in broad terms, for the treatment of oral cancer, and use radiotherapy, or surgery, or a combination of both. At present there seems to be no place for chemotherapy, though studies continue in an attempt to find effective agents.

In an attempt to standardize diagnostic and prognostic criteria for patients presenting with cancer, the TMN system has been developed. T refers to the tumour size, M to the presence or absence of distant metastases and N involvement of lymph nodes.

The system is used for all cancers and is modified to each particular region of the body. Unfortunately it has limited value in predicting survival in oral cancer. It should be recalled that if a death occurs from oral cancer, it is most likely to occur within the first two years and is commonly due to persistence of the disease at the original site of the primary lesion.

The TMN system does have some validity. For example, the presence of lymph nodes in the neck is a good predictor of a poor prognosis. Similarly, larger lesions generally do worse than the small lesions. The site of the lesion, however, is much more important and this is not included in the classic TMN system. For example, carcinoma of the lip has a far superior five-year survival rate compared to any other oral cancer. The depth of invasion of the tumour is also important as is whether the tumour spreads along vascular or neuro-vascular channels. The rate of growth also seems important and this may well be represented by the size of the tumour, although there seems to be tremendous variability in how long the patient has the tumour before they seek advice. Finally, less tangible factors play their part. For example, if the patient fails to respond to whatever primary modality of treatment is given, then the five-year survival is reduced by a further 50%. Thus, there is great variability in prognostic factors; and for example, the five-year survival of carcinoma of the tongue can vary between 24% and 51%. A recent paper on intra-oral cancer summarizes the prognosis well, and contains important criteria.[9] It assesses 542 cases of which 98% were followed up for five years. The authors showed a survival of 30% and 18% for stages II and IV respectively. Eleven per cent of patients developed distant metastases, and 14% developed second primaries in the aero-digestive tract.

Radiotherapy offers the overwhelming ad-

vantage of preserving normal gross anatomy and more or less normal function (Fig. 18.21). In addition, a general anaesthetic is usually not required. Consequently, every attempt is made to use radiotherapy whenever indicated, especially in the elderly. There are, however, some instances when some surgery is needed. Radiotherapy to bone which has been invaded by a malignant lesion is not as effective as surgery, and may result in osteoradionecrosis (Fig. 18.22). Large lesions and large lesions extending into the lymphatics are usually managed with a combination of radiotherapy and surgery. Surgical resection of tumour involving the jaws affords the best chance of curing these lesions. There are, however, difficulties in reconstruction and rehabilitation, particularly if the anterior mandible has to be resected (Fig 18.23). Surgery is also indicated for those lesions which have failed to respond to radiotherapy. The final important use of surgery is for those patients who present with lymph nodes in the neck.

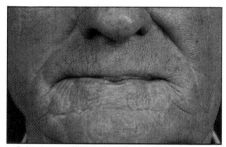

Figure 18.21 A small carcinoma of the lip treated by radiotherapy. Note the normal appearance and function. Unfortunately this patient developed spread of the tumour to the cervical lymph nodes and required a radical neck dissection

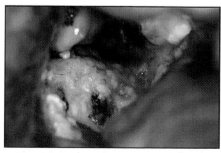

Figure 18.22 A painful osteoradionecrosis of the mandible. This followed a biopsy of a suspicious lesion at the site of a carcinoma treated by radiotherapy

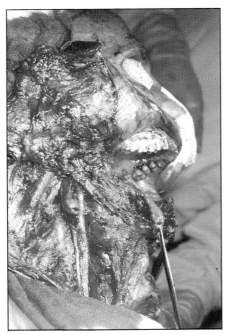

Figure 18.23 This view of a hemi-mandiblectomy and radical neck dissection, taken midway through the surgical procedure, demonstrates the extent of ablative surgery that may be required for cancer within the oral cavity

Radiotherapy

Briefly, radiotherapy consists of two basic techniques, external beam therapy and brachiotherapy.

External beam therapy

External beam therapy is commonly delivered from a very precise source, the linear accelerator. The beam is directed in a similar manner to a tomogram, striking the target area (the tumour) preferentially as a result of careful planning. The irradiation is normally up to 65 Gy, given in daily increments, over 6 weeks.

Brachiotherapy

Brachiotherapy uses a radioactive source, usually iridium, which is implanted, under general anaesthetic, into the lesion for a few days. This high dose of radiation, equivalent to external beam, is confined to the lesion and is particularly valuable for small lesions of the tongue and floor of the mouth.

At the time of the radiation the patient feels no discomfort. As the therapy proceeds, however, a mucositis may develop. In rare instances this may be so severe as to necessitate a pause in the therapy. The mucositis will often continue for about ten days after the therapy has finished. In the elderly, the symptoms may be exacerbated by a florid candidal infection. Symptomatic treatment, with dilute chlorhexidine or anaesthetic preparations such as Difflam, are helpful. Great care must be taken to ensure that old patients do not become dehydrated from fear of pain on swallowing.

An important late complication of radiotherapy is xerostomia in those patients in whom the major salivary glands have been irradiated. Although the symptoms reduce with time, they rarely totally disappear. Radiation caries may also follow from the xerostomia. The risk of osteoradionecrosis mainly affecting the mandible may occur after dental extractions or periodontal or periapical infections. This is an extremely painful condition which has recently undergone radical new techniques of management, in which the dead bone is removed and the patient subjected to hyperbaric oxygen. Using these techniques, healing is greatly improved, and can nearly return to normal.

Surgery

Surgery for oral cancer has two components, ablation and reconstruction.

Ablation

The ablation technique used differs for the primary disease and the secondary metastatic deposits in the lymphatics of the neck. The aim of surgery for the primary disease is to excise the cancer with a 2 cm margin of normal tissue. Resection of the cervical lymph nodes requires a different philosophy. For a lymph node to be palpated (and as yet this is the only reliable method of detection of tumour within a lymph node), it must be approximately 1 cm in size, and will contain many thousands of neoplastic cells. If one of the lymph nodes of the neck has clinical signs of tumour invasion, then it is assumed that others may be involved, although they are not as yet palpable. Matters are further complicated by the likelihood that the tumour may extend out through the capsule of the lymph node. Thus, simple enucleation of a single palpable node may leave other metastatic nodes in the neck and, in addition, may spill tumour cells if the capsule of the node has been penetrated. Consequently, surgery should involve a radical neck dissection removing sternomastoid, omohyoid, and often the digastric muscles. This radical surgery also removes en bloc the internal jugular vein, lymphatics and accessory nerve, as well as the cervical sensory nerves.

Ablative surgery to the primary lesion produces considerable functional deficit, affecting speech, mastication and deglutition. Neck dissection, apart from some weakness to the trapezius muscle due to its loss of innovation, has minimal deficit.

Treatment should also include advice about aetiological habits, particularly against the continuation of smoking. Nearly one-half of those who continue to smoke will develop a secondary primary of the aero-digestive tract. The advice should be given repeatedly and with conviction. There is some evidence that chemoprevention may help these patients.[10]

Reconstruction

The long-term prognosis for many patients with oral cancer is poor, and the tissue destruction caused by surgical removal of the lesion is substantial. A high standard of reconstruction can help both the patient and the surgeon to come to terms with the disease process. Different and ingenious methods of reconstruction abound, which greatly improve the quality of the patient's life.

Reconstruction must be considered in relation to soft and hard tissues. Soft tissue reconstruction may simply require direct closure after a small resection, but normally tissue must be brought into the region in order to close the defect (Figs 18.24–18.32). In small lesions of the tongue a simple split skin graft may close the resection. Pedicled axial pattern flaps are traditionally used for larger reconstructions. These flaps have an axial blood flow, often from unnamed vessels which allow them to have considerable length compared with the base width of the flap. This length allows flaps to be brought into the mouth from distant sites (Fig. 18.28).

Recently, myocutaneous flaps have been used for reconstruction.[11] These seem to have a better survival than some of the axial flaps. They often supply useful bulk, and can be carried out as one-stage procedures. These flaps still require an axial pattern blood supply to support the muscle, small perforating vessels supplying the skin. More recently, free flaps have been employed, in which vessels supplying the flap are anastomosed to vessels in the neck.

Reconstruction of the facial bones has always been a problem. Small lateral defects of the mandible can be left unrepaired, especially if the defect has been filled with a bulky myocutaneous flap. The maxilla is usually left deficient, an obturator being used to close the cavity. This has the advantage that regular inspection of the cavity can be made (Fig. 18.30).

If bone is required for reconstruction then, traditionally, free bone grafts from the iliac crest or rib are used. In a contaminated area like the mouth, or in a relatively avascular field as a consequence of irradiation, these grafts often survive poorly. Consequently, attempts have been made to improve the blood supply to the bone. An osteomyocutaneous flap, taking the underlying rib, with a pectoralis major flap, greatly improves the vascular bed for the graft. Some workers suggest these bone grafts are true vascularized bones. The next logical development is the ability to transplant a true free vascularized bone graft.[12] This will require the blood supply, both arterial and venous of the graft with the bone or skin to be disconnected at the donor site and anastomosed to vessels in the neck. These flaps have great benefits, but they can take a long time and usually require two operating teams (Figs 18.31, 18.32).

These general comments on the treatment of oral cancers apply to patients of all ages. However, it is easy to appreciate the significant morbidity to any patient let alone a geriatric patient following surgery for oral cancer. Such operations can take between one hour and nine hours. Thus, whilst the presenting cancer will define the nature and extent of ablative surgery, the reconstruction should be tailored to the patient's ability to cope with a long operation.

Reconstruction following an extensive surgical ablation may require specialist restorative support. For those few patients who

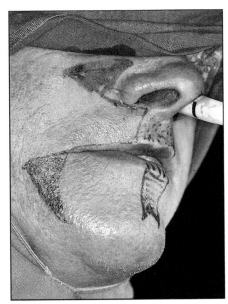

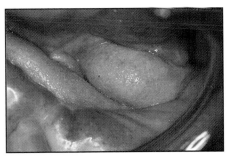

Figure 18.26 Two nasolabial flaps forming the anterior floor of the mouth

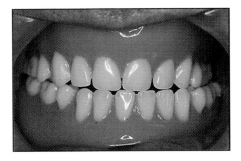

Figure 18.24 Local flaps can be useful in the elderly. Here a basal cell carcinoma is being excised and reconstructed using a variety of local flaps

Figure 18.27 The lower denture is resting on a single nasolabial flap covering the partly resected mandible

Chapters 7 and 8, are particularly apposite in this context.

Other neoplasias

Haematological malignancies may present in this age-group. They may be seen as spontaneous bleeding into the tissues or widespread ulceration. Diagnosis is usually made by haematological investigation.

Benign and malignant tumours of salivary glands also present in this age-group. Such tumours are rarer in the minor glands, but when they occur here have a higher incidence of malignancy. Unfortunately, they are not very radiosensitive, and surgery is often indicated.

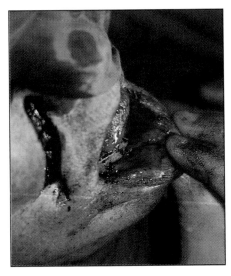

Figure 18.25 A nasolabial flap is being used to reconstruct the anterior floor of the mouth

require obturators, meticulous routine care for any remaining teeth is essential, and is usually the responsibility of the patient's General Dental Practitioner. The oral health procedures outlined for the treatment of periodontal disease and root surface caries, in

The facial skin may be affected with benign and malignant tumours. The lax skin of the older patient usually means that direct closure can often be made even following large resections. Again, the patients usually tolerate local anaesthetics for relatively large resections of face and lips.

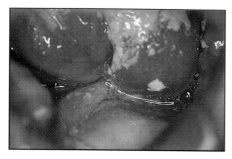

Figure 18.28 A deltopectoral pedicled flap from the chest, lining a larger area of the floor of the mouth. This traditional flap requires a second operation to divide the pedicle after 3 weeks

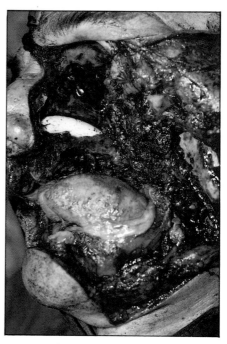

Figure 18.30 The primary obturator is fitted at the time of ablative surgery. In this case a hemimaxillectomy was carried out

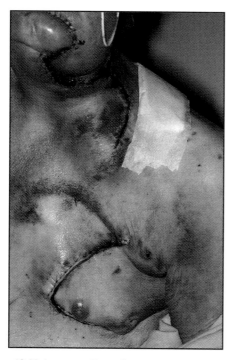

Figure 18.29 A pectoralis major myocutaneous flap has been used to reconstruct the floor of the mouth. This is a one-stage procedure and the muscle pedicle covers the carotid artery following the radical neck dissection. Note also that the donor site, the chest, is directly closed with only minimum distortion of the breast

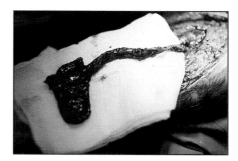

Figure 18.31 Skin is taken from the forearm, and its blood supply (radial artery and venae comitantes) seen in the pedicle will be anastomosed to the facial artery and vein

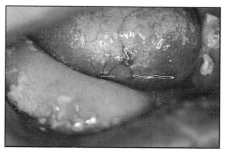

Figure 18.32 The radial free forearm flap provides good thin cover for the floor of the mouth

The lower lip and forehead are a common site of actinic change and frank malignancy. Basal cell carcinomas seldom metastasize, but at certain sites, such as the medial canthus of the eye and the alar base of the nose, they can be very aggressive, especially after they have been inadequately excised.

Aesthetic surgery

The view, commonly held by younger people, that the old should age gracefully is not always shared by the old! Macroscopic and microscopic changes in the tissues (discussed in Chapter 3) often result in marked skin creasing, and sagging of the skin which produces redundant tissue beneath the eyes and chin. The loss of buccal fat causes a hollowing of the face which further emphasizes the sagging skin.

Though most old people accept these changes, there is an increasing demand for correction. The 'face lift' operation involves tightening the skin. A pre-auricular skin incision is made extending into the hair line, and an incision is taken inferiorly and post-auricularly. The skin is mobilized from the subcutaneous tissues and redundant tissue removed. Care must be taken both to avoid damage to branches of the facial nerve, and post-operative haematomas. In the USA the operation is done as an outpatient procedure with local anaesthesia under sedation. In England general anaesthesia is more usual.

Local procedures such as blepharoplasty are sometimes indicated and, similarly, may on rare occasions be followed by complications such as blindness. Liposuction, in which fat is sucked and curetted from the tissues, is another technique that is available. It may be used to reduce submental fat collections usually in combination with skin reduction.

References

1 Kaplan H., The oral cavity in geriatrics. *Geriatrics 1971*; 26: 96

2 Ten Cate A.R., Age changes dentin-pulp complex, in: *Oral histology; development, structure and function*, C.V. Mosby, St. Louis 1985; 177

3 Starshak T.J., Shauders B., *Vestibuloplasty in preprosthetic and maxillofacial surgery*, C.V. Mosby, St. Louis 1980; 165–213

4 Larson H.D., Finger I.M., Guera L.R., Kent J.W, Prosthetic management of hydroxylapatite augmented ridges. *J. Prosthetic Dent. 1983*; 49: 461–9

5 Davis W.H. *et al.*, Long term ridge augmentation with rib grafts. *J. Maxillofac. Surg. 1975*; 3: 103–6

6 Stoelinga P.J.W. *et al.*, Interpositional bonegraft augmentation of the atropic mandible, *J. Oral Surg. 1978*; 36: 30–32

7 Stoelinga P.J.W. *et al.*, A reappraisal of the interpositional bonegraft augmentation of the atropic mandible, *J. Maxillofac. Surg. 1983*; 11: 107–12

8 Langdon J.D., *et al.*, Oral cancer. The behaviour and response to treatment of 154 cases, *J. Maxillofac. Surg. 1977*; 5: 221–37

9 Ilstad S.T., Tollerud D.J., Bigelou M.E., Remensnyder J.P., A multivariate analysis of the determinants of the head and neck, *Ann. Surg. 1989*; 209: 237–241

10 de Varies N., van Zandmijk N., Pastorion U., Chemoprevention in the management of oral cancer: Euroscan and other studies, *Euro. J. Cancer B Oral Oncol. 1992;* 28B(2): 153–157

11 Arivan S., Pectoralis major myocutaneous flap, *Plast. Reconstr. Surg. 1979*; 63: 73

12 Soutar D.S., Scheker L.R., Tanner N.S.B., McGregor I.A., The radial forearm flap: a versatile method for intraoral reconstruction, *Br. J. Plast. Surg. 1983*; 36: 1

19

Treatment planning

Angus Walls and Ian Barnes

Treatment planning for the older patient can be problematical. Often it requires a degree of foresight which can be assured only by the ability to see into the future. Pragmatism, which must not be confused with indifference, is sometimes the hard but necessary way to approach matters.

Difficult immediate decisions about treatment planning sometimes have to be made, for example, if a new elderly patient presents with a dentition in disarray, or if the dental, medical or physical condition of an established patient alters significantly. On the other hand the dental treatment of the old person who has been a regular attender is an ongoing matter which is unlikely to lead to a sudden need to face complex problems in treatment planning. Nevertheless, most dentists will have noted that the routine care of ageing patients often becomes increasingly difficult as the years go by, usually as a result of rapidly recurring root surface caries.

It is sensible, on occasions, to stand back and take stock. Therein is often a dilemma. Should increasingly irreparable broken down teeth be extracted and full dentures constructed before the patient becomes too old to be able to cope with the transition? Or should we continue to attempt to preserve the teeth, with the risk that when dentures are inevitable they cannot be tolerated? There is no clear-cut answer, other perhaps than to comment that only the Almighty knows our lifespan, and that the present comforts and quality of

life are more tangible than possible future problems. Certainly, when the options are put to them, most patients will opt to keep their teeth.

If a decision is made to render a patient edentulous, and the clinician believes that they will not readily adapt to the change, then the transition should be gradual. This can be achieved by the use of overdentures or transitional acrylic partial dentures.

The provision of dental care for the old patient may be made in the following sequence, as illustrated in Figure 19.1.

- Assessment and provisional treatment plan
- Primary care
- Definitive treatment plan
- Secondary care
- Tertiary care.

Assessment and treatment planning

In many cases assessment and treatment planning will be part of a longstanding ongoing treatment, and not the discrete excercise described, for clarity, below.

The basis of sound treatment planning is the recording of high quality clinical records at the initial assessment visit. These records should comprise the results of a detailed clinical dental examination, including a periodontal and occlusal assessment if appropriate, impressions for study casts, and a thorough radio-

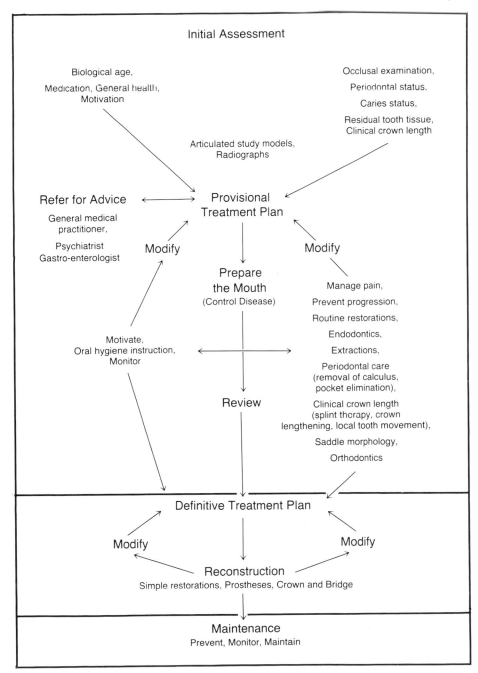

Initial Assessment

Biological age,
Medication, General health,
Motivation

Occlusal examination,
Periodontal status,
Caries status,
Residual tooth tissue,
Clinical crown length

Articulated study models,
Radiographs

Refer for Advice
General medical
practitioner,
Psychiatrist
Gastro-enterologist

Provisional
Treatment Plan

Modify

Modify

Prepare
the Mouth
(Control Disease)

Manage pain,
Prevent progression,
Routine restorations,
Endodontics,
Extractions,
Periodontal care
(removal of calculus,
pocket elimination),

Motivate,
Oral hygiene instruction,
Monitor

Clinical crown length
(splint therapy, crown
lengthening, local tooth movement),

Review

Saddle morphology,
Orthodontics

Definitive Treatment Plan

Modify

Modify

Reconstruction
Simple restorations, Prostheses, Crown and Bridge

Maintenance
Prevent, Monitor, Maintain

Figure 19.1 A schematic diagram of the process of treatment planning for an older patient

graphic investigation. When this has been done, three factors can be considered.

- What does the patient want?
- What can the patient tolerate?
- What can be achieved?

What does the patient want?

Some patients will ask for the impossible. For example, a deranged dentition such as that shown in Figure 19.2 cannot be reconstructed to be as aesthetic or functional as that shown

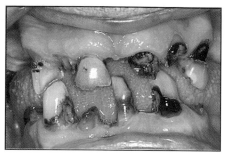

Figure 19.2 An ageing dentition in poor condition. The teeth are badly broken down and there is extensive periodontal disease. This patient's aspirations for his dentition need to be modified in the light of the condition of his remaining teeth

ın Figure 19.3. An old person may well be unaware of the significant benefits that can often be had, relatively simply, by the use of modern techniques. Or they may feel, wrongly, that it is not worth-while making an effort, or asking the dentist to make an effort on their behalf. The dentist may need to inform and encourage. Less often he may need to dissuade.

What can the patient tolerate?

A sensible treatment plan may well be insupportable because of the patient's frailty. The physiological and pathological changes associated with ageing must be taken into consideration when making a treatment plan. These changes are considered in Chapter 7.

What can be achieved?

What can be achieved partly depends upon the patient's tolerance. It is, perhaps, rather more dependent upon the condition of the

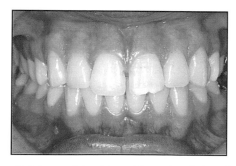

Figure 19.3 A sound dentition with good periodontal condition in a young individual. This sort of appearance may be desired by an older individual, but that aspiration is often impracticable

dental tissue that remains and the progression of disease. Regrettably, constraints of time and finance will sometimes prevent the implementation of a theoretically 'ideal' treatment plan for the grossly decrepit mouth.

The quality of the remaining dental tissue is of fundamental importance. This must be assessed from three standpoints, namely, the periodontal condition, the caries status, and the extent of the residual tooth substance.

Periodontal status

Periodontal breakdown is not an inevitable consequence of ageing. If an old dentition is so affected, there is a considerable body of evidence to show that provided the disease is controlled, long-spanned bridges can be supported on teeth with a marked loss of periodontal support.[1]

The ability of the old patient to maintain an adequate level of oral hygiene is paramount if the provision of either fixed bridgework or overdentures are to be considered. These types of treatment are likely to result in a dental architecture which is more difficult to maintain than that which the patient had at the outset of treatment. Consequently, if the patient cannot, or will not, keep their natural teeth clean, it is improbable that they will be able to cope with the more complex architecture of a fixed dental prosthesis. Having said this, the presence of plaque must not be seen as an absolute contra-indication to bridgework. Some old people will simply find it impossible to attain a scrupulous level of oral hygiene. In the absence of clinical evidence of active periodontal disease or decay one might ask which will do the most harm, a small well-made bridge or a denture?

Caries incidence

A high caries prevalence in an older patient will usually direct a treatment plan away from extensive restorative care, certainly until the causative factor can be identified and controlled. Assessment should include medical and dietary histories. Correction regimens will include the use of fluoride or remineralizing mouthwashes, modification of the diet, and alteration of a patient's drug therapy to reduce any tendency for drug-induced xerostomia.[2] Modifications of a drug regimen should be made only in collaboration with the patient's medical practitioner.

Teeth that are carious at the outset of treatment should be restored using conventional techniques prior to any further care. Alternatively, if an overdenture is planned, a policy of strategic extractions may be decided.

Residual tooth tissue

Aetiological factors that are identified as a cause of toothwear must be taken into account during treatment planning.[3] For example, a bruxing habit is likely to lead to the destruction of porcelain occlusal surfaces of bonded crowns. Metal occlusal surfaces would be a better option and also cause less damage to the opposing natural teeth. Similarly, advanced restorative treatment should not be offered until erosive factors have been identified and controlled. Failure to do this will result in further tooth tissue loss at the restoration margins, with the production of stagnation areas with a risk of plaque collection and recurrent caries. Also, most of the luting cements used for cast restorations are acid-soluble, and will be dissolved out of the crown in an acidic environment. This will result in potential loss of retention of the restoration, and a further space for plaque accumulation and recurrent decay. If it is necessary to place full coronal restorations in a subject with an ongoing erosive problem the crown margins should be placed subgingivally.

As a general rule as much tooth tissue as possible must be retained and utilized. Core preparations should be designed so that there is a collar of sound tooth tissue at the gingival aspect, which the crown margin will encircle and support. In this way lateral forces will not be entirely transmitted by pins and posts, and the likelihood of failure is reduced (Figs 19.4, 19.5).

Full veneer crowns are not always indicated; for example, when the whole of the lingual wall of a tooth has been replaced by a pinned core, which is relying upon the residual buccal cusps for mutual support and retention. Full crown preparation would substantially reduce and weaken the valuable tooth tissue of the buccal cusps. In such a case the construction of a three-quarter crown with

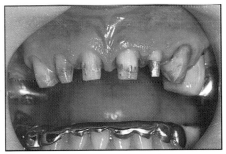

Figure 19.4 Pin-retained composite resin cores on 321|1. Note that the core on 2| extends down to the gingival margin of the preparation palatally

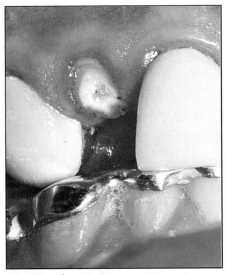

Figure 19.5 The 2| tooth five years later, the crown has failed as a result of fracture of the residual tooth tissue and loss of the pinned core

as much extension onto sound tooth-tissue as possible might be the treatment of choice (Fig 19.6).

It may often be difficult to assess the extent of any residual tooth tissue in a heavily restored tooth. Thus, large restorations should be removed and the extent of remaining tooth substance established prior to utilization of the tooth for an extensive reconstruction. This step is essential if the tooth is to provide major support for long-span bridgework. A useful guide to planning tooth preparation design is to record an impression of any teeth once the existing restorations have been removed to give a permanent record of the extent of the residual tooth tissue.

Much of the information that is required in order to establish the quality of the remaining

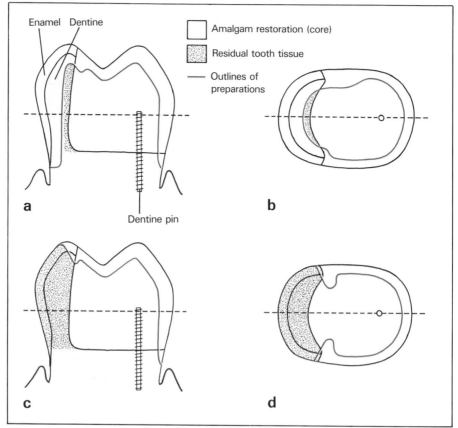

Enamel Dentine

☐ Amalgam restoration (core)

▨ Residual tooth tissue

— Outlines of preparations

a

Dentine pin

b

c

d

Figure 19.6 Diagrammatic representations of idealized preparations for a porcelain fused to metal (PFM) crown ((a) and (b)), and a three-quarter crown ((c) and (d)), on an upper premolar tooth with a large, pin-retained, amalgam core. Note the small quantity of residual tooth tissue on the buccal aspect of the preparation for the PFM restoration, compared with that for the three-quarter crown

dentition and to determine a definitive treatment plan is not available to the practitioner at the initial assessment visit. Consequently, it is usually necessary to draw up a provisional treatment plan initially, on the basis of the examination made on the first visit.

The provisional treatment plan

For many old patients, treatment will consist of the continuation of routine care, albeit with likely increasing problems of management. In those cases where progressive breakdown of the oral tissue necessitates a fundamental rethink, there are usually four possibilities for treatment.

- Fixed crown and bridgework alone
- The limited use of crowns in association with a partial denture to restore the edentulous spaces
- The construction of overdentures
- A clearance and the provision of complete dentures.

The appropriate choice will depend upon a number of factors including the concepts identified earlier, namely, the wishes of the patient, the state of the dentition, the experience of the operator and often, regrettably, financial constraints.

If a patient demands the removal of all of their remaining natural teeth, it is incumbent upon the practitioner to point out the disadvantages of this course of action, and he or she has the option to refuse to perform the treatment. Happily, patients usually seek advice, rather than demand specific forms of care.

Some examples of the types of decision that might be required to be made, are perhaps best illustrated. The patient shown in Figure 19.7 suffered a combination of marked tooth-wear, loss of posterior support with over-closure and poor periodontal status. This case could be managed by combining relatively simple restorative techniques with partial dentures or overdentures, or by a clearance and full prosthesis.

The dentition illustrated in Figure 19.8 is incomplete and worn. However, the oral hygiene and periodontal status are good. If complex rehabilitation techniques were to be used, they would probably be sucessful.

In other cases a simple treatment plan may be the sensible option, as for example in the case shown in Figure 19.9, where a partial overdenture was successfully made.

The principles of provisional treatment planning

Five principles may be borne in mind when making a provisional treatment plan.

- Teeth that have been reduced to gingival level as a result of wear, or caries, are often best used as overdenture abutments.
- In cases where the anterior teeth are extensively worn and there is a loss of posterior support, it is not practicable to attempt to increase the vertical dimension

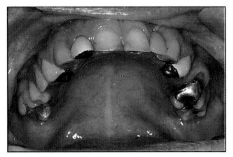

Figure 19.8 The dentition of a 56-year-old, who was concerned about her appearance. There was marked wear of the anterior teeth, associated with a clenching habit. The periodontal status was good and the patient was well motivated

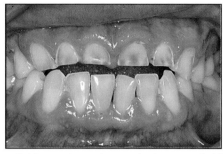

Figure 19.9 Loss of anterior tooth tissue, probably as a result of an erosive problem associated with nocturnal regurgitation. The patient has prepared his own overdenture abutments! (reproduced with permission of A.E. Morgan Publications)

upon the edentulous spaces alone, in order to create space for anterior reconstruction. If such an attempt is made, the edentulous spaces soon become uncomfortable, and there is a risk of accelerating the rate of alveolar bone resorption as a

Figure 19.7a, b The dentition of a 70-year-old: there has been extensive toothwear, with over-eruption of some teeth and loss of occlusal stability. The periodontal status is poor with deep pockets around the upper molars and gross mobility of the lower left first premolar

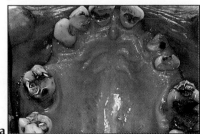
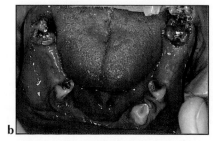

result of excessive loading. In such cases some temporary anterior support must be provided. This may be in the form of composite resin restorations, plastic crowns, or some form of overdenture.

- It is difficult if not impossible to achieve a good standard of colour match and aesthetics if the length of the worn front teeth is increased by means of a partial overlay denture (Fig. 19.10).
- It is inadvisable to use a severely periodontally involved tooth to support or retain a partial denture, other than as an electively root-filled abutment for an overdenture.
- The decision to render the patient edentulous is irreversible, and should be made with care.

Primary care

Primary care is the first stage of treatment, and is undertaken following the determination of the provisional treatment plan (see Fig. 19.1). Primary care includes the initial relief of pain, the management of periodontal disease and instruction in oral hygiene, the identification and treatment of factors causing deteriorations in the dentition, the treatment of active caries and the basic restoration of the teeth.

An examination of the temporo-mandibular joint and its associated musculature should be made and signs or symptoms of dysfunction identified. Dysfunction must be treated prior to commencing definitive treatment.

If a reorganized occlusal pattern is to be developed at an increased vertical dimension,

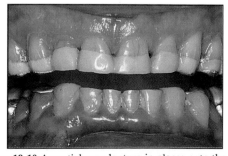

Figure 19.10 A partial overdenture in place; note the poor aesthetics of the junction between the anterior teeth and incisal facings (courtesy of Dr R.W. Wassell)

a hard acrylic splint should be made for diagnostic purposes and to assess the patient's ability to tolerate the change.

The definitive treatment plan

When primary care has been completed the clinician is able to make a more accurate assessment of the patient's oral status. It should now be possible to reassess and if necessary revise the initial treatment plan and to formulate a definitive treatment plan. For example, despite intensive instruction, a patient's oral hygiene may not have reached an appropriate level for crown and bridgework. Also, at this stage the clinician should be able to assess the type of restoration most appropriate for any tooth, and should be able to determine whether or not crown lengthening procedures will be necessary.

Secondary care (reconstruction)

The general principles of secondary care have been discussed in Chapter 10.

Tertiary care

The completion of a reconstruction is often perceived by the patient as being the end of treatment. It is essential that the need for regular recall maintenance is stressed. Tertiary care is a fundamental and often highly problematical stage in the long-term management of the ageing patient. It comprises three parts.

- Prevention
- Monitoring
- Maintenance.

Prevention

Preventative regimens will include the continuation of oral hygiene instructions to support the patients in their attempts to clean their restored dentitions to as high or a higher standard than that which obtained prior to reconstruction.

It may be necessary to teach the management of hygiene aids that have not previously been used, and to recommend the regular use of fluoride mouthwash or professional topical fluoride application so as to help prevent the development of root surface caries. It has been demonstrated that monitoring the salivary counts of *S. mutans* and lactobacilli may be of some benefit in assessing the risk of developing root-surface caries of patients with periodontally involved teeth with exposed root surfaces.[4] Kits which permit the estimation of salivary bacterial counts are available commercially, and may be of some benefit during tertiary care.[a]

Monitoring

Regular recall appointments are necessary for the old patient in order to ensure that an adequate standard of oral care is maintained. The commonly adopted six-month recall will in many cases be too delayed. In most old patients there will develop alterations in the pattern of dental disease with time. When this happens the practitioner should seek to ascertain whether there have been changes in the diet, medication or habits.

The integrity of all restorations should be checked at these regular recall visits. This is particularly important where large numbers of crowns and bridges have been placed. All cemented restorations should be monitored to ensure that the cement lute remains intact. The occlusal stability of a reconstruction should be assessed using shimstock and articulating paper. Minor occlusal adjustments at regular recall visits may assist in the maintenance of occlusal stability.

Maintenance

All restorative work requires to be maintained (Fig. 19.11), and this applies to all patients, including the edentulous. It is the clinical impression of the authors that for many elderly dentate patients there comes a time when disease develops or progresses, despite every effort of them or their dentist. Dentally aware patients pose particular problems. Their aspirations remain high but their ability to

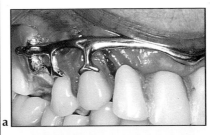

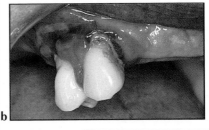

Figure 19.11 A failure of the maintenance phase of care. (a) A swinglock partial denture in place, the patient had been told that this was a 'permanent' partial denture which would be well retained, and consequently had not taken the denture out for two years. (b) The condition of the gingival tissues beneath the retainer

maintain complex work decreases, for various reasons (Fig 19.12). It can be very difficult for their dentist to explain that there is no alternative to an extraction.

In summary, planning a course of treatment for the old patient is the bedrock of successful treatment. It is also a stringent test of clinical acumen.

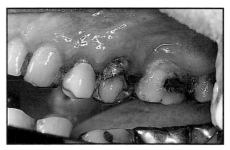

Figure 19.12 Plaque-laden teeth, despite conscientious efforts of a 78-year-old patient. Six years earlier his cleaning was effective, his teeth clean, and his incidence of root surface caries minimal. However, his dental aspirations remain the same

[a]Dentocult LB and Dentocult SM, Vivacare, Ivoclar, Vivadent 2, Meridian South, Leicester LE3 2WY

References

1 Nyman S., Lindhe J., A longitudinal study of combined periodontal and prosthetic treatment of patients with advanced periodontal disease, *J. Periodontol. 1979*: 50; 163–9

2 Sreebny L.M., Schwartz S.S., A reference guide to drugs and dry mouth, *Gerodontology 1986*; 5: 75–99

3 Smith B.G.N., Knight J.K., A comparison of patterns of toothwear with aetiological factors, *Br. Dent. J. 1984*; 157: 16–19

4 Ravald N., Hamp S-E., Prediction of root surface caries in patients treated for advanced periodontal disease, *J. Clin. Periodontol. 1981*; 8: 400–414

Domiciliary care for the elderly patient

John Christensen and Janice Fiske

The effects of ageing will vary from person to person and will be reflected in different needs for care and caring. The extreme of need is expressed in a requirement for the provision of domiciliary care.

Introduction

The need to maintain oral health does not cease with increasing age and impaired general health. On the contrary, it is well documented that poor oral health places an old and frail person at a higher medical risk. In addition, good oral health and the ability to chew food adequately adds to the quality of life in old age (Fig. 20.1).[1] Most old people live as independent, healthy individuals within the community, and have no specific problems in obtaining dental care. However, a minority are institutionalized or housebound as a result of debilitating physical, medical, mental or psychiatric conditions. In Northern Europe it is estimated that 4–7% of the population over the age of 65 live in long-stay residential care. The proportion of elderly people that are bedridden or housebound to such a degree that they cannot look after themselves is uncertain because there are no nationwide official statistics regarding this group of individuals. However, an estimated 12–14% of the elderly population falls into this categ-

ory. Whilst the proportion may seem small, the numbers of elderly people involved are significant. In the UK it is about one and a quarter to one and a half million people, and in the USA about six and a half to seven and a half million people.

The oral health of residents in nursing homes and long-term care facilities has in recent years been reported as poor in many European Countries.[2-7] These reports have revealed the need for dental care, both within long-stay accommodation and in the form of special programmes directed towards the housebound elderly, living in private homes or in sheltered accommodation.[8-10]

Although the need for treatment is described by dentists as great, the perceived need, the demand for dental care, and the utilization of dental services is, in general, low. There are a number of explanations for this disparity such as a lack of awareness of what modern dentistry has to offer; ageist attitudes of health professionals and elderly people themselves; the cost of dental treatment; and the simple fact that dental health is given a low priority compared with other health needs of elderly people. Another barrier to dental care for this frail and dependent section of the population is access to the dental surgery and the difficulty in obtaining domiciliary or home-based care.

There are a number of issues that have to be addressed during the development and provision of a domiciliary care service.

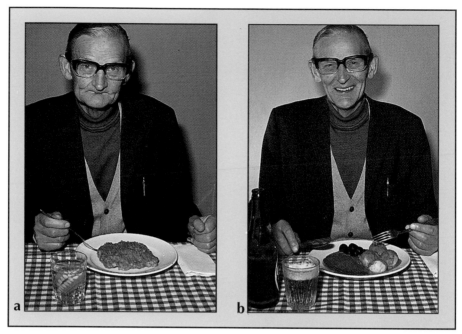

Figure 20.1 A meal may be the high spot of the day for an elderly institutionalized person. (a) The joy of eating will be impaired if they can only manage minced food as a result of poor oral status. (b) Dental treatment can improve their chewing ability and thus quality of life

The identification of housebound patients in need of care

Nursing and residential homes are usually occupied by that segment of the aged population which, because of frailty or illness, is totally dependent on help from professional staff. Sheltered accommodation allows frail, elderly people to continue to live independently, in a protected and supervised environment. These two groups are easily identified, because the local authorities keep records of institutionalized individuals and of those living in homes. In contrast, very few countries, if any, keep official records of housebound and bedridden individuals. Unless elderly people themselves ask for dental assistance, they are not identified to the profession. One common feature for these citizens is a dependence upon district nurses or other kinds of visiting carers to help change bandages, give injections or assist in personal hygiene.

Many housebound elderly people live alone. Some will receive help from home-care assistants with housework, shopping and cooking. Some will receive a daily hot meal from a 'meals on wheels' service. This group of health care and social workers can prove a valuable source of help in identifying housebound or bedridden individuals who may require dental care.

It has been the experience in Scandinavia and the UK that carers can enquire whether an individual has dental problems needing attention. A visiting dentist can then be notified that their services are required. This liaising or networking with other professional services is the basis for multi-disciplinary care. Not only can it bring the needs of an elderly person to the attention of the dentist, but the dentist can bring social, medical or nursing needs to the notice of another member of 'the team'.

Place of treatment

It is usually more convenient, and more cost-effective, for a dentist to treat patients in the surgery. However, transfer from home to a dental surgery of a frail elderly person by ambulance is expensive, and the cost of transportation can exceed the expense of the treatment.

Moreover, the elderly person often needs to be accompanied by a member of the family, a nurse or another carer, who is not always readily available. The dental surgery may be situated or equipped in such a way that access for a person on a stretcher or in a wheelchair is difficult. An older patient may suffer some discomfort during transportation, from the use of chairs without special padding or simply from being in an upright position for a considerable period of time. A lack of suitable toilet facilities at the dental surgery may pose another problem, as many old people suffer from incontinence, are catheterized, or take diuretics.

It may be most appropriate, therefore, to treat housebound and bedridden individuals in their own homes, despite the inconvenience that this method of delivering dental care may cause the dentist. Also, it may be best, on occasions, to treat an ambulatory person in their own home or environment which, because of its familiarity, feels safe and secure. Some elderly people with mental illness such as Alzheimer's disease become confused and disorientated when moved from familiar surroundings, others become distressed and may behave aggressively. The advantage of having a calm, relatively co-operative patient counteracts the inconveniences of providing domiciliary dentistry. The balance needs to be weighed carefully for each individual and for each item of treatment.

Essentially, domiciliary care requires the dentist to be able to transfer their dental skills from the dental surgery to the kitchen, sitting room or bedroom. Like any service it has advantages and disadvantages for both the service providers and users (see Tables 20.1 and 20.2). The main advantage for the dentist is that seeing someone in their home allows a more holistic view of them, and consequently a more realistic approach to their dental care. It allows an assessment to be made of the person's social circumstances and their priorities. It provides more immediate access to carers and supporting services. Also, it allows ready access to the patient's medication, and often to medical notes kept by the district nurse in the patient's home.

One of the principal benefits to the patient, that of remaining in their own environment, has both gain and drawback for the dentist. The gain is that the patient feels more relaxed, comfortable and in control than when in the dental surgery. Thus, they are more amenable to treatment, find it easier to remember information given to them, and are more likely to comply with preventive advice. The drawback is that the dentist has to learn to cope when away from their established environment. The fear of the unknown may

Table 20.1 Domiciliary dental care: advantages

Advantages of domiciliary dental care for the dentist
- an opportunity to learn more about the patient
- a person in their own environment is more relaxed and more comfortable
- the patient seems to be more interested in their treatment, thus motivation and compliance may be increased
- increased access to carers
- a change of environment
- valued and appreciated more
- an opportunity to develop or improve skills such as time management, planning, communication, liaising with other health workers, lifting and map reading

Advantages of domiciliary dental care for the patient
- increased access to dental care
- increased independence as she/he is no longer reliant on someone else to take them to the dentist
- being treated in their own environment
- decreased fear of the unknown
- increased control/power over events
- feels more important
- has a visitor/guest
- has peer group support in residential setting

Table 20.2 Domiciliary dental care: disadvantages

Disadvantages of domiciliary dental care for the dentist
- out of their own environment
- increased fear of the unknown
- decreased control/power
- lack of emergency back-up
- lack of hygiene control
- making compromises such as bad posture, poor lighting and lack of radiographic facilities
- can become involved in issues other than dentistry
- decreased time for patient care because of increased time spent travelling
- increased stress
- increased vulnerability

Disadvantages of domiciliary dental care for the patient
- service not widely known about
- limited scope of dental procedures
- limited choice of dentist
- difficult to miss appointments
- uncertainty of strangers visiting
- invasion of privacy/disruption of routine
- embarrassment regarding physical/social circumstances

be transferred from the patient to the dentist, who has to juggle with the problems of being a visitor in someone's home, taking enough control to be able to provide a professional service, yet respecting the individual's culture, wishes and property. On occasions, the dentistry may have to take second place to a social or health issue of more importance to the patient.

In terms of practical management, when trust has been gained it may be sensible to make contact with a good neighbour. Should communication be a problem, or access to the house be difficult, for example, because of the infirmity or deafness of the aged occupant. Such a person can be invaluable.

One of the difficulties in providing domiciliary care is the absence of the dental chair. Portable chairs are available but they add extra bulk and weight to the domiciliary kit. Also, handicapped elderly people can feel particularly vulnerable when receiving dental care in the reclined position, and physical disabilities may make this posture uncomfortable or impossible for some. For some types of dental work it is best for the patient to adopt an upright, seated position.

An upright chair with a cushion for head support against a wall may be adequate in some situations, although the dentist will have to stand and work in front of the patient. The dentist may be better off from an ergonomic point of view standing behind the seated

patient and supporting the patient's head against the dentist's body. It is better still if the patient has a wheelchair, with provision for the attachment of a headrest. When taking impressions of the lower jaw, kneeling puts the dentist at a good height, whilst maintaining comfort and posture.

If the patient is bedridden, it may be necessary for the dentist to bend over the bed. This is uncomfortable and may not be possible for the dentist with a back problem. Alternatively, the dentist may be able to sit on a chair next to the bed and work with the patient's head in their lap.

Dentists who provide routine domiciliary care can become vulnerable if they do not follow a protocol for ensuring personal safety. For example, they should undergo training in lifting before carrying heavy domiciliary kits and they must be chaperoned at all times.

Domiciliary care allows a person access to a service of which they might not otherwise be able to avail themselves. However, this service is not yet provided by all dentists, and this limits the patients' choice of service provider.

Attitudes of dentists to domiciliary care

The attitude of the dental profession to domiciliary dental care may be another explanation for the poor oral health so often found in housebound elderly people. For years, dentists have been used to a comfortable situation, where patients were abundant, and willing to come to the surgery. This is now changing as a consequence of the increase in the number of dentists and the reduction in the caries incidence in children.

It has recently been reported that only about one-fifth of dentists had ever provided dental treatment to residents in long-term care facilities[10,11] Of those who had provided domiciliary care, treatment was usually limited to extraction of teeth, and the provision and adjustment of dentures. Only about one-third of the dentists questioned indicated that they were willing to provide dental care outside the surgery. Most of this group were younger people who had some experience in domiciliary care.

The principal reasons given for the generally negative attitude to domiciliary care were a lack of suitable portable equipment, insufficient time, and inadequate financial remuneration. The negatively responding dentists were too busy treating ambulatory patients. This attitude was not, as it might seem, obstructive. Most of the dentists believed that there was no demand for domiciliary care, never having been asked to provide such a service. A negative attitude such as this has been reported of dentists who seldom or never treat old housebound and disabled people.[12] On the other hand, those with experience in such treatments usually express considerable professional satisfaction.

Lack of experience in, and training for, this special area of dentistry may be another explanation for dentists' reluctance to treat the old people with disabling conditions.[10,13] Apart from a change of attitude, it is essential that dental students and practitioners are better taught and trained, by including domiciliary dentistry in undergraduate curricula,[11,14] and setting up postgraduate courses in gerodontology. It would seem sensible that those dentists with an interest in providing domiciliary care should participate in these programmes.

Dentists who are prepared to provide domiciliary dental care should be identifiable to the general community. In Denmark the local branches of the dental association provide the social security department with lists of dentists interested in and capable of domiciliary dentistry. In England many Local Dental Committees do the same. The housebound patient may choose any dentist from this list. The Family Health Services Association (FHSA) maintains lists of all general dental practitioners working within the National Health Service in the UK, but usually these contain details only of the practice address and opening hours. However, in some districts additional lists of dentists prepared to make home visits, and of dental premises accessible to wheelchairs, are held by the managers of Community Dental Services and/or the FHSA.

The recent advent of a relative freedom to advertise has resulted in some practitioners in the UK publishing their willingness and ability to provide domiciliary care. Also, the requirement for NHS practices to make practice leaflets available to the public informing them of the dental services on offer will help to raise awareness about domiciliary care. This in turn will lead to an increased demand.

Elderly people of today belong to a generation where routine dental care was the exception rather than the rule. Dentistry was offered only at a dentist's surgery, and many older people are unaware that modern, portable equipment permits the diagnosis and treatment of most dental problems in their home. Elderly people of tomorrow will have higher expectations of dentistry and dentists, and will make greater demands on domiciliary services.

Equipment for domiciliary dental care

The simplest approach to on-site delivery of dental care is for the dentist to visit the patient in their home, bringing all the necessary equipment. The use of a mobile dental van equipped as a dental surgery is an alternative, treatment taking place within the van. The use of this type of self-contained van may seem appealing, because it offers the dentist the best facilities for all types of treatment, including the use of radiographs. However, a van has several significant drawbacks which may outweigh its advantages.[15] The initial cost and operating expenses are substantial. There are practical problems associated with access for some handicapped or bedridden individuals.

Currently, the majority of elderly people are edentulous, having some form of prosthesis as a replacement for the natural dentition. Impressions, jaw registration, adjustments of occlusion and peripheral extension of dentures are procedures that require relatively little equipment (Fig. 20.2). A rechargeable, battery-operated, portable motor, and a box with impression trays, materials and instruments are usually all that is needed (Figs 20.3, 20.4).

Mouth rinsing and the like can be done from a glass into a bowl. Lighting can range in sophistication from integral unit lights, surgeon's headlamps supported by a rechargeable battery pack, and the reliable Anglepoise. A portable clamp for use on a bedhead or chair is a useful standby, as may be two wooden wedges to allow a braked wheel-chair to be tilted backwards slightly.

The portable unit

In the future a growing proportion of the elderly population will retain some or all of

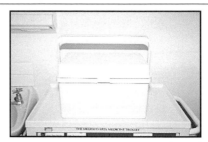

Figure 20.4a Babycare box – closed, ready to carry

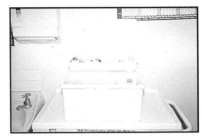

Figure 20.4b Babycare box – open, ready for use

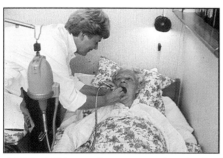

Figure 20.2 Bedridden patients can receive simple dental care in their home without the necessity for transferral to a dental surgery. This often involves a non-physiological working posture for the dentist

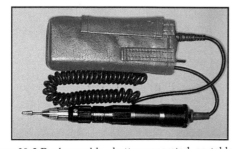

Figure 20.3 Rechargeable, battery-operated portable motor

their natural teeth. Every effort should be made to maintain these teeth, especially when the partially dentate person becomes physically or mentally disabled. Tooth extraction can no longer be justified on the grounds of age or general disease alone. Indeed, the converse is true. Age, disease and disability make it more difficult for an individual who becomes edentulous to cope with, and develop, the skills necessary to wear complete dentures. It will be easier to meet the expectations of the dentate elderly person than the one recently rendered edentulous.

The need for prevention of periodontal disease will result in an increased demand for hygiene measures such as scaling. All these types of treatment can require the use of a three-in-one water/air syringe, high- and low-speed handpieces, and possibly an ultrasonic scaler. Aspiration is mandatory when such equipment is used. There is also a need for adequate illumination, especially for cavity preparation in the mouth, and a high-intensity fibre-optic light is of benefit here. These facilities can be provided combined in currently available portable dental units, or as separate items.

In recent years, various designs of portable dental units have been available. Information on the individual units is obtainable from dental companies, dentists experienced in domiciliary care, or societies involved in the dental care of adults who are handicapped.

An example of a portable unit is illustrated in Figure 20.5. It contains a compressor that generates sufficient pressure to operate one high-speed, two low-speed handpieces and a three-in-one syringe, as well as providing adequate oral aspiration. The unit has an operating light, a fibre-optic light and a light for curing composite materials. An ultrasonic scaler and an amalgamator are included. An X-ray viewing box can be added. With the increased need for stringent cross-infection control, some manufacturers of portable equipment are excluding aspiration from the main unit and opting for separate aspirators.

Transportability, ease of assembly and disassembly and durability are some of the features that should be considered before purchase. The weight, available functions and cost of the unit are other factors to take into consideration. Units tend to be heavy, weighing anything between 11 and 35 kg, with the lighter ones generally requiring a source of compressed air. The weight and cost of a compressor must be included if choosing such a unit. If a compressor is not to be used, compressed air bottles will suffice, but need to be replaced or replenished.

Most units are costly. Prices range from approximately £2000 to £10 000. It is unlikely that a dentist will use one every day of the year, and it is probably sensible for a unit to be shared between colleagues. In Denmark some municipalities have purchased portable equipment which is at the disposal of dentists willing to enter into programmes of domiciliary dentistry. Another method of sharing the costs of the equipment is for local branches of the dental association or the local Community Dental Services to buy a portable unit and make it available, with or without a small fee, to dentists in the area. All these arrangements incur extra time for the dentist in the collection and return of the equipment, and consequently none is ideal.

Portable X-ray apparatus is available, but the legislation in many countries prohibits the taking of radiographs out of the dental surgery. In such cases a fibre-optic light may be useful for diagnostic purposes. However, it cannot replace the radiograph as a diagnostic tool.

A portable autoclave (Fig. 20.6) can be useful, particularly when dealing with patients with highly infectious diseases or compromised immune systems. However, its use is not essential, provided all equipment is sterilized and bagged before treating a patient, and

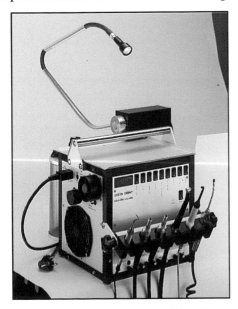

Figure 20.5 The Lysta-Dent Field Unit 2000. This portable unit has facilities for all forms of conservative dental care. When fully equipped it weighs approximately 18 kg excluding its carrying case. The unit is not now available in the UK. An alternative is the 'Mobident'. (Mobident Ltd, 36 Church Drive, Ilkeston, Derby DE7 8QB)

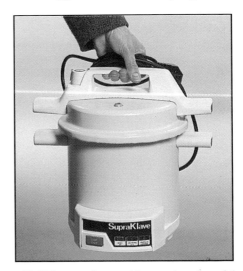

Figure 20.6 The use of a portable autoclave is useful when treating patients where cross-infection would be a hazard (Kavo lave)

a system of working is adopted such that clean and dirty instruments never meet.

Careful thought must be given to the disposal of clinical waste. Whilst this may not be an issue in a nursing or residential home where the disposal of clinical waste is part of the daily routine, it may be necessary for the dentist to take waste away from an individual's home for incineration or safe disposal of sharps. Throughout, the dentist must be aware of the primacy of the patient's home and property, and take all due care.

Oral hygiene procedures: a crucial barrier

Prevention is a fundamental element of dental care and includes daily implementation of oral hygiene. This concept is valid for all patients, including the full denture wearer, whose edentulous oral cavity must be kept clean in order to avoid infection. Neglect of oral hygiene is a common finding and a general experience at institutions for older adults, either hospitals, nursing homes or residential accommodation.[16] Figure 20.7 illustrates a dental catastrophe in a functionally dependent 80-year-old woman, who had been unable to maintain a proper hygiene regimen for a couple of years.

The most common reason for dental breakdown is a lack of knowledge of the needs for and techniques of oral hygiene on the part of the carers responsible for the health and welfare of residents in long-stay care. The curricula for the education of nurses and other staff dealing with the care of elderly patients rarely includes information on teeth and oral hygiene. Some carers have a relatively low level of education or are recruited from socioeconomic groups in which little or no emphasis is put on oral hygiene procedures. Other factors are lack of time and the stresses of an already heavy burden of work.

Many trained nurses and other staff express an aversion towards dealing with people's oral care and the cleaning of dentures. Mucus and food debris on teeth and dentures can be made more acceptable by advocating the routine wearing of gloves for such tasks, although this increases cost. Cleaning personal and intimate zones, such as the oral cavity, is generally disliked by nurses who are not only embarrassed by it themselves, but are concerned that it causes embarrassment to the recipient. Paradoxically, they cope, without comment, with the hygiene of all other parts of the body, including the removal of faecal matter. They are unlikely to find this any less distasteful, however, it is seen as a part of the role for which they have been trained to cope.

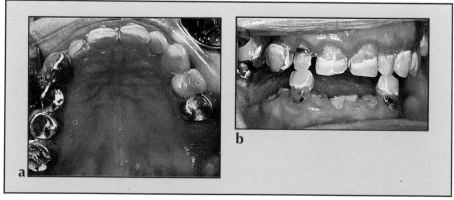

Figure 20.7 (a) An 80-year-old female patient with a number of remaining natural teeth. This patient was dentally aware, having been a regular dental attender throughout her life. After suffering a cerebral haemorrhage she was admitted to hospital in an unconscious state. The patient made a partial recovery and was transferred to a rehabilitation centre. She then took up long-term residence in a home for elderly people. Some two years later she complained of toothache, and a dental opinion was sought. (b) Her previously well-maintained dentition has undergone severe deterioration as a result of two years of neglect. The staff at the residential home were not aware of the need for adequate daily oral hygiene and the patient was in no position to maintain the required standard of self-care

Other fears, associated particularly with handling dentures, are more psychologically deep-seated. For instance, many nurses associate removing dentures from the mouth with death and the laying-out of the body. Some fears are realistic, such as the fear of being bitten or not knowing how much pressure can be used when cleaning someone else's teeth without hurting them yet still doing a good job. Education in oral hygiene measures has to acknowledge and address the fears of carers if they are to be overcome.

The situation is worse for the housebound and bedridden patient, for whom continuous supervision by professional staff is not available. Some old people may be aware of the necessity for oral hygiene but are not in a position to maintain it, because of their handicap. For others, oral hygiene has a low priority because of more obtrusive health and social problems. The dentist has to rely upon help from district nurses or home-care assistants to assist the housebound person with oral hygiene when necessary. These people already have heavy workloads, and although they may want to help, cannot always do so. The dentist responsible for the treatment must therefore educate the family or other informal carers in the need for, and methods of, oral hygiene. The appropriate regimens should be explained in detail and demonstrated on the patient (Fig. 20.8). For the dentate, bedridden elderly person, brushing with fluoride toothpaste is recommended. When this procedure is a physical impossibility, rinsing or swabbing the mouth with a chlorhexidine solution may offer an alternative.

It is important that the independence of an older person is not violated. The patient should be encouraged to participate as much as possible in oral hygiene, and any aids available should be used to make mouthcare an enabling rather than a disabling procedure. Toothbrush handles can be adapted in such a way that a person who was previously unable to grasp a brush, for instance because of arthritic deformity, can have some independence restored (see pages 65 and 66).

Initially, elderly people and/or their carers will require instruction and support. The results of their efforts should be evaluated regularly by the dentist. They should be provided with constructive feedback and modifications to oral hygiene procedure, reinstruc-

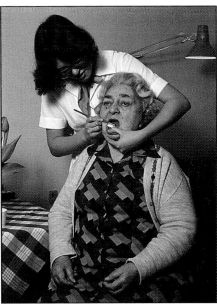

Figure 20.8 Nursing, auxiliary staff and family members need detailed instruction in the appropriate oral hygiene techniques for each individual in their care. It may be necessary for them to assist a handicapped elderly person to achieve the appropriate level of mouth care

tion, encouragement, and continued support given as appropriate.

In a small number of cases where it is impossible for the individual elderly person or the carer to maintain adequate oral hygiene, the dentist has a responsibility to instigate regular professional cleaning by a member of the dental team. Recent changes to the statutory regulations for dental hygienists in the UK mean that hygienists can undertake home visits to carry out care which the dentist has prescribed. This makes them ideally suited to provide continuing oral hygiene support for housebound elderly people.

The terminally ill patient (Angus Walls)

The dentist has a role to play in ensuring dignity and freedom from pain for the dying patient. To be able to meet with relatives and friends with stable dentures and apparently sound teeth is an important psychological boost for the patient and the family.

The dental problems experienced by terminally ill people are essentially similar to those of fit individuals, though the management strategy may differ. The principal goal should be to alleviate pain and correct an immediate problem in the most expeditious way. This may not result in a perfect, or permanent, end product. However, the impression that the treatment is simply palliative, though in truth it may be, should not be given to the patient. Thus, carious lesions are managed as conservatively as possible, exposed pulps being dressed with Ledermix. Glass-ionomer cements are useful. There are a limited number of problems which appear to occur with increased frequency amongst the terminally ill.

Ill-fitting dentures

There is no evidence that the quality of dentures worn by terminally ill people is any worse than in the population as a whole. However, a frequent reason for a request for help is the reported instability of a prosthesis. The most likely explanation for this is that while the individual is well, poor adaptation of a denture can be accommodated by oral gymnastics. This is a learned skill, which is often lost when the prosthesis is not worn for a period of time, particularly if the patient is ill at that time. Thus, when the patient tries to replace what was previously perceived to be a satisfactory prosthesis, it may now prove to be inherently unsatisfactory, with poor retention and stability. Loss of weight is often blamed, incorrectly, for this phenomenon. The use of a temporary soft lining material within the prosthesis provides a simple remedy. The lining will require to be maintained and replaced at intervals, or replacement dentures can be made using a denture copying technique.

Oral pain/ulceration

The thinned, friable oral mucosa of older people can be further compromised by chemotherapy, by general debilitation with poor oral hygiene, and by mouth dryness. The sensitive mucosa may be painful and may be subject to infective processes such as pseudo-membranous candidiasis. All of these problems can make eating and drinking uncomfortable. Despite the discomfort, oral cleanliness must be maintained and there are a number of agents that can be used with benefit.

Chlorhexidine

Chlorhexidine can be used as a mouth rinse, or on swabs for the severely debilitated. Unfortunately, the taste of a 0.2% solution (Corsodyl) is often unacceptable because it induces severe burning sensations from the mucosae. A 0.1% solution (Eludril) whilst less effective may be better tolerated.

Providone iodine

Providone iodine[a] can be used as a mouthwash, or on swabs for oral cleansing. It has a bitter taste. It may be a more efficient detergent than chlorhexidine and may provide improved cleaning for the severely debilitated subject.

Pineapple juice, or pineapple chunks

Pineapple contains significant quantities of proteolytic enzymes and induces a feeling of freshness in the mouth which can be a useful palliative. There is a risk of acid erosion/caries if its use is not controlled, and if the patient's level of oral hygiene is not up to the required standard. In the light of the circumstances for which it is being prescribed, this is perhaps of small significance.

Other palliative agents

Benzydamine hydrochloride oral rinse[b] is a pleasant tasting topical analgesic and anti-inflammatory rinse which can give symtomatic relief to some patients with sore mouths. Artificial saliva can be of benefit to those people with dry mouths, as can frozen tonic-water cubes.

The maintenance of oral hygiene and cleanliness for the terminally ill is important and may involve the active participation of carers. The problems that may be met have been discussed earlier in this chapter.

[a]Napp Laboratories Ltd, Milton Road, Cambridge CB4 4GW
[b]Difflam oral rinse, 3M Health Care Ltd, Morley Street, Loughborough LE11 1EP

An obligation of the dental profession

The improving dental health of the younger generation today will, over the coming years, spread to the older generation. The dental profession, and the individual dentist, have to realize that it is part of our professional obligation to ensure that the housebound and bedridden in the population receive proper dental care. Domiciliary dental care is an ethical obligation. As demand increases it will become an accepted part of practice.

References

1 Fiske J., Gelbier S., Watson R.M., The benefit of dental care to an elderly population assessed using a sociodental measure of oral handicap, *Br. Dent. J. 1990*; 168: 153–6

2 Manderson R.D., Ettinger R.L., Dental status of the institutionalised elderly population of Edinburgh, *Community Dent. Oral Epidemiol. 1975*; 3: 100–107

3 Smith J., Sheiham A., Dental treatment needs and demands of an elderly population in England, *Community Dent. Oral Epidemiol. 1980*; 8: 360–64

4 Hoad-Reddick G., Grant A.A., The dental health of an elderly population in North-West England: Results of a survey undertaken in the Halton Health Authority, *J. Dent. 1987*; 15: 138–46

5 Nordenram G., Bohlin E., *Dental status in the elderly: A review of the Swedish literature, Senior Citizen's Welfare Programme 1981*; 9: 1–66

6 Makila E., Oral health among the inmates of old people's homes III: Dentures and prosthetic aspects, *Proc. Finn. Dent. Soc. 1977*; 73: 99–116

7 Vigild M., Denture status and need for prosthetic treatment among institutionalised elderly in Denmark, *Community Dent. Oral Epidemiol. 1987*; 15: 128–33

8 Hogan J.I., A domiciliary dental service centre to the housebound from an Inner London health centre, *Community Dent. Health 1986*; 3: 117–27

9 Tobias T., Smith J.M., Barriers to dental care and associated oral status and treatment needs, in an elderly population living in sheltered accommodation in West Essex, *Br. Dent. J. 1987*; 163: 293–5

10 MacEntee M.I, Weis R, Waxler-Morrison N.E., Morrison B.J., Factors influencing oral health in long term care facilities, *Community Dent. Oral Epidemiol. 1987*; 15: 314–16

11 Fiske J, Gelbier S, Watson R.M., Barriers to dental care in an elderly population resident in an inner city area, *J. Dent. 1990*; 18: 236–42

12 Kiyak H.A, Milgrom P, Ratner P, Conrad D., Dentists' attitudes towards and knowledge of the elderly, *J. Dent. Educ. 1982*; 46: 273–7

13 Stiefle D.J, Truelove E.L, Jolly D.E., The preparedness of dental professionals to treat persons with disabling conditions in long-term care facilities and community settings, *Spec. Care Dent. 1987*; 7: 108–13

14 Christensen J, Introducing gerodontology to students in Denmark, *J. Dent. 1985*; 13: 184–91

15 Mulligan R., Considerations for using mobile dental vans to deliver dental care to the elderly, *Gerodontics 1987*; 3: 260–64

16 Berkley D., Improving dental access for the nursing home resident: portable dentistry interventions, *Gerodontics 1987*; 3: 265–8

21

Gerodontology – the future

Aubrey Sheiham

This book has considered the various practical problems encountered when treating the old patient or old dentition. There can be no doubt that such treatment has formed an increasing part of dental practice over the past few years. It is not surprising that this alteration in the pattern of the provision of dental care, as a result of a reduction in juvenile and adult caries, has been held up by some as being the long-term solution to the current under-utilization of some dental services and as the prospect of dental unemployment. This view is probably incorrect.

The improvements in dental health of children and young adults has led to a shift in the attention of dentists to the dental needs of older people. At present, most of the elderly population is edentulous. The level of edentulousness is decreasing, but in the short and medium term this decrease is unlikely to be dramatic. The succeeding age group will have many missing teeth and the maintenance of those teeth that remain, though posing undoubted technical problems, is in the overall pattern of things, unlikely to be unduly labour intensive. At the younger end of the age-range, dental caries and periodontal disease has decreased and if current trends continue, are likely to decrease further. What remains is the current group of middle-aged people with heavily restored teeth. They may well become heavy users of dental services, but nevertheless they constitute a relatively small percentage of the population.

Dental disease

The incidence of coronal and root caries increases slightly amongst older people. For example, in 1987 11% of 30–39-year-old Finnish adults had had root caries. The percentage increased to 19% in the age-group 40–49; to 28% in the group 50–59; and to 33% in those aged 60 and above.[1] However, although the numbers of older people that had had root caries is relatively high, the number of lesions per person is usually low, as is the attack rate. For example, Banting has reported an incidence of 2 lesions per 100 person months among institutionalized people.[2] The incidence rate among ambulatory people is probably lower.

It has to be considered whether the potential caries problem among older people has not been popularly overestimated. These findings suggest that there is not an 'explosion' in the incidence of root caries in older people, and that there is not therefore a great increase in the need for restorative dental treatment in the current middle to older age groups. Neither is there evidence that there will be more periodontal disease to treat because people retain more teeth for longer.[3]

Demographic trends

Currently there is an increase in the proportion of old people in the populations of industrialized countries, and amongst those old people there will be an increase in the numbers of the very old. Thus, the population pyramid is being transformed into a column.[4] Populations in developing countries are also ageing rapidly. By the year 2025, eight of the 11 countries with an elderly population greater than 16 million people will be in the Third World.[5]

The ageing of any population has a profound political, economic and social significance and adjustments have to be made to services, attitudes and social environments. Demands on the health services rise with advancing age. However, the demands for treatment do not increase simply in line with the increase in the age of the population. The proportion of people reporting long-standing illness increases as an exponential of age. The involvement of general medical practitioners and the use of institutions also shows an exponential increase throughout old age.[4] Thus, the basic facts relating to age and numbers fail to provide all the information that is required to plan for the needs of the old people in a population.

Stereotypes of old age

In industrialized societies the typical old person has in the past been, and even today is, sometimes thought of as suffering from poor health, poorly housed, living alone on an inadequate income, lonely, socially isolated, and often a burden to society (Fig. 21.1). Such images may be unthinkingly reinforced by those who primarily come into contact with old people who are chronically ill, or neglected.

It is now largely realized that these dated stereotypes are not correct. Most old people lead active lives and only a small percentage

(less than 10%) live in institutions. Most are independent, and of those that need care a high proportion are looked after in their own homes by a mixture of family, neighbours and 'professional carers'.

Old people are not clearly definable as a group, but as with younger groups, are distinguished by their diversity. It would be surprising were this not so. They are:

> an aggregation of a very large number of distinct or overlapping groups of individuals. . ., very different from each other in image, family circumstances, resources and living conditions; with a diversity of expectations, problems and pathologies. . . (These latter range from). . . a substantial majority whose problems are qualitatively no different from those of younger adults to a minority of extremely vulnerable sick or infirm persons needing total care.[6]

The concept of need

There is a commonly held assumption that the need for dental care can be objectively determined usually by means of clinical assessment. However, dental ill-health is open to wide interpretation, and similarly dental care needs require a wide definition. For example, any discussion of need must include reference to the perceptions and attitudes of the patients themselves. It must consider the degrees of disability and dysfunction that ill-health brings and it must assess the impact of ill-health upon individuals and the society in which they live (Fig. 21.2).[7]

In dentistry the assessment of needs has traditionally been defined in terms of technical procedures, manpower and resources. However, there is real danger that the assessment of need by a caring profession may not be entirely free of subjective judgements. It is professionally correct to monitor and con-

---

• Suffering from poor health
• Poorly housed
• Living alone on an inadequate income
• Lonely
• Socially isolated
• A burden to society

Figure 21.1 Popular stereotypes of old people

• Perceptions and attitudes of patients
• Degree of disability
• Degree of dysfunction
• Impact of ill-health on individual
• Impact of ill-health on society

Figure 21.2 Factors in assessing need for treatment

tinually assess concepts of normality and need. For example, we might ask the following questions:

- Is it essential for a person to be plaque free?
- Should all calculus be removed irrespective of the periodontal status?
- Is there a need to surgically treat all deep periodontal pockets?
- Do occlusally worn teeth necessarily require to be restored?
- Should missing molar teeth be replaced?
- Should technically imperfect full dentures be replaced if the patient is content with them?

Dental health goals

If there are no specified goals, it is impossible to know when you have succeeded. Surprisingly, until the Dental Strategy Review Group reported in 1981[8] formulating a goal for dentistry, there were no stated objectives for dental health care in the UK. Here are some examples for dentistry:

- Providing the opportunity for everyone to retain a healthy functional dentition for life[8]
- The maintenance of a healthy natural functioning dentition throughout life, including all the social and biological functions that relate to the personal well-being of an individual. These include such factors as aesthetics, chewing, taste, speech, and the freeedom from discomfort.[9]

A World Health Organization workshop, comprising chief dental officers for Northern and Western Europe, suggested a number of quantifiable goals relating to acceptable levels of dental health by age (Table 21.1).[10] These could be used when considering the provision of dental care for old people. The WHO recognized that 'dental health' does not imply that all 32 teeth need to be retained, nor is a periodontal attachment to the amelo-cemental junction a biological or social necessity.

Aiming to maintain a healthy functional dentition for life does not imply striving to save or replace, against all odds, a maximum number of teeth. It is realistic to aim to preserve strategic parts of the dentition. Thus, the goal for older people might be based upon the concept of the acceptability of a shortened dental arch (SDA). Käyser suggested that an SDA consisting of 12 front teeth and 8 premolars (20 teeth) was the minimum acceptable for people over 45 years of age.[11]

Changing needs and changing dental technology

Smooth surface caries is decreasing in prevalence, and currently the dominant type of new dental caries is that of slowly progressing pit and fissure lesions. Smooth surface and fissure lesions present as smaller lesions than 15 years ago, and if they require to be treated, this will be by means of sealants, glass-ionomer, composite or amalgam, separately or in combination.

Table 21.1 Suggestions for acceptable levels of dental health by age[10]

Age	Mean no. of missing teeth	DMF	Periodontal status
12	0	2	0 teeth with pockets > 3 mm
15	0	3	0 teeth with pockets > 3 mm
18	1	4	0 teeth with pockets > 3 mm
35–44	2	6	Less than 7 teeth with pockets > 4.5 mm
65–74	10	12	20 functional teeth

Note: In addition, an acceptable level of oral health would include:

1 satisfactory prosthetic replacement for any missing dental unit which obviously detracts from aesthetics

2 freedom from pain

3 freedom from unacceptable deposits

4 freedom from unacceptable intrinsic anomalies

5 an occlusion which is functionally and cosmetically acceptable

Root caries is not a major problem, even among the majority of old people. The pattern of dental disease in the old and middle-aged differs somewhat to that seen in the young. The older age-groups experience less secondary caries than in the past as a result of the same factors that have led to the reduction in primary caries, namely, the use of fluoride toothpastes together with a greater awareness of oral cleanliness, dietary changes, and possibly the use of antibiotics.

There can also be no doubt that recently developed dental materials and techniques, for example the adhesive and cariostatic glass-ionomers, have potentially greatly simplified some aspects of restorative dentistry, necessitating less destructive preparations, and allowing simpler, speedier clinical procedures to be undertaken at less frequent intervals.

Nevertheless, some complex work will continue to be needed, particularly in respect of cases of exaggerated toothwear, so as to improve aesthetics and maintain function. Such cases are increasingly presenting for treatment. Also, with the increased awareness of dental matters, many patients are being encouraged to have their dentures substituted by bridgework.

Periodontal health is improving and periodontal disease is not a major cause of tooth loss. In 90% of the population there is no or little loss of periodontal attachment.[12] Concepts of periodontal disease and the emphasis on surgical treatment have changed in the light of these facts.[13,14] However, oral hygiene and maintenance, but at longer intervals than at present, is still required, perhaps particularly so and more often for the very old and infirm.

Good oral cleanliness and freedom from halitosis will enhance an old person's self-image and dignity. Preventive dentistry in general, including the application of topical fluoride and control of sugar consumption, is widely associated with children. In the future these techniques will be more appropriately applied to people over the age of 60 years, especially in relation to the prevention of root caries.

The greatest contribution which dental care can make is the reduction of pain, discomfort, disability and handicap caused by untreated dental disease and ill-fitting unaesthetically designed prosthetic appliances and restorations. In future, demands of older people will rise more rapidly because of changing expectations. The present cohort of older people tend to be stoical, accepting deterioration in health with increasing age. This stoicism is being replaced by a greater desire for, and increased expectations of, independence and dignity.[15]

Health and disease trends among older people

People now remain physiologically younger for longer than in the past. Labelling them 'senior citizens' at 65, and writing them out of the social mainstream, is less defensible than ever.[16] On the other hand, ageing is associated with an increase in the prevalence of chronic disease and disability. A striking feature of disease in old people is the predominance of overlapping multi-system diseases which are degenerative in nature.[17]

Despite the high prevalence of chronic conditions, most old people believe themselves to be healthy. Less than 10% of people aged 65 years and over live in institutions. Of the non-institutionalized old people, some 5–10% are housebound, 5–20% are ambulatory only with difficulty, and less than 5% are bedfast.[18]

Dental care has a high priority for old people who are either living in institutions, are housebound or have impairment of mobility. A functional, aesthetically acceptable dentition improves the quality of their lives, socially as well as nutritionally.

An interdisciplinary approach to dental care for older people

Planning for dental care of older people, and in particular the priority groups, requires an interdisciplinary approach. The promotion and maintenance of an acceptable level of dental health for older people extends beyond the traditional confines of dentistry and medicine. In addition to the medical and paramedical professions, liaison with social service departments and voluntary agencies is essential. Also, strategies must be directed at and discussed with informal and professional carers. Dental health education is part of general health education and requires multidisciplinary participation, using existing networks.

The various groups involved with older people should be contacted so as to ensure that dental health is included in their programmes. In this respect the Community Dental Service is well suited to act as a focal point and co-ordinator.[19]

For many elderly people, one of the greatest needs is for someone to help clean their teeth or dentures. A hygienist is therefore an indispensable member of the dental team. She or he should encourage self-help, teach the carers to undertake mouth hygiene, monitor and modify diets, and inform them of how and when to contact the appropriate dental services.

The range of people included in the multidisciplinary team will depend on the requirements. Old people should not be viewed or treated as something 'special'. Nevertheless the services afforded to them will have to be modified in some important ways to meet their special requirements.[20] These will vary according to levels of dependency, which may be classified as:

1 independent
2 mildly dependent
3 moderately dependent
4 severely dependent (see Fig. 21.3)[21]

From the viewpoint of dental care, old people can be divided into three main groups:

- Mobile — of varying degrees of fitness who can visit a dental surgery on their own initiative, see classification 1 or 2 above
- Moderately dependent — housebound or living in an institution (medically or mildly psycho-geriatrically compromised)
- Severely dependent — people who require constant attendance and medical or nursing care in an institution or home.

- Independent
- Mildly dependent
- Moderately dependent
- Severely dependent

Figure 21.3 Levels of dependency of elderly people

General dental practitioners are well equipped to treat the mobile and many who are moderately dependent. The severely dependent should be treated by dentists and ancillaries with special training in dental care for older people.

Manpower and training implications in the future

The improvement in dental health of children and younger adults has resulted in a shift in the pattern of dental treatment. More old people are being treated and more complex work is being undertaken. In the short term there remain unmet dental needs among middle-aged and old people, but these are less than the decrease in the needs for dental treatment of young people. This reduced workload offers the valuable opportunity to review the piece-rate system of remuneration, which tends to encourage rapid work and can result in unecomomically short-lived restorations.

Dental schools

Even were the concept of working slower but doing treatment which is more effective and long-lasting to be accepted, there remains a body of opinion that there are currently too many dentists in industrialized countries. There is a common concern that unless the current numbers of dentists who are graduating are reduced in the near future an oversupply will lead to unemployment, underemployment, and a reduction in the legitimate and cost-effective appropriate delegation of dental care to ancillary workers.

Reeve and Watson suggest that dental curricula should stress the qualities of sympathy, and perseverance that are so essential in the treatment of older patients.[22] The need to treat old and worn dentitions, albeit limited in number, will also require the maintenance of high standards of treatment planning and clinical skill. It is encouraging that in many schools the emphasis on points for 'work done' is being superseded by assessment of the quality of treatment and the concept of total patient care. A similar evolution of attitude is increasingly being seen in post-graduate and vocational training.

It would be helpful for those dental schools who have not already done so, to set out aims and objectives in behavioural terms, in the context of ageing and community health goals, addressing the following issues.[23]

- An awareness of the general health (including dental health) needs of old people
- The development of communication skills (between dentist and patient and dentist and co-worker)
- The ability to generate co-operation between all carers and promote interdisciplinary and public participation
- An understanding of the social consequences of ill-health, based upon studies in social science and epidemiology
- Participation in primary care (combining general practice and community dentistry).

Ancillary workers

When the dental health goals described above have been determined, it should be possible to develop a policy on the levels of professional dental staffing required in the health services and the appropriate skills that these staff should have. Appropriate training programmes should be commissioned. In the light of an increased emphasis upon prevention and a relative increase in the proportion of less-skill-intensive treatments needed, such as prophylaxis and fluoride application, it would seem sensible and cost-effective to involve ancillary workers to a greater degree than at present. Such workers would include hygienists and dental health educators and dental therapists.

Continuing education

The change in the pattern of dental care and the need to further develop social skills in relation to the treatment of the old population, as well as the need fully to understand the scientific basis of ageing and its associated medical conditions, will require a programme of further and continuing education for the dental team. Health authorities and social services should have a commitment to providing the necessary resources to allow the appropriate dental advice to be relayed to non-dental workers, possibly through senior community dental health personnel.

The dental schools must take note of the changes, by constantly upgrading their academic and clinical training programmes, with an increase in emphasis on social care and communication skills.

Conclusions

A small proportion of older people will continue in the future to require technically complex dental care. Those who are disabled or severely dependent will require domiciliary dental care. The majority of old people will require levels of treatment similar to that of middle-aged people. In terms of dental manpower it is unlikely that the increasing numbers of old people will compensate for the reduction of dental treatment needs of children and young adults. The majority of future treatments are likely to be simpler than at present, and many could be done by ancillary personnel.

Dental services for old people may involve a wide range of formal and informal carers, and it is suggested that such care might best be co-ordinated by the Community Dental Service in co-operation and collaboration with general dental practitioners (including vocational trainers) and hospital dental staff.

Few people die healthy. Realistic goals for the dental status of people at the end of their lives should be defined. These might include the concept of the shortened dental arch. We should strive to reduce the frequency with which dental problems cause distress, and to increase the prevalence of socially and functionally acceptable mouths in old people. Dental care for old people requires an emphasis on social skills, which should be reflected in the dental education of student and dentist alike.

References

1 Vehkalahti M., Occurrence of root caries and factors related to it, *Proc. Finn. Dent. Soc. 1987*; 43: suppl. IV

2 Banting D.W., Dental caries, in: *Oral health and ageing*, ed.: A.F. Tryon, PSG Publishing, Littleton, Mass. 1986; 247–69

3 Sheiham A., Public health aspects of periodontal diseases in Europe, *J. Clin. Periodontol. 1991*; 10: 362–9

4 Paillat P., The ageing of populations, in: *The provision of care for the elderly*, eds J. Kinnaird, J. Brotherston, J. Williamson, Churchill Livingstone, London 1981; 3–13

5 Kalache A., Ageing in developing countries, *Critical Public Health 1991*; 2: 38–43

6 Illsley R., The contribution of research to the development of practice and policy, in: *Elderly people in the community: Their service needs*, HMSO, London 1983; 3–9

7 Sheiham A., Maizels J.E., Cushing A.M., The concept of need in dental care, *Int. Dent. J. 1982*; 265–70

8 DHSS, *Towards better dental health – Guidelines for the Future*, HMSO, London 1981

9 Pilot T., Analysis of the overall effectiveness of treatment of periodontal disease, in: *Efficacy of treatment procedures in periodontics*, ed.: D. Shanley, Quintessence, Chicago 1980; 213–31

10 WHO A review of current recommendations for the organisation and administration of community oral health services in Northern and Western Europe, *Report of a WHO workshop*, Copenhagen, WHO Regional Office for Europe 1982

11 Käyser A.F., Minimum number of teeth needed to satisfy functional and social demands, in: *Public health aspects of periodontal disease*, ed.: A. Frandsen, Quintessence, Chicago 1984; 135–47

12 Sheiham A., The epidemiology, etiology and public health aspects of periodontal disease, in: *Periodontics – In the tradition of Orban and Gottlieb*, sixth edition, eds: D.A. Grant, I.B. Stern, F.C. Everett, C.V Mosby, St. Louis 1987; 216–51

13 Socransky S.S. *et al.*, New concepts of destructive periodontal disease, *J. Clin. Periodontol. 1984*; 11: 21–32

14 Kieser J.B., *Periodontics: A practical approach*. Wright, London 1990

15 Finch H., *Health and older people. Research report no. 6*, London, Health Education Council, 1986

16 Fifer, A. Bronte, L. eds, *Our aging society – Paradox and promise*, London, W.W. Norton & Co, 1986

17 Avorn J.L., Medicine: the life and death of Oliver Shay, in: *Our aging society – Paradox and promise*, eds: A. Fifer, L. Bronte, W.W. Norton & Co, London, 1986; 294

18 Heikkinen E., Waters W.E., Brzezinski Z.J., *The elderly in eleven countries, Public health in Europe*, Copenhagen, WHO Regional office for Europe, 1983

19 Age Well, *Dental health education initiatives for older people. Report of a Workshop*, London, Health Education Council, 1986

20 Brotherston J., Policies for the care of the elderly, in: *The provision of care for the elderly*, eds: J. Kinnaird, J. Brotherston, J. Williamson, Churchill Livingstone, London, 1981; 14–23

21 Hermanova H., Identification of high-risk groups in Prague, in: *The provision of care for the elderly*, eds: J. Kinnaird, J. Brotherston, J. Williamson, Churchill Livingstone, London, 1981; 148–54

22 Reeve P.E., Watson C.J., *Dental students' personality*, *J. Med. Educ. 1985*: 119: 226–37

23 Plamping D., Sheiham A., *Strategies for improving oral health in Britain*, Monograph Series, London. Joint Department of Community Dental Health and Dental Practice, University College London and The London Hospital Medical College

INDEX